Psychosocial Occupational Therapy

Frames of Reference for Intervention

Second Edition

Mary Ann Bruce, MS, OTR
Saddleback Memorial Rehabilitation Center,
Laguna Hills, CA

Barbara Borg, MS, OTR
Colorado State University, Fort Collins, CO

SLACK Incorporated, 6900 Grove Road, Thorofare, NJ 08086–9447

Psychosocial Occupational Therapy

Frames of Reference for Intervention

Second Edition

Editorial Director: Cheryl D. Willoughby
Publisher: Harry C. Benson

Psychosocial occupational therapy: frames of reference for intervention/
  Mary Ann Bruce, Barbara Borg—2nd ed.

p. cm.
Includes bibliographical references and index.

ISBN 1-55642-203-2

1. Occupational therapy.   2. Mentally ill—Rehabilitation.
I. Borg, Barbara.   II. Bruce, Mary Ann. Frames of reference in psychosocial occupational therapy.   III. Title.

RC 487.B78 1993
616.89′165—dc 20   93-8444

Printed in the United States of America

Published by: SLACK Incorporated
              6900 Grove Road
              Thorofare, NJ 08086-9447

Last digit is print number: 10   9   8   7   6   5   4   3   2   1

Contents

About the Authors

Mary Ann G. Bruce and Barbara Borg have been friends and colleagues since 1970. They have shared clinical and academic views, held similar positions in occupational therapy practice and education, and more recently collaborated on numerous scholarly projects. They co-authored *The Group System: The Therapeutic Activity Group in Occupational Therapy* published by SLACK Inc., in 1991.

Mary Ann Bruce holds a bachelor of science in occupational therapy from Colorado State University and a master of science degree in counseling from Southern Connecticut State University. She has been an associate professor and department chair at Quinnipiac College, Hamden, Connecticut, and an associate professor and interim program director at the University of Texas Health Science Center, San Antonio. Currently, she is in private practice and pursuing a doctoral degree in cognition and human learning.

Barbara Borg graduated from Colorado State University with a bachelor of science degree in occupational therapy and from the University of Northern Colorado with a master of arts degree in counseling. After working in adolescent and adult psychiatry as a staff occupational therapist and administrator, she worked in a private agency doing individual, couple and family counseling. Ms. Borg has just recently returned to the Occupational Therapy Department at Colorado State University, where she previously taught for several years. She also currently contracts with several agencies in the Denver area and pursues her interest in professional writing.

Acknowledgments

The authors wish to express their appreciation to family and friends who have offered encouragement during the writing of this text, and to patients, students and colleagues who have shared life, treatment and educational experiences with us.

Introduction

In some ways it seems that we began work on this second edition on the very day the first edition was completed. Many new ideas have been presented since 1986 and new information gathered, much of which we have been anxious to comment on or include in our text.

In our estimation, an important function of a frame of reference is that it helps us as therapists to identify, select and organize the principles that give coherence to our practice. In the same spirit, the function of a text such as this is to identify viable frames of reference in occupational therapy and present their position clearly, without overwhelming the reader with information. This has been our goal in both the first and this edition.

At times, our goal has felt like a formidable task. The more we have explored the literature in support of the various frames of reference that are discussed, the more striking is the extent to which information and certain beliefs are shared among the frameworks. When Ann Mosey published her book *Three Frames of Reference for Mental Health* (1970) she identified the psychoanalytical, the behavioral, and the developmental positions. Although some concepts were shared, the stands taken within each framework were quite opposite. The situation was not unlike that in psychology in which one contrasted the ideas of Freud, a psychoanalyst, against those of Skinner, a behaviorist.

These polarities seem to be lessening, however, and the commonalities shared by the frameworks become evident in the updated information presented in this second edition. Many of the programs, assessments and theories that we encountered in the literature, while identifying themselves with a specific frame of reference, draw from concepts or ideas that are similar, even identical to those cited by proponents of other frameworks, although the final product or emphasis is distinct. This perhaps reaches its pinnacle in the development of the model of human occupation.

We expressed unequivocally in the first edition our belief that as a profession occupational therapy profits from having multiple and diverse frameworks with which to meet the changing needs of the patients and clients whom it serves. We continue to stand firmly by this belief, but recognize, too, that no one can or should want to sit on both sides of the fence on opposing theoretical and practice issues. Thus it is important for the therapist to recognize that, despite some similarities, guiding paths of departure distinguish one framework from the others.

The reader is encouraged to evaluate each one of these frameworks carefully, not only for their surface appeal, but to better understand where paths diverge, and what that means in terms of the application of each framework. One thing seems to stand out—the conviction, common to all these frameworks, that it is through participation in *activity* that the person learns, changes feelings and perceptions, and finds meaning and purpose in life.

Although our format in this second edition is very similar to that in the original text, we have added many subheadings, in part to make it easier for the reader to recognize themes and contrast frameworks. We have added study or focus questions to help bring the reader's attention to the commonalities and distinguishing features of each of the frameworks. We have also indentified significant terms with boldface type. These terms have been left in the context of the chapter so that they may be more easily understood.

This edition has also been rewritten to reflect the profession's and our commitment to a nonsexist, nonprejudicial attitude. We appreciate the editors' cooperation in giving priority to the individual. We encourage the reader to join us in the movement to speak of our patients or clients as persons with depression or chronic problems and not label them as "the chronic," "the anorexic," or "the depressed."

Additonally, we have added a chapter on the cognitive disabilities framework of Allen and her associates and another on research and practice in the movement-centered approaches that originated with the work of Ayres and Lorna King. Based on recommendations of colleagues we have included an appendix on the problems of suicide and have reorganized some information to form the holistic frame of reference.

Over the past seven years we have informally monitored the literature for research and treatment discussions that pertain to psychosocial occupational therapy, in part to assess the direction of practice and in part to identify changing priorities. We have found discussions representative of all the frameworks identified in this text. It is interesting to note, however, that research in the past several years has been predominantly in the areas of cognition, cognitive disabilities and human occupation, whereas practice (as discussed in relation to individual programs and case studies) has been across frameworks.

Chapter 1

HISTORICAL OVERVIEW OF PSYCHOSOCIAL OCCUPATIONAL THERAPY

Focus Questions

1. How has humanistic philosophy influenced occupational therapy?
2. Cite some beliefs on which occupational therapy is based.
3. Describe how social changes have affected occupational therapy.
4. What differences are suggested by the use of the term *patient* versus *client*?
5. What is a frame of reference? How is it used?
6. Which official documents of the American Occupational Therapy Association influence mental health practice?

Introduction

This historical overview of psychosocial occupational therapy is presented to highlight marker events within the occupational therapy profession as well as those in the mental health field. These events have influenced the boundaries of psychosocial occupational therapy, have affected theory and practice in occupational therapy and in mental health, and have influenced the guidelines for education and research. Understanding the history of our profession, as it reflects on each of our personal histories, gives us insight into where we have come from and why we value what we do, and helps us appreciate our paths in relationship to the larger society.

The following events and trends should not be approached as facts to be memorized. Rather, the reader is given a flavor of the events and trends that have become a part of occupational therapy as a profession. The reader is reminded of this history when proceeding through the chapters in this book, as this text is organized chronologically from the earliest Freudian-based practice to the most recent frameworks of cognition and model of human occupation.

Occupational Therapy in Psychiatry and the Mental Health System

Humanitarian Care

Throughout occupational therapy's history, whether viewed from within psychiatry or mental health systems, the profession has been influenced by the philosophy of humanism. From the early writings to the present, the humanistic philosophy is either directly acknowledged or its influence is evident in the manner in which the patient is described, in the importance given to the therapeutic relationship and the patient's contributions to the therapy outcome, and in the types of intervention strategies described to increase the patient's quality of life. This text presents humanism as a philosophy that is evident in or influences each frame of reference practiced in occupational therapy. Therefore, it is not treated as an individual frame of reference, as has been the orientation in some other occupational therapy literature.

Occupational therapy arose out of a "moral" concern for the mentally ill in the late 1800s and early 1900s. During this time, two hospitals in the East, McClean Hospital and Frankfort Asylum, are noted for having treatment programs based on a holistic philosophy in which patients were treated kindly and were involved in activities that were believed capable of helping them adapt to their culture.

Founder's Beliefs

From these initial roots come the approaches of the founders of the profession: Meyer (concerned with the complex biological and psychological interactions of persons which influence their social performance in daily life); Slagle (concerned with using purposeful activity to develop habits); Dunton (concerned with forming habits to help the patient work and socialize in the community); Haas (concerned with achieving competence and a sense of pride from activities completed in the workshop); and Bryan and Marsh, who used industrial therapy to help patients continue to be productive members of society.[20] These philosophies continued to be used and refined throughout the 1920s and 1930s and have remained influential into the 1990s as noted in current literature.

Role of Occupation and Activity

After World War I, occupational therapy was developed to provide occupations for the men-

tally ill and to help them resolve "problems of living."[16,43] The occupational therapy used in this period was developed by Meyer and others who were humanistic and sought to help the patient identify his or her capabilities and use them productively. This form of therapy was practiced in the medical setting and was seen as augumenting medical treatment.

During the 1930s and 1940s the occupational therapist provided services through the use of activities selected to aid in diagnosis, to facilitate adjustment to the hospital, to supplement other therapies that the patient received, and to develop constructive habits.[16,43]

Expansion of Theory and Practice

During the late 1940s and throughout the 1950s, there was minimal legislation for mental health. The occupational therapy profession invested energy primarily in developing more scientific approaches to treatment and in expanding the services to the physically disabled.[16,43] Some viewed this scientific movement as a negation of humanism and a movement away from the original philosophic base of the profession. Alternatively, this trend was viewed theoretically as an expansion of theory and practice to include principles of both science and humanism in a holistic or biopsychosocial approach.

In psychiatric occupational therapy during the 1950s the understanding of psychodynamics and principles of interpersonal psychology influenced occupational therapy practice. The incorporation of information from psychiatry and psychology has broadened occupational therapy's understanding of the therapeutic relationship and strengthened our understanding of the meaning of activities for patients. As a result of findings from interpersonal psychology, occupational therapists have an increased sensitivity to nonverbal communication and its potential for increasing understanding, and increased awareness of how social and interpersonal communication can influence and benefit the treatment process.

Symptom-Activity Match

The major negative outcome of the scientific movement was to categorize patients and activities in a way that attempts to match a particular activity to the treatment of a particular diagnosis or to relieve specific symptoms. Activities began to be used in a restricted manner, and often an unrealistic attempt was made to cure a patient who had an illness rather than help the individual use capabilities to solve problems in living and adapt to his or her life situation.

The symptom-activity match process tends to eliminate the personalization of treatment and the appreciation of the interpersonal context in which activities occur; however, this negation of the interpersonal context of activity is minimized in contemporary practice. Although certain activities may be seen as more appropriate given the limitations related to symptomatology, activities are not like pills given to cure symptoms.

Medications

The influence of science was also felt in psychiatry as psychopharmacology evolved and psychiatrists sought to control patient symptoms through the use of medication. Since the 1940s, medications have been used in moderation or extensively depending on the philosophy of the attending physician or care setting. The type and dose of medications are controversial, and these issues are not elaborated in this text.

The occupational therapist is sensitive to the effects of medication on patient performance and reports findings to the attending physician and other treatment team members. In some situations the use of medications minimizes patient symptoms and makes patients more amenable to treatment. In other cases, however, such as with overly or heavily medicated patients or patients medicated for long periods of time, detrimental side effects may occur.

Remedicalization of Psychiatry

As medical technology makes possible the increasingly sophisticated study of the brain, there has been a decided reembracing of the belief that many psychiatric problems are tied to structural or chemical brain abnormalities, including those carried genetically. Therefore, many hope to better remediate or even prevent symptomatology through the identification of effective medication. More recently this trend has been referred to as the **medicalization** or **remedicalization** of psychiatry.[34,37]

Occupational Therapy in the Community

From 1943 to 1954 there was increased support from the community at large and from within occupational therapy to develop vocational rehabilitation programs for psychiatric patients. This support promoted prevocational evaluation and programming and led to patient employment within treatment settings.[8] The employment of patients in treatment settings was furthered by the development of sheltered workshops and through contractual agreements made between mental health settings and community businesses during the 1960s. However, patient work programs were called into question during the 1970s as patient advocacy grew and as work unions classified jobs and limited the boundaries of employment to the confines of the institutional setting.

Patient's Rights

During the 1960s, the community mental health movement was a strong force that contributed to the growth and development of mental health practice, occupational therapy practice, and applied psychology in general. The community mental health movement introduced new terminology, expanded treatment settings and treatment strategies, suggested new responsibilities for mental health professionals (with some role blurring), heightened public awareness of mental health issues, and requested an empathetic response from the general public to the "mental" patient. These changes helped bring about federal, state and local legislation that called attention to patient's rights, legal responsibilities of institutions, and standards criteria for patient care and quality assurance.[24]

Psychosocial Occupational Therapy

The impact of the community mental health movement is evident in the professional journals published since the 1960s. One of the first observations made from a review of the occupational therapy literature is a change in the terminology used for defining the realm of practice. Early writing refers to **psychiatric occupational therapy**, a term tied to psychiatry, a medical specialty. Writings of the last 25 years have continued to reflect psychiatric-medical ties, but have also suggested an expanded concept of theory in the use of the terms **psychosocial occupational therapy** and **occupational therapy in mental health**. The change in terminology reflects the expansion of practice beyond the traditional hospital or medical setting to the community mental health, school and home settings.

Expanded Role for Occupational Therapists

In mental health practice, occupational therapists were asked to develop occupational therapy services for day treatment programs and for residential community living or transition centers and to design prevention programs. The occupational therapist's role evolved to include that of educator and consultant, and the responsibilities and expertise that the therapist offered in these new roles allowed the therapist to be viewed as a peer with other professionals on the treatment team rather than as an aide to the psychiatrist.

> Being an aide to the psychiatrist was the predominant role for the occupational therapist as well as for other health professionals who worked in psychiatric hospitals during the 1950s.

The broadening of the occupational therapist's role to include patient education and prevention influenced the philosophical base of practice. Some old concepts were renewed, and new ideas were incorporated to form health concepts and treatment approaches that would strive to use the patient's healthy side or strengths, remediate psychosocial problems, treat symptoms, promote adaptation, provide patient education, and increase the patient's quality of life.

Activities Therapy

One outcome of this expansion was the evolution of activities therapy. In an activities therapy program, occupational therapists, recreational therapists, dance therapists, art therapists, music therapists, and sometimes horticultural therapists were employed. These therapists came with their own professional training and offered a particular specialty, as suggested by their titles, which contributed to treatment within the therapeutic milieu. The therapists used creative-expressive media, work-oriented experiences, recreational activities, activities of daily living, and interpersonal communication experiences to improve psychosocial functioning.

The activities therapy movement has had great impact on the growth and development of psychosocial occupational therapy as well as on other specialties such as recreational therapy. It also continues to influence and perhaps limit occupational therapy's future. Although each of the therapies listed may be viewed as one kind of activities therapy, there is no professional training specific to an individual calling himself or herself an "activities therapist." Economic constraints and the limited resource pool of qualified occupational therapists has in some instances promoted the hiring of activities therapists rather than occupational therapists.

Expansion of Practice

In spite of the shortage of occupational therapists practicing in mental health, this speciality area continues to broaden. The literature of the last decade suggests that mental health practice is expanding to meet the psychosocial needs of children,[38,15] the homeless, and persons with HIV disease.[13,33,40]

Throughout the history of occupational therapy, the expansion of practice has not only given rise to a proliferation of therapeutic approaches and called into focus multiple frames of reference, but also has led to a diverse use of terminology and created controversy. There has been a lack of consensus about the role of the occupational therapist, what qualities are unique to occupational therapy, and how the profession can best be unified. Specific to mental health practice, the question has been raised as to how the profession can recruit and retain therapists in mental health and whether psychosocial occupational therapy will survive.[3,4,5,6]

Deinstitutionalization of State Hospitals

Up to and throughout the 1950s, most illness was treated in inpatient settings: state hospitals, general city and county hospitals, and a few private institutions.[35] The most severely disturbed individuals were institutionalized in state psychiatric hospitals, many for years or even most of their adult life.[24]

Bowing to economic and philosophical pressure, state agencies began to release these individuals: In 1955, 560,000 residents were in state institutions; by 1988 only 115,000 individuals lived in these facilities.[24] Unfortunately, most of these residents were not prepared to live independently. The burden of caring for those who reappeared in need of mental health services fell largely to community mental health and other local service agencies. Persons in acute crisis were often hospitalized, but whenever feasible, outpatient treatment was used.

Economic Constraints

Private insurers such as Blue Cross-Blue Shield and Mutual of Omaha have historically covered inpatient psychiatric care only to a limited extent.[35] They have been even more restrictive in their coverage of outpatient treatment. Additionally, state and federal reimbursing agencies such as Medicare and Medicaid have felt the economic crunch and have demanded more careful accountability in the use of state and federal institutions.[11,14,35] Professional peer review and a plethora of cost accounting systems evolved in an effort to contain costs and ensure that treatment providers delivered the outcomes promised.

One result has been a move toward an acute care model of hospitalization. Acute inpatient hospitalizations are intended for individuals in severe crisis, for example those who are psychotic or suicidal. An **acute** hospitalization period is typically defined as lasting 30 days or less. The goals for the patient are the clarification of diagnosis, plus other assessment, stabilization on medication, and the beginning of a psychotherapeutic relationship.[11,25]

Impact of Health Care Changes

Occupational therapy has been tremendously affected by these changes in mental health care. Health care costs continue to skyrocket, consumers are more knowledgeable, and reimbursement is more limited. The occupational therapist, along with other health care professionals, has been called on to demonstrate and document the effectiveness of intervention and to contain costs. In years past, occupational therapy services were covered as part of the inpatient room rate. Occupational therapy services are now often identified and paid for separately by the reimbursing party. With the patient in treatment for shorter periods and fewer available dollars, there is increased competition among service providers.

One response from the profession has been to consult more closely with the consumer in professional policy making.

The reality is that many individuals suffer chronic or recurring psychiatric problems. Given the mandate to keep inpatient treatment as brief as possible, there is a double-pronged impetus to occupational therapy to build functional skills that will enhance the ability of these persons to care for themselves.[9,22]

As summarized by Foto,[11] insurers and reimbursement payers (and we would add patients, their families and the community at large) want health delivery systems that "promote wellness, provide appropriate care, reduce hospital days, treat patients at the lowest level of care appropriate, return patients to the healthiest state and most functional level possible and keep patients satisfied and served."

Other Social Influences

Countless other socioeconomic events have influenced and continue to affect mental health practice. Examples include the civil rights movement, the women's movement, changes in criminal law and an increased use of the "insanity" plea; and society's changing view about disease, mental health and illness, and deviance. These trends have led to legislation and legal decisions in support of patient rights and patient advocacy. Many witnessing the growing number of homeless and displaced persons and an increase in the number of single-parent families predict an acceleration in the number of persons who will need psychiatric care or transitional support. These changes have contributed to the heightened social conscience of occupational therapists as they strive to respond to the greater interests of society.

Defining Terms in Occupational Therapy

Paradigm, Model, Frame of Reference

The profession of occupational therapy holds multiple definitions and interpretations for the terms **model, paradigm** and **frame of reference**. Rather than repeat these definitions, we summarize the terms as they have been used in the recent professional literature.

Paradigm

The work of Kuhn[21] is often cited in the discussion of the term **paradigm**. As applied to occupational therapy, a paradigm would contain the guiding premises and theories behind the profession as a whole. As such, a paradigm identifies the theories that have been or need to be tested and that will lead to the creation and organization of knowledge.

Model

Using the literature from education and the professional fields of social work, medicine and law, Mosey[32] summarized a **model** as follows: ". . . A profession's model is the typical way in which a profession perceives itself, its relationship to other professions, and its association with the society to which it is responsible. The model of a profession is characterized by a description of the profession's philosophical assumptions, ethical code, theoretical foundation, domain of concern, legitimate tools, and the nature of and principles for sequencing the various aspects of practice."

The models of practice in psychiatry are identified in the sixth edition of *Willard and Spackman's Occupational Therapy*: 1) biophysical, 2) intrapsychic, 3) behavioral, 4) sociocultural, 5) phenomenological, and 6) integrative.[17] These models are based on knowledge from the biological and social sciences. From these models occupational therapy has developed the major frames of reference in the profession.

Frame of Reference

A **frame of reference** refers to principles behind practice with specified patient or client populations. It includes a description of the population to be served, guidelines for determining adequate function or dysfunction, and principles of remediation.

Psychosocial occupational therapy has multiple frames of reference that have been organized in numerous ways. Llorens[23] presented a chronological discussion of occupational therapy frames of reference and common theories on which they are based. She identified the following frames of reference applied in occupational therapy practice: "humanistic, psychoanalytic, behavioral, developmental, acquisitional, neurodevelopmental, neurobehavioral, spatiotemporal adaptational, occupational behavior, occupational performance, and neurorehabilitation."

The frames of reference presented in this text were selected because collectively they are a diverse representation of the body of knowledge in psychosocial occupational therapy. When reflecting on the evolution of practice, recent theoretical developments that broaden or change the emphasis of current practice can be seen. Given the multiple arenas of practice, we have chosen frameworks that are applicable in multiple psychosocial settings in occupational therapy with patients with varied diagnoses, and patient problems. The frameworks are presented in a manner that allows the reader to see the evolution of psychosocial thinking in occupational therapy, and thereby shows how each successive framework incorporates some of the important ideas of the preceding frameworks.

Patient or Client?

An outcome of the community mental health movement was to call into question the use of the term **patient**. Many mental health professionals felt that the term patient reinforced the sick role of the individual and supported the idea of pathology or illness and the individual's need to be taken care of by health professionals. Mental health professionals, wishing to minimize the sick role, chose the term **client** to focus on problems of living not illness, and to encourage the individual to assume responsibility for his or her own health and care. A client is someone who "seeks a

service but not a medical service."[12] The reader should note that the use of the term client is not supported by most psychiatrists who continue to treat patients.

In occupational therapy both terms, client and patient, are used depending on the treatment setting or perhaps the preference of the occupational therapist or the treatment team with which the therapist works. In the mid-1980s, however, a controversy developed over the use of the two terms. Before then, the choice of the term patient was probably made with little consideration given to legal, ethical and moral issues. These issues, as well as the far-reaching implications for the profession, were brought to the occupational therapists' attention by Reilly and were researched and summarized by Sharrott and Yerxa.[36,39]

Sharrott and Yerxa justify the continued use of the term patient for the following reasons: 1) The term is based on a moral-ethical tradition rather than an economic-legalistic foundation and the occupational therapy profession has a moral-ethical base, 2) the term is compatible with the Meyerian philosophy of the profession, 3) the term connotes the ethical stance of moral treatment of the nineteenth century, and 4) the term supports opportunity for health care regardless of the patient's ability to provide financial renumeration.[39]

Covenant Code

For those therapists who support the use of the term client to equalize the responsibilities in treatment, Sharrott and Yerxa use Veatch's conceptualization of medical ethics to identify how responsibilities can be equalized in the patient-therapist relationship. Briefly, Veatch[44] proposes that medical ethics be based on a **covenant code**. "A covenant is a contract that emphasizes moral bonds and fidelity and requires right action by both health professionals and the lay public." Medical ethics are designed to apply to "patient-health professional relationships."

The fundamental principles of the covenant are as follows:

1. Keeping promises and commitments to one another;
2. Treating one another as autonomous members of the moral community free to make choices that do not violate other basic ethical requirements;
3. Dealing honestly with one another;
4. Avoiding actively and knowingly the taking of morally protected life;
5. Striving for equality in individual welfare and equality in the right of access to health care;
6. Producing good for one another and treating one another with respect, dignity, and compassion.[39,44]

Terminology in this Text

This text uses the term patient. The term is congruent with occupational therapy's philosophy and history. It supports a moral-ethical base for practice. It is compatible with mutuality of respect and responsibility vital to the patient-therapist relationship, and it supports occupational therapy's advocacy role for quality care for those we treat regardless of the disability or the treatment setting. We recognize, however, the need to function within one's environment and are aware that the use of the words client, student, or resident may be dictated by the setting in which the occupational therapist works. Regardless of the term applied, the material presented in the text is viable in practice.

Marker Events in the Occupational Therapy Profession

We have briefly considered some of the changes within society, medicine and the mental health community and their influence in the history and development of psychosocial occupational therapy. Next we review briefly the administrative decisions made by the governing body of the occupational therapy profession that have influenced theory, practice, education and research in psychosocial occupational therapy. In general, the administrators and governing body of the American Occupational Therapy Association have supported, individually or jointly with other organizations, educational and research activities that promote the growth and development of psychosocial occupational therapy.

Grants for Theory Development and Continuing Education

In the 1950s the Mental Health Study Act (1955) and the Grant to the American Occupational Therapy Association from the National Institute of Mental Health provided funds that led to the Boiling Springs Pennsylvania Conference (1956). Leaders in the field of psychiatric occupational therapy met to discuss the influence of recent developments in psychiatry and psychology on occupational therapy. In the published proceedings, West (1959) notes that the conference heightened the awareness of the benefits of a holistic approach to treatment, of occupational therapy as a component of the therapeutic milieu, of the collaborative efforts of the occupational therapist and other members of the treatment team, and of the increasing use of groups in occupational therapy treatment.[43]

One event that occurred within the profession and simultaneously within the community mental health movement was the Social Rehabilitation Services Grant (1964), which led to the establishment of 14 regional and 21 national institutes for the purpose of providing continuing education experiences in group process, object relations theory, and principles of administration and supervision.[43]

Funded Research for Community Program Development

In 1966, the National Institute of Mental Health funded research to study and design occupational therapy programs in comprehensive community mental health. The study indicated that there had been a shift from in-hospital to community settings for treatment, a decrease in the average number of treatment days used per patient, an expanded role for the occupational therapist that required him or her to assume more leadership responsibility and use administrative-supervisory and consultation skills, and a change in the activities used (e.g., activities that were shorter term and that required fewer heavy tools and equipment and more portable tools because of the multiple settings in which occupational therapy occurs).[18]

Symposia on Theoretical Discourse

In 1967 at Albion, Michigan, seven leaders in the field of psychosocial occupational therapy met to consider the theories in psychiatric occupational therapy and to try to integrate them into a mind-body theory that would be meaningful and applicable to occupational therapy. Those at the symposium concluded that 1) the seminar had unrealistic expectations, 2) educators and clinicians needed to study the existing body of knowledge and to identify the relationships within this knowledge, 3) the relationships identified needed to be researched, 4) a frame of reference was needed that used a holistic approach, and 5) occupational therapy had two major paths of theoretical development—one for physical disabilities and one for psychiatry.[28,29]

The next marker event in 1968 occurred when the American Occupational Therapy Association's Consult in Psychiatric Rehabilitation extended an invitation to clinicians to submit papers describing frames of reference used in psychiatric occupational therapy. Several papers were selected for publication in the *American Journal of Occupational Therapy*. Three theories were presented: 1) a theory that combined ego psychology and learning theory,[7] 2) a learning based theory,[41] and 3) a developmental theory.[28,29,31]

Evaluation of Theory and Policy Governing Practice

The 1970s were characterized by workshops and task forces that met to study occupational

therapy in mental health and by further administrative decisions designed to govern practice. Investigation sought to identify the status of practice and the underlying theories in practice, to refine the standards and ethics of practice, to identify the boundaries of practice, and to identify the assessment and intervention strategies used—all with the intent of unifying the profession. Among the events identified was a symposium held in Boston in 1970, "The Skill Continuum from Play Through Work." The major goal of the symposium was to "develop a philosophy . . . for viewing human activity as a continuum and the productive behavior of later life as a development from the foundations established during childhood."[19]

The papers presented at the Boston meeting were published in the September, 1971 issue of the *American Journal of Occupational Therapy* and emphasized the following: 1) the patient's desire for competence as a motivating force for behavior;[45] 2) the relationship between intrinsic motivation and the growth and development of the child through play;[10] 3) the necessary elements in a milieu that promote play;[42] 4) the value of play in treatment to promote learning, coping, and adapting to change;[30] 5) the relationship between the play of a child and the creativity of the adolescent and the adult;[30] 6) the role of work and play in the development of occupational behavior;[26] 7) the childhood and adolescent experiences that influence work behavior;[2,27] and 8) the relationship of work to the broader concept of "activity" and the role of activity in the rehabilitation process.[19]

Professional Policies

During the 1970s the Representative Assembly became a policy-making body for the profession. This Assembly approved documents such as the Ethical Statement of the profession in 1976 (see Appendix A for 1992 document), Standards of Practice in Mental Health in 1978 (see Appendix B for current Standards of Practice), and Uniform Terminology in 1979. These documents continue to be reviewed and updated.

Assessment Institute

From the beginning the profession has expressed concern about the lack of valid and reliable assessment tools in mental health practice. This concern resurfaced in 1977 by the Mental Health Specialty section of the American Occupational Therapy Association. As a result, an assessment institute was held in 1979 before the annual conference in Detroit. Occupational therapists were invited to present the assessments that they used in practice. Assessments were reviewed and recommendations were made regarding their further development and research potential. One of the outcomes of this institute was the presentation of the Bay Area Functional Performance Evaluation (BaFPE) and the recommendation for its further development and research design. Today this assessment battery is used in many mental health settings and continues to be researched to determine validity and reliability standards. (See the description of the BaFPE in Chapter 6.)

Philosophical Base of the Profession

In 1978, at a special meeting of the Representative Assembly in San Diego, leaders in the profession were invited to discuss the profession's philosophical base, the status of practice, and education and credentialing issues. From the discussions that occurred a philosophical base of the profession was identified and "occupation" was identified as the common core of occupational therapy.[17]

Development and Revision of Education and Practice Policy

The events, concerns, and ideas that characterized the 1970s into the 1980s and now shape current discussion, legislation, theory development, practice, education, and research. During the 1980s and 1990s the American Occupational Therapy Association adopted and revised several key documents, all of which continue to be reviewed and updated as warranted. These documents include the Occupational Therapy Code of Ethics (1980, 1992), Uniform Terminology for Occupational Therapy (revised 1989), the Essentials and Guidelines of an Accredited Educational Program for the Occupational Therapist (revised 1991), Essentials and Guidelines of an Accredited Educational Program for the Occupational Therapy Assistant (revised 1991), Guidelines for Occupational Therapy Documentation (1986), and Work Hardening Guidelines (1986). Practice papers delineate the roles and functions of the occupational therapist working in the area of adult day care (1986), long-term care (1983), Alzheimer's disease and related disorders (1986), cognitive impairment (1991), hospice (1986), and as a case manager (1991).

One other significant position taken by the American Occupational Therapy Association was to encourage the use of gender-neutral language in professional publications and documentation.[1]

The documents cited reflect the growing need to provide uniformity of documentation and treatment. In keeping with the demand to improve cost-effectiveness while maintaining quality of care, the American Occupational Therapy Association, through its constituent bodies, provides educational opportunities and materials to its members. Therapists practicing in the area of mental health may also function within the guidelines for practice established by other professional organizations such as the National Association of Private-Practice Hospitals, the National Institute of Mental Health, the National Mental Health Association, and Medicare Guidelines for Occupational Therapy Services (Department of Health and Human Services).

Effect of Specialization on Psychosocial Occupational Therapy

Education, research and practice in the field are also reflected in and influenced by the literature. Many textbooks and juried journals that focus on practice as well as research have contributed to occupational therapy's body of knowledge. When reviewing the list of publications in psychosocial occupational therapy, one is struck by the vast increase in the number of texts now available as compared to 20 years ago. The increase in publications reflects the growth of the profession and its knowledge base as well as paralleling the trend toward specialization in the occupational therapy profession and the movement in professional education to master's and doctoral level preparation for therapists.

The introduction of multiple journals, such as *Occupational Therapy in Mental Health* (1980), the *Occupational Therapy Journal of Research* (1981) and the Mental Health Specialty Section Newsletter broadened the arena for professional exchange. These additional publications are another indication of the expanded role of psychosocial occupational therapy within the profession, and they provide one means to disseminate the growing body of knowledge pertinent to psychosocial practice.

Summary

From this cursory review of occupational therapy history and from the professional literature, major theoretical and practice issues have emerged. Posed as questions these issues include the following:

1. What are the legitimate boundaries of occupational therapy mental health practice?
2. What are the legitimate tools for evaluation and treatment?
3. Do we treat patients, clients, residents, or students?
4. How can we best organize occupational therapy's body of knowledge? As a model? As a frame of reference? As a paradigm?
5. How should we categorize the models of practice in the field?
6. Should there be only one frame of reference for practice?

7. Is there a unifying theory of occupational therapy?
8. What is unique to occupational therapy?
9. How can we best standardize assessment?
10. Can and should we unify the treatment strategies used in the field?
11. Where are the greatest needs for research in psychosocial occupational therapy? Quantitative, qualitative, or both?
12. What will enhance further needed research in education and in practice?
13. How can the profession meet the demands of psychosocial practice with the limited number of occupational therapists in the professional pool?
14. How do we best assure and document quality care?
15. How do we prepare for the future needs of the mental health profession and ensure the continued endorsement of psychosocial occupational therapy practice within funding constraints and the changing environment of the health care system?

There is no simple solution to any of these problems, and perhaps some of these questions do not or should not have a definitive answer. This text summarizes the body of knowledge in psychosocial occupational therapy and encourages the reader to carefully consider the wealth of theory and practice that exists. Question it; discuss it with colleagues; propose research; or just think about what you read. Most importantly, avoid making a hasty decision or giving a quick answer to one of the preceding questions when such an answer would limit patient care under the guise of professional unity.

References

1. American Occupational Therapy Association: Association policies. *Am J Occup Ther* 45(12):1112, 1991.
2. Bailey D: Vocational theories and work habits related to childhood development. *Am J Occup Ther* 25(6): 298–302, 1971.
3. Bailey D: Reasons for attrition from occupational therapy. *Am J Occup Ther* 44(3):23–30, 1990.

4. Bailey D: Ways to retain or reactivate occupational therapists. *Am J Occup Ther* 44(3):31–38, 1990.

5. Burnette-Beaulier S: Occupational therapy profession dropouts: Escape from the grief process. *Occup Ther Mental Health* 2:45–55, 1982.

6. Cottrell RF: Perceived competence among occupational therapists in mental health. *Am J Occup Ther* 44(2):118–124, 1989.

7. Diasio K: Psychiatric occupational therapy: Search for a conceptual framework in the light of psychoanalytic ego psychology and learning theory. *Am J Occup Ther* 22:400–414, 1968.

8. Dunton D: Psychiatric occupational therapy. In Willard H, Spackman C (Eds:) *Occupational Therapy* Ed 3. Philadelphia, JB Lippincott, 1963, pp. 57–74.

9. Fine S: 1988. Working the system: A perspective for managing change. *Am J Occup Ther* 47(7):417–419, 1988.

10. Florey L: An approach to play and play development. *Am J Occup Ther* 25(6):275–280, 1971.

11. Foto M: Managing change in reimbursement patterns. *Am J Occup Ther* 42(9):563–565, 1988.

12. Gillette N: Occupational therapy and mental health. In Willard H, Spackman C (Eds): *Occupational Therapy*. Ed 4. Philadelphia, JB Lippincott, 1971, pp. 51–132.

13. Gutterman L: A day program for persons with AIDS. *Am J Occup Ther* 44(3):234–238, 1990.

14. Hanft B: Prospective payment for pscyhiatric services. In Robertson S (Ed): *Mental Health Focus: Skills for Assessment and Treatment*. Rockville, MD, American Occupational Therapy Association, 1988, pp. 3.10–3.15.

15. Hatje Kaufman C, Daniels R, Laverdure P, et al: Pediatric occupational therapy within a cognitive-behavioral setting. In Scott D, Katz N: *Occupational Therapy in Mental Health: Principles in Practice*. London, Taylor & Francis, 1988.

16. Hopkins H: An historical perspective on occupational therapy. In Hopkins H, Smith H: *Willard and Spackman's Occupational Therapy*. Ed 6. Philadelphia, JB Lippincott, 1983.

17. Hopkins H, Smith H: *Willard and Spackman's Occupational Therapy*. Ed 6. Philadelphia, JB Lippincott, 1983.

18. Howe M: The role of occupational therapy in community mental health. *Am J Occup Ther* 22(6):521–524, 1968.

19. Johnson J: Considerations of work as therapy in the rehabilitation process. *Am J Occup Ther* 25(6):303–308, 1971.

20. Kielhofner G, Burke J: Occupational therapy after 60 years: An account of changing identity and knowledge. *Am J Occup Ther* 31(10):675–689, 1977.

21. Kuhn T: *The Structure of Scientific Revolutions*. Chicago, University of Chicago Press, 1974.

22. Lang S, Cara E: Vocational integration for the psychiatrically disabled. *Hosp Community Psychiatry* 40(9): 890–892, 1989.

23. Llorens L: Theoretical conceptualizations of occupational therapy: 1960–1982. *Occup Ther Mental Health* 4(2):1–14, 1984.

24. Marcos L: Taking issue: Who profits from deinstitutionalization. *Hosp Community Pscyhiatry* 40(12):1221, 1989.

25. Margo G, Manring J: 1989. The current literature on inpatient psychotherapy. *Hosp Community Psychiatry* 40(9):909–915, 1989.

26. Matsutsuyu J: Occupational behavior: A perspective on work and play. *Am J Occup Ther* 25(6):291–294, 1971.

27. Maurer P: Antecedents of work behavior. *Am J Occup Ther* 25(6):295–297, 1971.

28. Mazer J (Ed): Toward an integrated theory of occupational therapy. Seminar Aug.26–31, 1967, Albion, MICH. *Am J Occup Ther* 22(5):451–456, 1968.

29. Mazer J, Mosey A (Eds): Special section—Theories of psychiatric occupational therapy. *Am J Occup Ther* 22(5):398–450, 1968.

30. Michelman S: The importance of creative play. *Am J Occup Ther* 25(6):285–295, 1971.

31. Mosey AC: Recapitulation of ontogenesis. *Am J Occup Ther* 22(5):426–438, 1968.

32. Mosey AC: *Occupational Therapy—Configuration of a Profession*. New York, Raven Press, 1981, p. 50.

33. O'Rourke GC: The HIV-positive intravenous drug abuser. *Am J Occup Ther* 44(3):280–293, 1990.

34. Palmer F: The present context of service delivery. In Robertson S (Ed): *Mental Health Focus : Skills for Assessment and Treatment*. Rockville, MD, American Occupational Therapy Association, 1988, pp. 1.28–1.36.

35. Peters M: Reimbursement for psychiatric occupational services. In Robertson S (Ed): *Mental Health Focus: Skills for Assessment and Treatment*. Rockville, MD, American Occupational Therapy Association, 1988, pp. 3.3–3.9.

36. Reilly M: The importance of the client versus patient issue for occupational therapy. *Am J Occup Ther* 38(6): 404–406, 1984.

37. Robertson S: Factors influencing service delivery. In Robertson S (Ed): *Mental Health Focus: Skills for Assessment and Treatment* Rockville, MD, American Occupational Therapy Association, 1988, pp. 1.24–1.27.

38. Sholle-Martin S, Alessi NE: Formulating a role for occupational therapy in child psychiatry: A clinical application. *Am J Occup Ther* 44(10):871–883, 1990.

39. Sharrott G, Yerxa E: Promises to keep: Implications of the referent "patient" versus "client" for those served by occupational therapy. *Am J Occup Ther* 39(6):401–405, 1985.

40. Sladyk K: Teaching safe sex practices to psychiatric patients. *Am J Occup Ther* 44(3):284–285, 1990.

41. Smith A, Tempone V: Psychiatric occupational therapy within a learning theory context. *Am J Occup Ther* 22(5):415, 1968.

42. Takata N: The play milieu: A preliminary appraisal. *Am J Occup Ther* 25(6):281–281, 1971.

43. Tiffany E: Psychiatry and mental health. In Hopkins H, Smith H: *Willard and Spackman's Occupational Therapy.* Ed 6. Philadelphia, JB Lippincott, 1983, pp. 267–334.

44. Veatch R: *A Theory of Medical Ethics.* New York, Basic Books, 1981, pp. 327–328.

45. White R: The urge towards competence. *Am J Occup Ther* 25(6):271–274, 1971.

Chapter 2

THE FRAMEWORK OF THERAPY IN OCCUPATIONAL THERAPY

Focus Questions

1. Describe briefly the elements that contribute to the framework of therapy.
2. What contributes to the boundaries of the therapeutic relationship?
3. How is therapy defined?
4. In what kinds of situations are people more likely to risk change?
5. What is the difference between group content and process? Describe and give examples of each.
6. What is the primary advantage of situational leadership?
7. How does a therapeutic group differ from a social group?
8. In what ways can the therapist help a patient feel safe within a treatment group?
9. How do purposeful activities contribute to the boundaries of treatment? How do they contribute to the attainment of patient goals?
10. What is meant by the activity process as contrasted with the activity product?
11. What is the art of therapy as compared to the science?

Introduction

As we journey through this text and travel the major routes of occupational therapy practice, we use a framework that has the common elements in the therapy environment that form the framework of the occupational therapy process. These common elements (patient, therapist, activity, and environment) are similar to the landmarks of a map that guide a journey and the choices made to reach a specific destination.

In occupational therapy practice, the therapist uses a frame of reference or map to guide choices and decisions (clinical reasoning) that support the patient's pursuit of goals and arrival at a specific destination. During the every day encounters between 1) patient and therapist, 2) patient and activity, and often 3) among several patients and treatment staff within a group milieu, the framework for therapy is formed. This framework has a therapeutic relationship, a group or individual milieu, meaningful (purposeful) activities, and a clinical reasoning process. These four framework elements exist and interact within each frame of reference and must be understood because they are the landmarks that influence each patient's destination. They are discussed in this chapter to help the reader understand the contribution that each makes to the occupational therapy process. How these elements emerge and interact within a particular frame of reference is discussed in the chapters of this text.

Therapeutic Relationship

As educators, we have stood before eager students early in the semester, seeking to convey not only fact but also our feelings about the significance and special nature of the therapeutic relationship. Enthusiastic ourselves, we nevertheless were in something of the same dilemma as a person trying to talk about a melody. We spoke about rhythms, characters and intonations that admittedly fell far short of the actual experience of the melody in the relationship.

Here, again, we wish to discuss what for us have emerged as essential dimensions of the therapeutic relationship, recognizing that we have been selective in the attributes we choose. We know, too, that like the notes in a song, the elements in a personal relationship must be heard in relationship to each other.

As you read, we hope that you will recognize in the values and behaviors described reminiscences of relationships you have known in your own life. From your own experience you bring both intuitive and well-formed ideas about the kinds of interpersonal conditions you find helpful, and those you do not. Pausing to reflect on your own experiences may help bring to life the discussion that follows.

Defining the Therapeutic Relationship

The therapeutic relationship is a unique coming together of two people for the express purpose of one assisting the other to manage internal or external stress, to mature, and to meet personal needs in a more satisfying way. The therapeutic relationship is between those two persons whom we refer to here as patient and therapist; other terms may be used in a context that is not medically oriented. In the therapeutic relationship, the patient is at the center. It is the mutual understanding of a patient's thoughts, values, fears, needs and aspirations that is the focus; and it must be his or her goals that ultimately define treatment.[2,19]

After familiarizing oneself with the major frameworks in which therapy is conceptualized, it becomes clear that opinions differ about what is therapeutic, and the role of the therapist can be coined in quite different terms, depending on the treatment framework. Particularly evident, however, is that professionals from a variety of helping disciplines and treatment models recognize that effective treatment requires a sound relationship between patient and therapist. Further, whether the primary therapeutic agent is seen as physical exercise, leisure activity, verbalization, or medication, many commonly held beliefs regarding the therapeutic relationship cut across the so-called boundaries of differing treatment philosophies and modalities.

We have selected for elaboration here therapeutic conditions that, in some instances, were given initial emphasis within the humanistic-existential movement (see Chapter 3). However, these conditions are consistent across the frameworks elaborated in this text. To look further at what constitutes a therapeutic relationship we need to pause and reflect, "What is therapy?"

What is Therapy?

Therapy is a process by which patients in distress can come to experience themselves in new ways that are more personally satisfying and that help them to relate more positively in the environment. At its heart, therapy facilitates change—be it a change from dis-ease to increased "ease" or physical well-being; expanded ideas, attitudes or skills; or changed ways of approaching events and tasks. A person seeks therapy when he or she is ineffective in independently making desired changes.

In occupational therapy, activities are seen as an essential therapeutic agent. Through involvement with activity patients learn new skills, mobilize physical energy, and learn more about themselves and others. They not only talk about what they wish to change (although reflecting upon personal experiences may enhance the ability to learn from them) but also try out and practice new behaviors.

Risking Change

Many of the activities in occupational therapy are not unusual or new; they are often the stuff of life. In both mental health and physical medicine, however, we see patients who cannot imagine themselves trying, much less succeeding, at the activities that are so familiar and available to them. For these patients, therapeutic activity remains inaccessible until they are able to picture themselves in a new role or they are willing to risk change, or a combination of both. The therapeutic relationship opens windows and widens pathways when risks are taken within its support, encouragement, caring and guidance.

Occupational Therapist's Role in the Therapeutic Relationship

When we risk change, we risk failure as well as success. We risk upheaval and uncertainty; we move to unfamiliar ground. To let go of the old and familiar, a person must first feel safe, and it is an essential role of the therapist to ensure safety.

Safety

Think for a moment about the situations in which you were willing to test a new idea or experiment with an activity that was quite foreign to you. We suspect that you needed to feel emotionally safe. Few of us have so much self-assurance that we will easily risk ridicule or tempt criticism. Perhaps someone with you assured you that if you faltered, they would be there to offer support.

Patients need to know that they will not be shamed or shame themselves. Beyond that, they need to know that they will not be forced into going further than they wish, that the boundaries they set will be respected. Sometimes that means allowing the patient to go very slowly even when we might want to get the ball rolling quickly. Patients must also feel physically safe. If they fear loss of control or physical harm, they need to know that they will not be allowed to harm themselves or others.

Coming from and providing a firm knowledge base enables the therapist to establish an environment of safety. Being knowledgeable about the patient's physical and emotional needs and about the demands and limitations within a broad range of human endeavor is requisite if a patient is to feel safe within our care. Providing the patients with information helps them gain power and control in relation to their own safety or well-being and is an important part of the continuing effort to enhance the patient's ability to be effective and appropriately self-reliant.

While we cannot predict the outcome of therapy, when we as therapists behave in a manner that is consistent and predictable, others tend to feel more safe with us, for they know what they can expect from us and what is expected of them.

We all hear about professionalism and may mistake it for starched shirt stuffiness or distancing maneuvers. In fact, as professionals, we strive to be consistent, ethical, dependable and knowledgeable and we make a statement of our commitment to the best of care. Such a commitment helps establish the sense of safety necessary for another to entrust us with his or her efforts to change.

Trust

An essential part of the therapeutic relationship is the ability of the therapist to foster trust, which is integral to the sense of safety we have just addressed. Three kinds of trust between two persons are emphasized here: respecting confidences, congruency and valuing ourselves.

Respecting Confidences. Respecting confidences relates to one person knowing that another will be honest—that his or her conduct is based on moral integrity. We have probably all been in situations in which we were not certain if our confidences would be kept, or perhaps we have been unsure if someone had been truthful. In such situations we tend to close up rather than open up, feeling a need to protect ourselves, our thoughts and our feelings.

Being Congruent.   There is also trust based on finding the other person to be authentic or "real." That is, there are certain values and characteristics that emerge consistently in the person's interactions. We do not encounter a chameleon. Our patient is more likely to experience us as real when we are, as described by Rogers, congruent.[32] **Congruent** in this usage means that our words, affect and actions go together to give a clear and consistent message.

Being congruent requires that as therapists we be aware of our beliefs and values. As stated by Rogers, ". . . if I can form a helping relationship to myself—if I can be sensitively aware and acceptant toward my own feelings—then the likelihood is great that I can form a helping relationship toward another."[32] Knowing what we ourselves believe helps us to keep our needs separate from those of our patients, helps us to be clear about our own boundaries and limitations, and allows us to behave in a manner that is consistent and establishes trust.

Valuing Ourselves.   Trust is nurtured also when we as therapists behave openly, as if we trust ourselves and believe in the worth of our therapy and in our own worth. This behavior includes acknowledging when we don't have all the answers and showing that we are willing to risk our own failures. When patients can see that we are willing to be vulnerable and open to learning, they find that they do not have to be perfect to be trustworthy and they have a model of self-acceptance from which they can learn.

Caring

Another important facet of trust is ensuring patients that we give their well-being the highest priority. They trust that we care about them. Devereaux[8] describes caring as the heart of the therapeutic relationship and notes ". . . its presence enriches all other aspects of the relationship." As she states, being cared about is the opposite of anonymity within and disconnectedness from the rest of the world. If you ask prospective or practicing therapists about their desire to be therapists, they will very often cite their wish to help or care about others. Brammer[4] refers to the need to care as a valuing of altruism. He reminds us that in our reaching out to others we fulfill our own need to feel valuable and connected to others. In recognizing that as therapists each of us gains something important for ourselves, we are better able to keep our motives and beliefs separate from the aims of our patients.

Valuing Our Patient.   Each of us has personal ideas about how caring can best be expressed, and, indeed, each human relationship will bring special circumstances and unique opportunities for caring. At its core, caring means that we believe that our patient is valuable, that we desire to know each person in a real way, and that the individual's needs, feelings and aspirations direct our service. Caring is not to be confused with mothering or infantilizing our patient. Rather, in caring for our patient we try to help the person become more independent and better able to meet the challenges of life.

Ironically, many patients who seek or come reluctantly into treatment state that they have no need to change because, as they say, "No one cares about what I do." When we let our caring show, we do not act as a substitute for friends, parents, spouses, or others; but we do provide a person-to-person relationship in which someone *does* care. At times, this approach is an evocative challenge to long-held suppositions as the patient may confront the possibility, "Perhaps someone does care? Perhaps I am worthy of being cared about?"

Open Communication

Safety, trust and the confirmation of caring all depend in their vitality on open communication within the therapeutic relationship. Where there is open communication, both patient and therapist can express themselves, state their concerns, clarify areas of doubt or ambiguity and move toward the common goals of therapy.

Much has been written about specific skills and therapist attitudes believed to enhance communication. Some of the more frequently cited books that describe helping behaviors are listed in the Recommended Reading List at the end of the chapter. For example, when we maintain good eye contact, indicate verbally and nonverbally our interest, and avoid a judgmental stance, we increase the likelihood that our patient will trust us with his thoughts.

Permission To Be Genuine. Open communication implies something deeper than encouragement to talk. It depends on an attitude of true permission for our patient to be genuine with us. Can you recall any instances where a parent, teacher, friend or other said, "Tell me what you really feel," or "Be yourself." Yet, when your response was received as challenging, the permission to be honest was rescinded. An essential part of open communication is allowing the patient to experience negative as well as positive feelings and to share those that he or she chooses to share with us. That approach is not always as easy as it sounds.

Patients may be angry with us when we feel they have no cause; they may express romantic feelings; they may behave unpredictably and threaten our personal need for order and control. While not making ourselves targets of abuse, when we listen to those feelings that may make us uncomfortable, we let patients know that our caring about them does not come and g with their ability to please us, and we increase the likelihood that patients can better understand their own concerns and feelings. In the process, we may learn more about who we are. We do not have to agree with or feel the same way that our patient does.

In fact, communication is a reciprocal process, and often includes our stating when and how things look different from our perspective. Open communication depends on both the patient and therapist having a respect for the right of the other to feel as each does, and it provides an opportunity for each to gain insight into the perceptions of the other.

Understanding. Open communication is necessary if patients are to believe that they are understood, that the therapist really knows the patient. Depending on the conceptual model, we as therapists may seek specific kinds of information from the patient, but it is important that we gain not only information that we believe is necessary from our viewpoint, but also that the patient knows that we understand what he or she thinks is important.

Often, a patient who is going through a particularly difficult time may feel isolated. For example, a woman newly divorced might say, "No one can know how I feel." Or, an amputee being encouraged to put pressure on a painful stump might say "It's easy for you to tell me to bear down; you don't feel the pain I do." In a way, both patients are correct. We cannot know exactly how each feels. But, if we can draw on our own experiences and attempt to look and listen for the purpose of understanding, we can go a long way toward appreciating the frustration and pain each experiences. In so doing, we increase our ability to communicate caring and to serve the best interests of our patients. Further, our encouragement to the patient to take risks does not become an insensitive demand.

Valuing Change

In the therapeutic relationship, the patient sees the therapist as someone who values change and who believes in a person's ability and potential for positive change. While each individual is ultimately responsible for taking risks, each of us is encouraged when someone we trust says, in essence, "I really believe you can do this."

The recent literature emphasizes the devastating effects of parenting in which a child is told over and over again, "You are inept." "You'll never amount to anything." And, as therapists we are unlikely to imagine ourselves making such statements. Yet, in our efforts to care or help we may give our own detrimental messages. When, for example, we overprotect patients to prevent them from failing, or because their reliance on us makes us feel important, we communicate, "I don't believe in your ability to take care of yourself, or to be successful."

At times we must use careful clinical judgment to determine the presence of an actual risk of physical harm and to assess how it can best be managed. Much of the changing and risk taking in the psychosocial setting, however, relates to emotional risk taking. We may find ourselves wishing to protect our patient from disappointment, failure or rebuffs. The clinical judgments we make in these instances are some of the most difficult. If we have established a sound therapeutic relationship, however, we enhance the ability of our patient to handle disappointments or experience them as more manageable. When we let patients know that we value them regardless of what they have accomplished, then we facilitate risk taking.

Accepting Tentativeness

For the relationship to be therapeutic, both the patient and therapist must accept some tentativeness in therapy. A patient may understandably try to limit ambiguity and perhaps ask for assurances that everything will go according to plan. This desire is not unlike the wish that most of us have had at some time for life to go according to plan. Learning to cope with the everyday vicissitudes depends on the confidence that each of us, patient and therapist, has in ourselves, our knowledge and skills, and on the degree to which we are

aware of the uncompromising values that give us our bearings.

As therapists we need to realize that while treatment plans give us direction, some of the most memorable learning occurs when we and our patient can respond spontaneously to unscheduled events or unexpected feelings. If we remember our initial premise that therapy facilitates change, we can better realize the essential need to accept tentativeness as part of the therapeutic process.

Relationship Boundaries

Finally, the therapeutic relationship is one in which the therapist recognizes and abides by its limitations. Some of the limitations in therapy relate directly to the nature of the patient's problems and the extent of resources. The following more general limitations are integral to the nature of the relationship itself.[2]

Time Limits. Therapy is a temporally bounded process: It cannot and will not go on endlessly. Helping a patient be aware of the probable length of treatment enables patient and therapist to establish reasonable expectations for what can be accomplished. If therapy facilitates change, we might speak metaphorically of therapy serving as a bridge into unfamiliar terrain. The therapist is the guide. Once the bridge is crossed, however, there is a point at which the guide departs, and the patient continues independently. Therefore, the patient and therapist must always consider ways in which, as Devereaux states, we can "create opportunities for reconnecting the patient with other human beings and the environment."[8]

Other limitations are related to the structure of therapy: mutually agreed upon boundaries regarding the length of each treatment session, the therapist's availability at times other than those scheduled, and the responsibilities specific to patient and to therapist as they work together in therapy. Whether the structure of therapy is negotiated informally or formally (e.g., through verbal or written contract), it is important to recognize the purpose of such structure. In part, the creation of this structure enhances predictability in therapy and increases the level of safety, as discussed earlier. It also provides expectations by which we can judge if the goals of therapy are being met.

Dependency. Just as important, such a structure provides a mechanism that helps keep us from slipping into patterns of relating that could keep our patient perpetually and increasingly dependent on us. In special instances, dependency will appropriately be fostered, especially, for example, where a patient has had extreme difficulty in asking for or accepting any help from anyone. What we caution against here are those times in a therapeutic relationship when a therapist becomes so involved in helping that she loses sight of the others in the patient's world who could effectively, and better, relate to the patient around given needs.

Friendship. Beyond the obvious ethical boundaries prohibiting the therapist from compromising the emotional or physical well-being of the patient, the therapist must also understand that he or she is not a friend. Although our patients may understandably feel friendly toward us and we may feel friendly toward them, a friendship is not created for the purposes of therapy, nor therapy for the purpose of friendship. We will like many of our patients very much, but when therapy ends, so does the therapeutic relationship. If patients can be helped to recognize the qualities that have made it possible for them to feel good about themselves with us, then they can begin to see in themselves the potential they have to build friendship. They do not need to feel cheated when therapy ends. Rather, they are better able to relate meaningfully in the environment.

Summary of Therapeutic Relationship

In his description of self-actualization, Arthur Combs asked:

"How can a person feel liked unless someone likes him? How can a person feel acceptable unless somewhere he is accepted? How can a person feel he has dignity unless somewhere someone treats him so? How can a person feel able unless somewhere he has some success?"[6]

The answers to these questions, said Combs, contain the guidelines to the "... encouragement of growth and development everywhere," and the basis for the conditions of therapy.[6]

In this brief review, we have tried to illustrate that each therapeutic condition is related to the integrity and substance of the whole relationship. When one therapeutic element is lacking, the entire relationship is jeopardized. As you read further in the text, try to identify the way in which the therapist operating within each of the different frames of reference affirms the therapeutic conditions described and operationalizes these in occupational therapy practice.

Role of Group Dynamics

The discussion of group treatment and group dynamics in this chapter briefly reviews the more general theoretical principles that are applicable in occupational therapy practice. This general overview identifies the characteristics that make a group therapeutic, highlights the process for forming a group, identifies the role of the occupational therapist in the group, and describes the function of group dynamics in occupational therapy groups.

The coverage of group treatment and dynamics in this chapter does not provide expertise in skills necessary for leading or for processing a group, but it will give direction for further study in this area. The reader is encouraged to research the psychology, sociology and occupational therapy literature pertaining to group development and process, leadership styles and their impact, roles within a group, group strategies and responses, and the use of treatment groups in the multiple arenas of occupational therapy practice. The material available that pertains to group theory and application merits a text in itself. Although not covered in depth, group principles are exemplified throughout this text. Sample activities, skills and techniques used by the occupational therapist during treatment groups are described within the context of each of the major frames of reference presented.

Since the early 1900s, social scientists have been interested in groups and how people function in group situations. In the late 1930s, the study of groups became an identified field of inquiry and Kurt Lewin[26] popularized the term *group dynamics.* In 1945, an organization was established for the research and study of group dynamics. Since then, the application of group theory and dynamics in treatment and education has evolved to form the multiple group treatment formats and educational strategies that are available today. In addition to the academic interest in group theory and its clinical application, the development of group treatment has been fostered by the community mental health movement, the increased patient load and scarcity of mental health professionals, including occupational therapists and the expansion of psychological and sociological theories that support the use of group intervention.

Occupational Therapy Groups

In occupational therapy, patients have been treated in groups since the profession's origin. However, the systematic application of group dynamics in activity groups for the purpose of heightening therapeutic progress became popular during the 1960s. Gail Fidler and Ann Mosey have made major contributions to the application of group theory in occupational therapy. In addition to publications by these therapists, numerous other articles and books provide examples of how occupational therapy groups are used in in mental health and other specialty areas of the profession.[3,9,15,19,20,22,23,34]

Task Groups

In 1963, Fidler[11] called attention to the group phenomenon in occupational therapy treatment and in the working relationships that occupational therapists maintained with other professionals. In her book she identifies the relationship among patient groups, staff groups and the family group. She gives an overview of the roles and functions of the occupational therapist within the treatment group and suggests therapeutic responses that the occupational therapist can make, which help to establish rapport between the therapist and patients. Fidler acknowledges the influence of group development, leadership styles, group characteristics and therapist and patient responses on the activity process and the outcome of the treatment experience. Six years later, Fidler expanded further her initial discussion of group treatment and identified the task-oriented group and its purpose in occupational therapy. The theory that supports task groups was described as a meld of sociological, psychoanalytical and learning theories.

Activities for Exploration. Fidler's theory could be summarized as follows: Interpersonal, intrapsychic and environmental forces influence affect, learning and behavior. Therefore, these forces are explored in a here-and-now atmosphere to identify patient stresses, explore conflict and problems, elicit interaction among patients, and facilitate learning and change. Exploration and learning in the here-and-now occur in occupational therapy task groups. During group activities, the psychosocial forces and their influence are evident. Thus activities can be used to explore stresses and conflicts to remediate problems and to increase learning through doing. In other words, when we participate in an activity group, we learn not only specific tasks related to the activity's completion, but we have an opportunity to learn about how we approach tasks and how we get along with fellow group members. Occupational therapy is described as a "learning lab" in which the patient develops skills for life and the work world through task experiences.[12]

Task-oriented treatment groups as described by Fidler were developed at the New York Psychiatric Institute. The original group was composed of eight patients who were selected because they were unable to be productive in life, they had limited independent function, and the therapist determined that they were ready for the group experience, although readiness criteria are not identified. The group met for 1.5 hours, four times per week, and worked on a common task that was to be achieved through group effort and concensual decision making. Fidler stated that the task could be "any activity or process directed toward creating or producing an end product or demonstrable service for the group as a whole and/or for persons outside of the group . . . ." Some examples are "publishing a newspaper, cooking, gardening, a patient council, [and] ward decorating . . . ."[12]

Emphasis on Group Process. The purpose of the task-oriented group is to "provide a shared working experience wherein the relationship between feeling, thinking and behavior and their impact on others and on task accomplishment and productivity can be viewed and explored. Alternate patterns of functioning can be considered and tested within the context of the here and now, to the end that such learning may induce ego growth and improve function. Task accomplishment is not the purpose of the group but hopefully the means by which purpose is realized."[12] Stated another way, the task group as described by Fidler has a strong emphasis on group **process**, a term we will encounter again in the discussion of an object relations treatment framework.

The term **task group** has frequently been used by other writers to connote a task-centered group, or one whose primary aim is to create an end product or solve a problem, and not one primarily concerned with group dynamics or therapy.

In accord with the model of groups dis-

cussed by de Mare and Kreeger[7] in Great Britain, we have distinguished a group category between a verbal psychotherapy group, which is concerned mostly with member interaction, and a task group, which is concerned primarily with the group's end product. This group is referred to as the therapeutic activity group but in substance is similar to the task group, as Fidler uses the term.[3] By looking at how group members accomplish the task, one learns about the group's cohesiveness, group problem-solving strategies, the group and individual patient's view of reality, cause and effect relationships, the communication patterns in the group, and the relationship between the roles and functions in a group and the patient's community responsibilities.

Developmental Groups

Mosey's views on group treatment in occupational therapy were published in 1970, 1973 and 1981. She discussed developmental groups, roles within a group, group skills, group process, activity groups and a tentative taxonomy for activity groups.

The concept of developmental groups originated with Wilbauger and was further developed and presented by Mosey[27] in *Three Frames of Reference for Mental Health*. The developmental groups identified are 1) parallel group, 2) project group, 3) egoecentric-cooperative group, 4) cooperative group and 5) mature group. The groups are correlated with developmental age spans and necessitate identifiable, interaction subskills. Each group is briefly defined in Appendix C.

Activity Groups

In 1973, Mosey[28] further contributed to the occupational therapy body of knowledge regarding groups through her discussion of group dynamics and group processes in her book *Activities Therapy*. In this publication, she defined a group and discussed group membership roles (task and social-emotional roles); decision making in groups; the communication process; and group goals, cohesiveness and group norms. She provided this information to increase the activities therapist's understanding of small groups and the way in which groups can be used to help prepare the patient to live more independently in the community.

In an activity group, individuals relate around a specified task or activity to assess patient function and to implement treatment goals. To understand the interaction within the group as well as its outcome, one must look at the characteristics of the activity, both medium and process, as well as be acquainted with the principles of small group interaction.

Mosey stresses that what an individual can do within an activity group is representative of what can be accomplished within other nontreatment groups in which the person participates. As such, the activity group acts as a microcosm of the larger environment, as we shall examine further in our discussion of the object relations framework for practice.

Group Taxonomy.   Mosey noted that activity groups tend to be classified according to the goal of the group but proposed that this "leads to confusion."[29] As an alternative, she suggested a tentative taxonomy of activity groups. Identified in the taxonomy are evaluation groups, task-oriented groups, developmental groups, thematic groups, topical groups and instrumental groups.[29] The groups are defined briefly in Appendix D. The reader is referred to the original source for the discussion of these groups.

Functional Groups

The functional group model of treatment, described by Howe and Schwartzberg,[20] is based on the ideas and experiences of many occupational therapy educators and clinicians. The model integrates group theories from the social sciences and occupational therapy theory. Purposeful activities or occupations are used in a functional group to influence a person's health and well-being and to develop adaptive strategies to meet environmental expectations. The group has a here-and-now focus and provides a structure that will encourage self-

initiated action with a group-centered focus. The group activities provide opportunity for experiential learning to increase independence and competence in work, play, and self-maintenance. The group experience provides an opportunity for interpersonal and intrapersonal learning as well as skill development.

The sample groups described in this model are similar to those traditionally identified in occupational therapy practice: project group, energy conservation/time management group, art and creative groups, craft groups, and cooking groups. The reader is referred to the original source for theoretical details and group protocols for functional groups.

Organizing Information Through a System Model

After studying the relationship between system and group theories and evaluating the groups used in occupational therapy, Borg and Bruce[3] conceptualize the therapeutic activity group as a group system. The authors describe system theory as an organizing framework for conceptualizing, planning and implementing therapeutic activity groups. System theory is *not* identified with a specific frame of reference because the theory accommodates the beliefs of varied theory and practice models in occupational therapy. When using the group system framework, the therapist need not discard preferred or current theoretical endorsements.

Group System

The group system consists of a leader, participants, activity and environmental elements that interact dynamically. Anything that affects one element in the system necessarily affects everything else in the system, and the best way to understand how a group can bring about therapeutic gain is to investigate how all the elements in the group work together. Figure 2.1 depicts the Group System and its dynamics. For details regarding the relationship between system theory and group treatment, as well as multiple examples of therapeutic activity groups, the reader is referred to the original work.

Occupational therapy groups have been referred to as task groups, therapeutic activity groups, activity groups and functional groups. A key concept, however, is that the group's interactive process is viewed as important as what task the group might accomplish.

What is a Group?

Groups have been defined generally as a coming together of two or more people for a specific purpose. Psychologists and sociologists has expanded this definition. Cartwright and Zander[5] developed the following definition. A set of people constitutes a **group** when "one or more of the following statements will characterize them: a) they engage in frequent interaction; b) they define themselves as members; c) they are defined by others as belonging to the group; d) they share norms concerning matters of common interest; e) they participate in a system of interlocking roles; f) they iden-

tify with one another as a result of having set up the same model-object or ideals in their superego; g) they find the group to be rewarding; h) they pursue promotively interdependent goals; i) they have a collective perception of their unity; j) they tend to act in a unitary manner toward the environment."

Knowles and Knowles[25] depict the difference between a collection of people and a group. The schematic representation of a collection of people depicts the lack of boundaries, lack of a shared goal, lack of group consciousness, undefined membership and multiple directions of its members. There are no lines of interaction and interdependent communication. See Figure 2.2, a schematic adaptation of the Knowles and Knowles group model.

Therapeutic Group Characteristics

We each belong to a number of groups. We are members of a family and may be members in religious, social, political or community

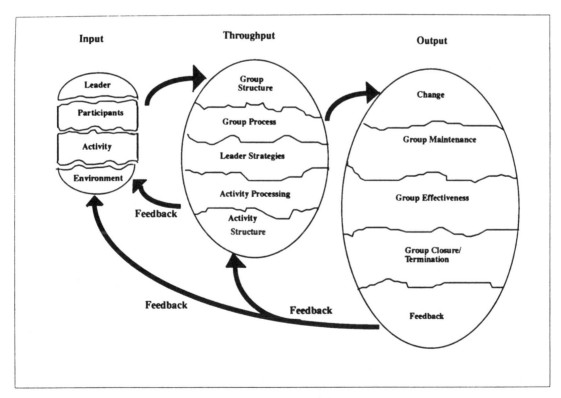

FIGURE 2.1.   Therapeutic Activity Group as a System. Reproduced from Borg & Bruce (1991). *The Group System: The Therapeutic Activity Group in Occupational Therapy*, Thorofare, NJ. SLACK Inc.

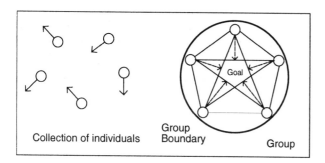

Collection of individuals   Group Boundary   Group

FIGURE 2.2.   Group model. Adapted from Knowles, M and Knowles, H: *Introduction to Group Dynamics*. Cambridge Adult Education Co., New York, NY.

groups. Although we benefit from these interactions, these groups differ from therapeutic groups. Treatment groups usually have more specific objectives, usually within the framework of learning, remediation or change; and they have an identified time period for existence. In therapy, a group consists of persons who come together because of common concerns and stresses or problems in living. The goals for remediation, learning, coping or change may be formulated by the group members, or they may be established by the treatment staff. In occupational therapy, patients come together daily or several times a week for the specific purpose of changing the way they think, feel or behave in their daily life. Patients may work on individual projects within a group, work collectively on a particular task, participate in role playing experiences or learn from academic tasks presented and processed in small groups. Because particular activity groups are exemplified throughout the book, we will speak generally of the role of the therapist and the manner in which a group experience can be used to enhance the goals of therapy.

The Role of the Occupational Therapist in the Group

The responsibilities previously identified in the discussion of the therapeutic relationship apply to the therapist's participation in group treatment but are expanded beyond the patient-therapist dyad by the complexity of in-

teraction that occurs among patients during the group experience. The occupational therapist continues to assure physical safety for all patients in the group and reflects an attitude of acceptance, caring, understanding and valuing change. The therapist also promotes and facilitates these attitudes among patients within the group and tries to elicit expression of caring, acceptance and support for change by patients for each other. How this is accomplished is influenced by the therapist's leadership.

Styles of Leadership

Authority.   The occupational therapist has a choice of leadership style. The therapist can chose to be an authority in the group, plan and present the activity, and set and enforce the boundaries for interaction. In general, as an **authority** the leader assumes the responsibility for determining the activity, delegating the task procedures, identifying the patient roles, controlling the group process and limiting interactions to achieve an outcome that she has determined desirable.

Democratic Role.   In contrast, the leader may assume a **democratic role** by facilitating group member interaction and a sharing of leadership. Consistent with the democratic style of leadership, the therapist delegates to the patients shared responsibility for selecting the activity, implementing the task, and processing the experience. When patients are encouraged to participate in the decision-making process, and to identify the roles they wish to assume, the free exchange of ideas among patients is facilitated.

Situational Leadership.   Hersey and Blanchard[16] use the term **situational leadership** to describe the role taken when the leader adapts to the maturity level of the group participants. According to them, no one style of leadership is best. Rather, certain styles are more likely to be successful given the ability and desire of the members to be responsible for organizing the group and keeping it on course. In other words, the leader must be flexible from day to day. A given group of participants might, for example, be able to be self-directed on a certain day given one task, but floundering on another day when attending to a different activity.

Gatekeeper

Regardless of the leadership style the occupational therapist is a **gatekeeper**. In this role, the therapist is available to provide safety and facilitate trust, caring, communication, understanding, acceptance and change—all key elements in the therapeutic relationship, which can be enhanced by group interactions. This task is not easy and its importance should not be underestimated. The therapist must rely on a knowledge of group dynamics and an understanding of individual patients in accordance with the chosen treatment frame of reference.

Safety and Trust

When the occupational therapist initiates a group, he or she establishes a sense of safety by identifying the purpose and boundaries of the group, ethical standards related to group interaction and rules of confidentiality. Additionally, the therapist identifies the group structure and any formal rules for group interaction. Some rules for group interaction can be conceived as less formal because patients learn from observing each other and the therapist, and they learn acceptable ways to provide positive or negative feedback and constructive means to gain attention.

Not only must patients trust the therapist, they need to trust each other if they are to learn from each other. The occupational therapist continually encourages patients to respond to each other constructively without channeling communication through the therapist.

For example, when a patient indicates that he or she has felt slighted by another in the group, the therapist might ask the patient to redirect the communication to the appropriate other. Or, when a patient states that he or she felt clumsy or inept doing the group task, the therapist might ask the group to respond, asking, "Who in the group has felt this way?" or, "What have others done in similar situations?"

Universality

As patients interact during treatment groups, they learn that others have had similar experiences, problems, needs and feelings. They realize that they are not alone. When patients share and learn from each other, they develop a sense of mutual caring and concern; a lessened feeling of isolation; and an increased confidence in one's own ability to cope with life, accept oneself and accept stress. Many social scientists believe that the ability of a group experience to make the individual more aware that his or her concerns and problems are universal makes a group activity particularly effective.[39]

Communication

Trust, caring, safety and understanding depend on the verbal and nonverbal communication among group members during the group and activity experience. The occupational therapist, at times acting as a model, facilitates interactions that promote acceptance among patients and open communication which results in a constructive outcome, although patients may not always be happy and comfortable during the occupational therapy groups. However, the therapist and patients will provide the support necessary for patients to take risks and make change and to cope with the discomfort that is experienced during learning and the group activity.

Content and Process. When looking at the interpersonal communication that occurs during occupational therapy groups, the therapist is aware of the content and process of a group. The **content** refers to the statements that patients make and to the specific behaviors that occur as the outcome of the identified task.

One might think of the content as the **what** of the group activity. The **process** of the occupational therapy group is the **how** of the activity or the dynamics that occur as the group ensues: for example, the interactions among patients; the nonverbal behaviors that occur in response to the activity, other patients, the occupational therapist or the setting, and those unspoken elements that seem to influence individual patient behavior, the activity and the group outcome.

General Group Format

The manner and extent to which the occupational therapist chooses to discuss the group and activity process depends on the needs, skills and limitations of the patients; the goals of the group; and the skill and expertise of the therapist. Regardless of the depth of or manner of processing, however, the following general format can serve as a guide for the therapist leading a group. This format is organized around three stages in the group process: 1) preparation, 2) developing the group experience and 3) closing a group.

Preparation

During the initial or preparatory phase, patients are given the information they need to participate in the day's planned activity. It also is a time when members have a chance to relax, anticipate, or otherwise become more receptive to the activity. Preparation can include any of the following: introduction of new members, a statement of the group's goals or goals of individual members, a review of norms of behavior within the group, the giving of didactic information, an explanation of the planned activity, or warm-up exercises. To illustrate, the therapist might begin by saying:

OTR: "Welcome! Today in occupational therapy we will be together for the next hour and a half to learn about how we use time and how we manage time. First we

will draw a 'pie of life,' " (an experience described by James and Jongeward, in *Born to Win*).[21] The therapist then asks a patient to give to group members the materials needed to complete the task.

Development Phase

After the pie is drawn, the therapist facilitates discussion of how patients use their time. A round robin format may be used; for example, each patient is allowed to tell how he or she uses time. Or, the therapist may ask for patients to volunteer to talk about their drawing.

As patients describe the way they use their time and the feelings they have about the way their time is spent, the therapist may highlight the similarities among group members. The therapist may say for example, "I notice several of you have indicated that you spend 80% of your time with nothing to do. Perhaps learning to use our unstructured time would be a useful goal in future group activities."

Patterns of Participation. During the group activity and the discussion that follows, the therapist notes patterns of participation. No single pattern is best; in general the broader the interaction pattern the better. In other words, it is generally desirable to have many patients actively participate. Although individuals can learn by listening or watching, when many or all members actively participate in the group, a greater pool of ideas is generated from which all can draw, patient interest tends to be greater, and participants tend to feel a stronger investment in the group. The therapist will help patients communicate both their ideas and feelings in an effort to increase understanding.

Nonverbal Communication. The therapist takes note of **nonverbal communication** such as that reflected by the patient's posture, facial expression, gestures and physical location within the group. He or she observes how the patients work together, and at times, the therapist reflects personal observations back to the group in an effort to make the group more aware of its own process. As the activity continues, the therapist typically promotes cooperation and participation, which often result in a cohesive or team feeling.

Enhancing the Activity Process. The leader tries to minimize subgroup formation or cliques such as adults versus teenagers or old members versus new members. Cliques can interfere with the activity process and group outcome, decrease cohesiveness, and lessen the likelihood that patients will feel that they can learn from the experiences of others. The therapist is exhorted to promote an atmosphere of warmth, helpfulness, responsibility, friendliness and cooperation. Toward this goal, the therapist frequently needs to help patients set standards for courtesy, productivity, tolerance and support.

Periodically, the therapist also may need to help the group identify procedures that will enhance the activity process and facilitate goal accomplishment. Goals must be clear and understood by each member in the group throughout the activity experience and in relation to the time left to complete the group task.

The content of the group in the preceding example includes the completed drawings, plus the ideas and feelings shared by patients as regarding the way they spend their time. The process in the group includes the participation pattern (who participated and who responded to whom), the nonverbal behaviors of the group members, the style of leadership that the group required, and the group's general reaction to the experience.

Group Closure

To achieve closure, the occupational therapist summarizes the group experience. When summarizing, the therapist might restate the purpose of the group, identify or clarify the learning outcome of the experience, or emphasize the therapeutic benefit of the experience. The therapist allows patients to share with each other their perceptions of the experience and

to give each other feedback, as well as suggestions about future group activities.

In addition to summarizing and reflecting on the group experience, the occupational therapist tries to connect the experience to the environment outside the treatment setting. He or she may refer to past experience, analogous experiences in the patient's natural environment, or expected similar future situations.

An example summary of group closure may be similar to the following "pie of life" group summary:

OTR: "Today in occupational therapy, we have drawn a 'pie' to help us look at how we use our time (goal restatement). During the discussion of our drawings, we learned that most of us don't know what to do with our free time (a statement of the *learning outcome*). Learning to use our free time can be one of the benefits of your hospital stay and can help you when you return home (a statement that identifies the *link* between hospital and community). In future occupational therapy groups, we will do activities that can help you develop new interests and learn about your community and the resources that you can use to fill your free time when you return home (a statement that sets the stage for *future* treatment activities)."

Documentation of Occupational Therapy Groups

Once the group is completed, the occupational therapist documents the experience in each patient's chart or in a more central location, such as a staff or department communications notebook or log. The purpose of this documentation is to communicate patient progress and to keep other treatment team members informed of the significant patient interactions and learning that occurs in occupational therapy. The sample group note shown in Figure 2.3 provides a possible format for documenting groups. However, the documentation format may vary to meet the needs of the health

---

Date November 28, 1993

Group Title Activities of Daily Living / Time Management

Group Goals

1. Each patient will draw a "pie of life."
2. Each patient will identify how he or she uses time; the proportion of time used in self-care, work and leisure activities.
3. Each patient will communicate with group members regarding the use of time as depicted in the group drawing experience.
4. Each patient will identify one change each wishes to make regarding the use of time.

Occupational Therapy Activity

The "pie of life" is a paper and pencil task. The patients met for 50 minutes. They were instructed to draw a circle and divide it into pieces that represent the portion of time during the week that is devoted to being alone, with friends, with family, at work, doing recreation activities and doing self-care activities.

Patients in Attendance

(Here the therapist lists the names of those patients who attended the occupational therapy group.)

Summary of the Group Experience

(Content and process observations are noted): Ten patients participated in the Daily Living Group. All in attendance completed the "pie of life" drawing. John J. and Mary S. refused to describe how they use time but listened to others' comments. During the discussion, "How to use free time while in the hospital and at home" emerged as the primary concern among the majority of participants. Other themes that emerged were that 1) participants have few interests, 2) they are unfamiliar with resources in the community, 3) they lack sufficient funds for transportation to community recreation facilities and 4) they would like more in-hospital activities on weekends. Karla N. and Brian G. volunteered to plan weekend activities with staff assistance.

The occupational therapist suggested that future daily living groups could be used to plan weekend events and will also provide activities to help patients develop interests, contact community resources and incorporate activities to assist patients in learning to use free time.

In general there was a spirit of cooperation and sharing in the group. The two new group members, Jack K. and Beth W., were introduced by Karla N., who throughout the group experience showed initiative and promoted group interaction.

FIGURE 2.3. Sample Occupational Therapy Group Note.

setting and the established documentation protocol.

Summary of the Role of Group Dynamics

Not all occupational therapy is carried out within a group context. When therapy does occur in a group setting, there can be greater opportunity for patients to function in every day social experiences. Within these group experiences, the patient has increased resources from which he or she can learn, gain feedback and elicit support. For the group to be a helpful learning experience, the therapist must maintain the therapeutic relationship he or she has established with each patient, while assisting patients to relate to each other in a way that is honest, yet accepting of individual differences, and in a manner that supports risk taking and change.

Purposeful Activity

The third component of the framework for therapy is the activity in which the patient and therapist participate. In the occupational therapy literature, multiple terms are used to describe activities that bring about change and among them multiple definitions of purposeful activity. Some of the terms used in the literature to describe activity include purposeful activity,[12,24,29] therapeutic activity or treatment activity,[38] goal-directed activity and purposeful task,[37] activity experience,[1] and occupation.[10,18]

Goal Directed

In each of the preceding definitions, with the exception of occupation, the existence of a goal is implied. That is, the activity used in treatment has a specific objective. The term **occupation** also has many definitions, but in general it has been defined as the way in which an individual occupies time. Until recently, neither goal-directed behavior nor purpose is necessarily implied in the term occupation. In 1983, however, in a paper approved by the Executive Board of the American Occupational Therapy Association regarding practice, Fine[14] quotes a 1972 *American Journal of Occupational Therapy* article and writes, "Occupation in the title [Occupational Therapy] is in the context of goal-directed use of time, energy, interest and attention to foster adaptation and productivity, to minimize pathology and to promote the maintenance of health."[1] In this text, however, we use the term *purposeful activity* with its goal-directed focus, rather than the term *occupation*, which is used in varied contexts and is popularly identified with the model of human occupation.

In addition to the Fine paper, the American Occupational Therapy Association submitted a position paper to clarify the use of the term **purposeful activity**. The paper states that an activity becomes purposeful when it has unique meaning for the patient; when it utilizes the patient's abilities; when it helps the patient fulfill life roles; when it helps the patient achieve personal goals; and when it increases the patient's feeling of competence and mastery in self-care, work and leisure. Purposeful activities are tasks or experiences used in occupational therapy evaluation and treatment to assess, facilitate, restore and maintain physical, emotional and cognitive function.[17]

As used in this text, purposeful activity is conceived in accordance with its definition as presented by Fidler and Fidler,[13] supported by the American Occupational Therapy Association, and reiterated by Mosey.[29] "An activity is purposeful only if it is congruent with 'the individual's sensory, motor, cognitive, psychological and social maturation . . . developmental needs and skill readiness . . . and recognized by (the individual's) social and cultural groups as relevant to their values and needs.' Purposeful activities are doing processes that involve 'investigating, trying out and gaining evidence of one's capacities for experiencing, responding, managing, creating and controlling.' "[1,13,29]

We are not advocating one definition of purposeful activity as best. We do want the reader to be aware that multiple definitions exist that have and will continue to influence the theory and practice of occupational therapy.

In the following discussion, we highlight the contribution made by activity in the framework of therapy, identify activity as an agent of change, and emphasize that activity becomes purposeful when it is used within the context of the person and his or her environment. Further discussion of the ways in which activities are used puposefully in treatment are presented in relation to each of the frames of reference presented in this text.

Purposeful Activity in the Framework of Therapy

In the therapy experience, the patient is the center within the group or activity experience. The dynamic interaction of the patient with other patients, with the occupational therapist, and with the activity brings about change. Through this dynamic process, the activity becomes a change agent. More specifically, activities can facilitate change because they allow a patient to gain knowledge, acquire new skills, relearn to use his or her capabilities, identify individual abilities and limitations, change or develop personal interests, learn to use time effectively, broaden opportunities for recreation and work, and increase the network of people with whom the individual interacts.

Role of the Occupational Therapist

The role and responsibilities of the occupational therapist identified for the therapeutic relationship and in group treatment also apply when the occupational therapist uses purposeful activity to facilitate change. The therapist communicates that activities have value; that activities provide a safe vehicle for learning and change; that participating in activities can increase self-knowledge and knowledge of others; that activities can facilitate understanding, communication and problem-solving with others; and that activities in treatment can serve as a bridge to the community. The therapist may also teach specific activities or activity components to patients and help patients to identify which activities are more likely to help them to achieve personal goals.

Safety and Purposeful Activities

When the occupational therapist provides a safe environment for activity, he or she is concerned with both the physical and emotional safety of the patient. For instance, the therapist is alert to the precautions necessary for for fire prevention and general safety when ensuring a safe physical environment. He or she provides a clean and organized environment; informs the patient about how to safely use materials and equipment; and provides the necessary supervision mandated by the patient's abilities, cognitive level and psychological state.

The therapist supports the patient's emotional safety by guiding the patient's choice of activity. Patients are helped in choosing an activity that is sufficiently challenging to allow them to learn and change and that will not be beyond their ability and capability. Generally, the therapist tries to avoid a failure experience and promote success. However, the degree to which the therapist actively intervenes to promote success will vary according to the patient's needs and the practice frame of reference.

Valuing Purposeful Activity

An especially important role of the occupational therapist is to communicate to the patient his or her belief in the value of purposeful activity. As discussed previously, many individuals who seek treatment find it difficult to see themselves trying new activities or succeeding at familiar activities. This problem may be especially evident when a patient lacks confidence, has limited information and skills, or has diminished energy due to a history of stress, conflict, failure or depression. Different

therapists prefer different kinds of activities (e.g., crafts, activities of daily living, or activities that stimulate sensory integrative function) due in part to personal preference and in part to biases related to their chosen frame of reference. Whatever activities are selected, the therapist must value the activities that are made available to patients. Sensing that the therapist believes in the ability of given activities to help patients achieve their goals encourages patients to expend the energy and take the risks involved in active participation.

Boundaries Created by Purposeful Activity

Activities provide boundaries that can serve to increase the patients' sense of safety, as well as make more evident the successes they have achieved. This occurs because inherent in many of the activities used by occupational therapists are concrete or specific guides for behavior and interaction. These boundaries may be more readily apparent to patients when a given activity is familiar to them, when the activity is around a tangible object or stair-stepped task, or when an activity has definable rules. When patients can conceptualize the skills required in a given task, there is less ambiguity and uncertainty, and they can more easily anticipate what may be gained from activity participation. Many activities provide their own instantaneous and consistent feedback to patients. For example, with sewing, making a clay pot, and potting a plant, patients can see the results of their efforts. Activities also provide a vehicle around which patients can receive immediate feedback from peers, staff and friends about their performance.

The inherent structure in most activity groups can also ease the discomfort patients feel as they try to learn social skills. For example, it may be more comfortable to practice social skills and work with others around planning a patient party or organizing a game of softball than to attempt socializing in a patient day room. In the dayroom, patients may feel unsure about which topics are safe or wonder if others even want to interact with them.

Purposeful Activity and Treatment Outcome

In addition to the specific goal of the activity relative to the individual patient, how the therapist uses purposeful activity influences the treatment outcome. The occupational therapist may choose to emphasize the use of activity to produce a specific end product such as a woven wall hanging, a homemade cake, a painting, a wood project, a successful party or a well-written resume. Or, the therapist may choose to focus on the learning and the process that occurs during the activity. The activity process is analogous to the process that occurs during a group experience.

Processing Activities

The process of the activity refers to the personal meaning the activity has for the patients, the insight patients gain about how they work with others, the problem-solving and work skills they acquire as they participate in the activity, the interactions that occur between the patient and therapist or the patient and other patients as the activity ensues, and the relationships they form between the treatment experience and the knowledge and skills needed to interact in daily life.

The activity process may not be readily evident to the patient. The occupational therapist shares the patient's observations regarding the activity process to highlight the benefits of the activity experience, to facilitate change and to provide the bridge between treatment and their daily environment. The sharing of these observations, also called **processing the activity,** is accomplished in a manner that is sensitive to the patient's cognitive, social and emotional abilities and needs.

Purposeful Activities as a Bridge to the Community

When activities are purposeful, they serve as the bridge to the community. That is, the activities have meaning to the patient because they relate to a goal the individual has for the future, or the activity relates to the roles he or she assumes in the community and the tasks that the patient wishes to accomplish. In addition to relating to specific roles or tasks, the person gains confidence in his or her ability to deal successfully with new challenges outside the therapeutic milieu.

Clinical Reasoning

Since the publication of the first edition of this text, increased attention has been given to the decision-making process in occupational therapy practice. We view this process of clinical reasoning as a final contributor to the framework of therapy, quite unlike those we have described so far. **Clinical reasoning** acts as an internal guide or structure by which the therapist selects from all available information and uses it to understand the patient and make treatment decisions.

When discussing the clinical reasoning process, occupational therapists have consistently referred to the work of Pelligrino and Schon.[30,35,36] Clinical reasoning is viewed as encompassing the initial and ongoing, deductive and inductive reasoning processes. When engaged in clinical reasoning, the occupational therapist integrates scientific knowledge, ethical principles and the "artistic" elements of the occupational therapy intervention.[31,33]

Scientific Knowledge

To frame problems and generate treatment options, the therapist relies on his or her scientific knowledge base. Knowledge of medicine, social sciences and occupational therapy theory support the deductive reasoning process used to solicit and evaluate assessment data, compare the individual to the classical diagnostic or medical picture, and then generate hypotheses about presenting problems and problem solutions. In this text, the frames of reference provide the knowledge base for framing evaluation data and hypothesizing treatment.

Humanistic and Ethical Principles

Concurrently, the therapist uses humanistic and ethical principles to establish and maintain a therapeutic relationship. Within the therapeutic relationship, the therapist can gain the subjective viewpoint needed to understand the patient and personalize a patient's specific problems, needs and strengths within the context of scientific data.

By being sensitive to the patient's subjective view, the therapist can help the patient formulate treatment goals and understand treatment options and their consequences. When the patient has adequate understanding of the available treatment options, the therapist helps the patient make choices that are compatible with personal goals.

The Art of Therapy

Given all that the therapist might know about a specific clinical problem and all the treatment strategies he or she might hold, there is no cookbook for the actual implementation of therapy and dealing in an ongoing way with the everyday dilemmas and victories inherent in therapy. Yet some therapists consistently can think on their feet and seem to know intuitively what actions are best at a given time. It might be said that they have skill in the art of therapy. The art of therapy is that elusive yet powerful ability to bring information, caring and skills together in a way that fosters positive treatment change. It is what patients and clinicians refer to when they say a particular therapist seems to know what to say or do, even when there has no been time to pre-plan. Although surely a cognitive process, the art of therapy seems to encoporate skills that have become automatic and can be drawn on without a great deal of conscious attention.

Summary

The therapeutic relationship, group experience, purposeful activity, and clinical reasoning have been identified as framing the process of therapy. Although each has been treated as a separate dimension, the reader recognizes that these therapeutic elements engage and develop simultaneously during the therapeutic process. No two therapeutic experiences can ever be identical. The remaining chapters explore how the interaction of these therapeutic elements takes on a special character in accordance with the values and beliefs imposed by each frame of reference.

Recommended Reading List

Avila D, Combs A, Purkey W: *Helping Relationships: Basic Concepts for the Helping Professions*. Boston, Allyn and Bacon, Inc., 1971.

Bandura A: *Principles of Behavior Modification*. New York, Holt, Rinehart and Winston, 1969.

Benjamin A: *The Helping Interview*. Boston, Houghton Mifflin, 1969.

Brammer L, Shostrom E: *Therapeutic Psychology: Fundamentals of Actualization Counseling and Psychotherapy*. Ed 3. Englewood Cliffs, NJ, Prentice-Hall, 1977.

Brammer L: *The Helping Relationship: Process and Skills*. Englewood Cliffs, NJ, Prentice-Hall, 1979.

Carkhuff R, Berenson B: *Beyond Counseling and Psychotherapy*. New York, Holt, Rinehart and Winston, 1967.

Carkhuff R: *Helping and Human Relations*. New York, Holt, Rinehart and Winston, 1969.

Egan G: *The Skilled Helper*. Monterey, CA, Brooks/Cole, 1975.

Huss J: Touch with care or a caring touch. *Am J Occup Ther* 31:11–18, 1977.

Ivey A: *Microcounseling: Interviewing Skills Manual*. Springfield, Ill, Charles C Thomas, 1977.

Krumboltz J, Thorenson C: *Counseling*. New York, Holt, Rinehart and Winston, 1969.

Mayeroff M: *On Caring*. New York, Perennial Library, Harper and Row, 1971.

Perls F: *Gestalt Therapy Verbatum*. Lafayette, CA, Real People Press, 1969.

Rogers C: *Client Centered Counseling*. Boston, Houghton Mifflin, 1951.

Truax C, Carkhuff R: *Toward Effective Counseling and Psychotherapy*. Chicago, Aldine, 1967.

References

1. American Occupational Therapy Task Force: Occupational therapy: Its definition and functions. *Am J Occup Ther* 26(4):204–205, 1972.
2. Avila D, Combs A, Purkey W (Eds): *The Helping Relationship Sourcebook*. Boston, Allyn and Bacon, Inc., 1972.
3. Borg B, Bruce MA: *The Group System: The Therapeutic Activity Group in Occupational Therapy*. Thorofare, NJ, SLACK Incorporated, 1991.
4. Brammer L: *The Helping Relationship: Process and Skills*. Englewood Cliffs, NJ, Prentice-Hall, 1979, pp. 30–32.
5. Cartwright D, Zander A: *Group Dynamics—Research and Theory*. Ed 3. New York, Harper and Row, Publishers, 1968, p. 48.
6. Combs A: Some basic concepts in perceptual psychology. In Combs A, Avila D, Purkey W (Eds): *Helping Relationships: Basic Concepts for the Helping Profession*. Boston, Allyn and Bacon, Inc., 1971, pp. 121–122.
7. de Mare P, Kreeger L: *Introduction to Group Treatments in Psychiatry*. London, Butterworth and Company, 1974.
8. Devereaux E: Occupational therapy's challenge: The caring relationship. *Am J Occup Ther* 38(12):791–798, 1984.
9. Duncombe L, Howe M: Group work in occupational therapy: A survey of practice. *Am J Occup Ther* 32(5): 317–319, 1985.
10. Fairman C: Response to Smith and Tempone, psychiatric occupational therapy within a learning context. *Am J Occup Ther* 22 (5):422, 1968.
11. Fidler G, Fidler J: *Occupational Therapy—A Communication Process in Psychiatry*. New York, Macmillan, 1963, p. 43.
12. Fidler G: The task-oriented group as a context of treatment. *Am J Occup Ther* 23(1):43–48, 1969.
13. Fidler G, Fidler J: Doing and becoming: Purposeful action and self-actualization. *Am J Occup Ther* 32:305–310, 1978.
14. Fine S: Occupational Therapy: The Role of Rehabilitation and Purposeful Activity in Mental Health Practice. White Paper. Rockville, MD, American Occupational Therapy Inc., 1983.
15. Gibson D (Ed): Group Process and Structure in Psychosocial Occupational Therapy. Special Issue. *Occup Ther Mental Health* 8(3):1–164. NY: Haworth Press, 1988.
16. Hersey P, Blanchard K: Situational leadership. In Tubbs S: *A Systems Approach to Small Group Interaction*. Ed 2. New York, Random House, 1984, pp. 201–204.
17. Hinojosa J, Sabari J, Rosenfeld M: Purposeful activities. *Am J Occup Ther* 37(12):805–806, 1983.
18. Hopkins H: A historical perspective on occupational therapy. In Smith H, Hopkins H (Eds): *Willard and Spackman's Occupational Therapy*. Ed 6. Philadelphia, JB Lippincott, 1983.
19. Hopkins H, Smith H (Eds): *Willard and Spackman's Occupational Therapy* Ed 6. Philadelphia, JB Lippincott, 1983.
20. Howe MC, Schwartzberg SL: *A Functional Approach to Group Work in Occupational Therapy*. Philadelphia, JB Lippincott, 1986.
21. James M, Jongeward D: *Born to Win: Transactional Analysis with Gestalt Experiments*. Reading, MA, Addison-Wesley Publishing, 1971.
22. Kaplan K: The directive group: Short-term treatment for psychiatric patients with a minimal level of functioning. *Am J Occup Ther* 40(7):474–481, 1986.
23. Kaplan K: *Directive Group Therapy: Innovative Mental Health Treatment*. Thorofare, NJ, SLACK Inc., 1988.
24. King LJ: Toward a science of adaptive responses. *Am J Occup Ther* 32:429–444, 1978.
25. Knowles M, Knowles H: *Introduction to Group Dynamics*. New York, Association Press, 1972, p. 41.
26. Lewin K: *Field Theory in Social Science*. New York, Harper and Row, 1951.
27. Mosey AC: *Three Frames of Reference in Mental Health*. Thorofare, NJ, SLACK Inc., 1970.
28. Mosey A: *Activities Therapy*. New York, Raven Press, 1973.
29. Mosey A: *Occupational Therapy—Configuration of a Profession*. New York, Raven Press, 1981, pp. 99, 110–112.
30. Pelligrino ED, Thomasma DC: *A Philosophical Basis of Medical Practice*. New York, Oxford University Press, 1981.
31. Robertson S: Reasoning in practice. In Robertson S (Ed): *Mental Health Focus: Skills for Assessment and Treatment*. Rockville, MD, American Occupational Therapy Association, 1988, pp. 1.48–1.50.
32. Rogers C: The characteristics of a helping relationship. In Avila D, Combs A, Purkey W: *The Helping Relationship Sourcebook*. Boston, Allyn and Bacon, 1972, pp. 13–14.
33. Rogers J: Clinical reasoning: The ethics, science, and art. In Robertson S (Ed): *Mental Health Focus: Skills for Assessment and Treatment*. Rockville, MD, American Occupational Therapy Association, 1988, pp. 1.51–1.66.
34. Ross M: *Integrative Group Therapy: The Structured Five-Stage Approach*. Ed 2. Thorofare, NJ, SLACK Inc., 1991.
35. Schon D: *The Reflective Practitioner*. New York, Basic Books, 1983
36. Schon D: *Educating the Reflective Practitioner*. San Francisco, Jossey Bass Publishers, 1987.
37. Willard H, Spackman C (Eds): *Occupational Therapy*. Ed 3. Philadelphia, JB Lippincott, 1963.
38. Willard H, Spackman C (Eds): *Occupational Therapy*. Ed 4. Philadelphia, JB Lippincott, 1971.
39. Yalom I: *The Theory and Practice of Group Psychotherapy*. Ed 2. New York, Basic Books Inc., 1975.

Chapter 3

OBJECT RELATIONS FRAME OF REFERENCE

Focus Questions

1. What themes do existential humanism and occupational therapy hold in common? Describe them.
2. How does the object relations frame of reference help the occupational therapist understand the subjective experience of the patient?
3. How do the original and current Freudian theoretical views differ? How are these currently applied in mental health settings?
4. What guidelines does this framework provide for giving feedback to patients regarding their behavior and activity performance?
5. What is the purpose of processing activities? Describe how the occupational therapist does activity processing during evaluation and treatment.
6. What are the guidelines for interpreting drawings and symbols? How should they be used?
7. What has the object relations frame of reference contributed to occupational therapy theory and practice?

Introduction

Some of the most commonly accepted as well as soundly criticized beliefs about the nature of personality, the function of activity and the therapeutic relationship have their basis in the tenets of object relations framework. Key figures in the evolution of this framework include Freud, Jung, Alexander, Rogers, Maslow, May, and Perls in psychology and Yerxa, Azima, Fidler and Fidler, and Mosey in occupational therapy.

Although this text cannot describe the work of any single theorist in detail, we have selected related postulates and have tried to illustrate how theorists have built on the work of their predecessors and ideas evolved. At its heart, the object relations framework strives to legitimize personal, subjective experience and challenges the premise that any experience can be understood apart from the bias of its beholder.

Definition

The object relations frame of reference, an eclectic frame of reference, is the theoretical approach that views persons, media and activities as objects invested with psychic energy. Interaction with these objects is necessary to satisfy personal needs. Once basic needs are satisfied, energy is available to move the person toward a goal of personal expression and balance. Activities are selected for their utility in enhancing interpersonal communication and facilitating healthy emotional experiences and are designed to lead to an understanding of patient needs, conflicts, feelings and behavior.

Theoretical Development

The object relations frame of reference is an outgrowth of the early psychoanalytical and communication process approaches in occupational therapy that were developed and described by Azima and Fidler and Fidler.[2,24] In 1970, Ann Mosey took a Freudian term, **object relations** and used it to describe an eclectic approach in occupational therapy that included Jungian, neo-(new) Freudian, humanistic-existential, as well as classical Freudian influences in medicine and psychology.

In an **eclectic approach**, several theories are integrated to formulate a new and disciplined approach. It provides a rationale for evaluation and treatment based on identified theoretical concepts and clinical techniques. It is not a license of total freedom for the clinician to do as he or she pleases, nor is it a simple common sense approach.

In the Beginning: Freud

Because the mental health field as a whole and object relations theory in particular continue to owe so much of their practice to the ideas professed by Sigmund Freud, a brief summary of these principles is provided to highlight some key concepts that influenced early psychoanalytically oriented occupational therapy and that continue to bear on current object relations practice. For those students who need a further review, Hall's *Primer of Freudian Psychology*[37] is recommended. We must stress, however, that Freud lived and wrote many years ago, and his ideas have been subject to change, as new information is gathered by contemporary theorists. Object relations theory is *not* a mere recitation of Freud's thinking.

Society and mental health treatment have come a long way since Freud first elaborated his beliefs in *The Interpretation of Dreams*.[27] If his peers and eventually the citizenry were outraged then by his emphasis on the role of sexual feeling in unconscious thought and conscious behavior, they nonetheless were given a new way to conceptualize human thought, feeling and behavior.

Today we talk about our feelings as if they have a value and substance of their own; we describe thoughts as being *conscious, unconscious,* or *subconscious* and expect others to understand what we mean by these terms. We may substitute our term *hang-up* for Freud's *complex*, but we discuss our *hang-ups, neuroses,* and *paranoias* and those of our friends as if they have influence, purpose and some basis in our personal history.

Although Freud might be accused of opening a Pandora's box of self-examination, one can see that he and those who followed gave us the concepts, the vocabulary and the license to talk about and understand ourselves in a way that we now take for granted. Further, Freud expanded the domain of the medical profession beyond physiology where aberrant behavior had to be treated with medication or, typically, not at all, to include a psychological approach in which a patient's thoughts and feelings could be dealt with in and of themselves.

Libido

Freud saw the person as a closed energy system, the energy which he labeled **libido**. He viewed this energy or libido as limited—as directed inward (to self) or outward (to other persons or objects). In everyday terms, we may hear someone say, "This project is important to me; I've put all my energy into it," or, "I'm so worried about my children's problems, I have no energy left for anything else." Libido was believed to be instinctual in origin and pleasure-seeking. To extend an analogy suggested by Hall,[37] we might think of a newborn infant, exemplifying ourselves, as having 16 ounces of libido. (Be aware, one cannot actually see, touch or weigh libido!)

The newborn infant experiences hunger, thirst and pain and will cry vigorously when uncomfortable. Our rather typical infant will have caring parents who act to meet the child's needs and the infant can literally picture the kind of people and nonhuman objects that give comfort and satisfaction. Soon, the child is able to imaginatively long for mother, bottle, soft toys and any other objects experienced as enjoyable. Unfortunately, the 16 ounces of libido can only be used for reflexive physical activity and for wishing or picturing. Although libido is pleasure-seeking, it is not, of itself, able to distinguish between a real object (baby bottle) and fantasy (thoughts about the bottle). Thoughts about bottle will not stop hunger pangs, and our infant is confronted with the need to develop greater powers of differentiation and control. To describe how this process occurs, Freud conceptualized the ego as emerging from the id.

Ego Emerges from Id

That portion of the mind or psyche that was unable to differentiate between reality and fantasy was said to reside in a portion of the self Freud called the **id**. The id is present at birth and houses the instincts, including those related to survival. The id experiences intolerable tension when biological needs are not satisfied and pleasure when needs are met and tension is released. However, id-energy or id-libido knows what it wants but not how to get it. Out of necessity, some id energy leaves the id and develops into another intrapsychic area Freud termed the **ego**.

Ego-libidinal energy also tries to satisfy, or bring pleasure, but it has the advantage of being able to realistically assess the outside world. As Freud said, ego functions help the individual perform a task by "becoming aware of stimuli, by storing up experiences about them (in memory), by avoiding excessively strong stimuli (through flight), and ... by learning to bring about expedient changes in the external world to its own advantage (through activity)."[79] The reader should be aware that there are no actual boundaries in the brain or elsewhere between the id, ego and superego. Rather these terms are a shorthand way of conceptualizing and identifying different processes within the personality.[37]

Ego Functions

The ego is considered to be the organizer of the personality. It is that part of the person able to state and feel "I am myself," "I am real," and "I am not part of anyone else." It is the logician and the mathematician. It can focus attention on one part of experience (the foreground), while putting the rest into the background. The ego is aware of time and sequence and is given the job of postponing gratification. The ego can also use libido to plan actions capable of removing obstacles to satisfaction in a function Freud called **aggression**. When the ego collects data, establishes priorities for it, and puts a plan of action into effect to see if the plan works, the ego is said to be doing **reality testing**.[37]

> Aggression as an innate human drive in addition to the drive for pleasure was proposed by Freud in his later writing. It was viewed as neither more nor less important than other drives, being described rather matter-of-factly as influencing human behavior. According to both Menninger[60] and Stafford-Clark[79] the therapeutic community has not generally focused on this drive in their work with patients, perhaps themselves uncomfortable with the whole concept.

Thus the ego uses its share of libido to decide which needs will be satisfied and when and how. Our developing child, now two years old, has some sense of self as separate, calls that self by a name, knows what he or she wants, and possessing a functioning, does not need to cry on the hopes that a bottle will magically appear. With determined ego direction, the child can use one-fourth ounce of libido to crawl up to mother with an empty bottle, pull the family cat out of mother's lap (aggression), and ask for the bottle to be filled, (using a primitive form of sign language or insistent whines typical of the young child). Because libido is limited and our child has only 16 ounces to invest, should he or she direct too much effort to satisfying daily needs, such as those for the bottle, there might be too little left to meet new challenges.†

Psychological Influence in Occupational Therapy

Applying an understanding of id and ego functions, the occupational therapist working within this frame of reference was concerned about flexibility and broadness when looking at a patient's object relationships. Did the patient have energy invested in a wide enough variety of objects so that a full range of needs was being met? When an object (thing, event, person) was no longer need-satisfying, could this patient pull back energy from it and reinvest the energy in a productive, socially acceptable way? When the patient was involved in tasks, was the ego in control or was the id need for immediate gratification leading to impulsive, chaotic behavior? The occupational therapist was concerned about the patient's ego function, for it was that part of the psyche that helped identify needs, weigh alternatives, circumvent or remove obstacles, and act on decisions in daily life. Stated another way, the ego enabled adaptation.

Superego

If the individual were not a social being, the id and the ego might be effective in carrying our child into adulthood. However, libidinal energy had to be extended to one other intrapsychic area, the area that Freud called the **superego**. Because the child's survival depends initially on the love and approval of parents and ultimately of peers, some energy is used in assessing which objects and courses of action will be approved of and which actions his or her parents will think are "bad." The child develops what is commonly called a **conscience**, that inner voice that influences actions by evoking guilt, when he or she has displeased others, and pride, when he or she does what is right.

The Unconscious

The id, ego and superego must share that "16 ounces" of original libido. All three portions of the psyche want pleasure for the person and must find a way to work together in relative balance and harmony so that each part can do its necessary work. For what one might call efficiency of operation, some knowledge that our infant has gained—knowledge that might be interesting but of no practical value—may be pushed out of current awareness or consciousness into the area Freud termed the **unconscious**.

It is interesting to compare Freud's constructs of id-ego and conscious-unconscious to more recent studies of the lateralization of brain function. For the right-handed person, the left hemisphere is considered primarily (but not solely) responsible for the ability to verbalize, do mathematics, think logically (that is, in terms of cause preceding an effect), and to deal in ordinary time-space constructs. The right, or nondominant, hemisphere has more responsibility for the ability to intuit, visualize and deal with affect. The right hemisphere lives in timelessness, does not see events proceeding logically one before another and, therefore, is acausal. The reader is referred to Ornstein's *Psychology of Consciousness*[67] and *Left Brain, Right Brain*, by Springer and Deutsch.[78]

---

†In his earlier writing, Freud emphasized the role taken by the ego when managing id or biological demands and looked at pathology as primarily a breakdown in the ego's ability to control id impulses. In later work, however, he emphasized that role of the ego in normal behavior, adapting to the environment to establish social relationships, not just to reduce tension, but in pursuit of social and creative goals. This is not, according to Hartmann,[41] what Freud is most remembered for.

Likewise, knowledge or thoughts that our child's evolving superego deems as shameful may be pushed from consciousness into the unconscious or may never have been allowed into conscious awareness at all. Much material that is held in the area of the unconscious includes thoughts one would be ashamed of, were he or she conscious of them. Although it is in an area of nonawareness, the unconscious continues to exert a powerful influence over behavior. Freud believed that only a small part of the mind lay in the realm of the conscious.

Identifying an in-between area of awareness, Freud suggested that some thoughts reside in the **preconscious** where they are not in current awareness but able to be recalled.[27]

Development of the Personality

Complementary to his theories about id-ego-superego and conscious-unconscious, Freud conceptualized that while a person is pleasure-seeking in essence, the objects and events that would be experienced as especially pleasurable would change as the individual matured. Freud began with the newborn and outlined stages of psychosexual and psychosocial development that moved a person into adulthood. He attributed special importance to the first three developmental stages, which span the first five years of life, citing prototype object choices and key patterns of psychosexual interaction that he believed influenced the individual's interactions for a lifetime. In large part, this belief led Freudian therapists to focus extensively on a patient's very early history.

In *Three Essays on Sexuality*[28] and in subsequent works, Freud noted that as the child develops, specific areas or zones of the body become especially sensitive to touch or stimulation and that touch to that zone is very pleasureable. Freud termed all bodily pleasure as sexual pleasure and did not limit his use of the term sexuality to genital sexuality as we tend to do today.[28]

The first area to be significantly pleasure-related is the mouth and surrounding area or the oral zone. This zone is followed by the anal zone, which is then followed by the genital or phallic zone. Activities that stimulate these various zones, or which come to be associated with these zones and the way they function, will be experienced as need-satisfying. As the person matures and new body zones take on special importance, the old pleasure zones are still pleasure-related, but have less relative importance.

Stage Theory

As each of the body zones is experienced as a focus of pleasure and sensitivity, significant persons and social interactions become associated with the way in which pleasure is achieved.

Oral Stage. For the newborn infant to about the age of two, the oral zone is the focus of pleasure and the child is in the **oral stage**. For these children, activities that stimulate the mouth, such as those involved in sucking at mother's breast, or biting are favored. Mother is the most important person-object, and the ability to receive nurturance and to learn to trust that needs will be satisfied are important social developmental tasks.

Anal Stage. For the child about age one to three years, the anal zone is especially sensitive. Activities associated with excreting, particularly in terms of mastering control over excrement, will be satisfying. At this **anal stage**, mother and father are important as nurturers, but the child's relationship with them is changing. He or she has learned to say "No!" and tries to gain a sense of autonomy and control over the environment, while not alienating parents.

Phallic Stage. When the child is three to five years of age, he is in the third stage of development, the **early genital or phallic stage**. Freud viewed the early genital stage as the key period for appropriate gender identification.[23] He considered the male and female child as essentially bisexual (demonstrating traits of both sexes) until this stage, when young children become physiologically and cognitively more aware of their own genitals.

Freud saw the boy child as becoming desirous of mother, and therefore in conflict with father, and now a rival for mother's affection. The boy resolves this potentially disastrous rivalry by identifying with (seeing himself like) father, repressing his wish for mother, thereby moving further away from mother in increased independence, and laying the foundations for his own eventually heterosexual relationship with a woman of his own.

The girl-child, Freud postulated, sees herself as like mother, and disappointed in the discovery that she has no penis. Therefore, she moves further from mother, and substitutes the wish for a penis with a wish to bear children, at first for father, and then for a man of her own.

The early genital phase was especially important for Freud in three areas: 1) the emotional distancing from mother, called **separation-individuation**, 2) the child's translation of a longing for the parent of the opposite gender into an eventual wish for a heterosexual adult partner, and 3) the identification of the child with the same-gender parent and the suitable incorporation of "masculine" or "feminine" behavior.

Freud saw the intrusive, sexual action of the male as prototypical of masculine activity: outgoing, aggressive commanding. The female, whose sexual role or function was seen as receptive was by extension viewed as feminine when her behavior was passive and subservient to the male. This conceptualization of social role as derived from sexual function—and a Victorian interpretation of function at that—has led to some of the most severe criticism of Freud's psychology. Clearly, this belief that women needed to be passive if they were to be feminine influenced the field of psychology for decades and has since been challenged as an incomplete, biased understanding of the female.[21,23]

In addition, during the early genital phase the child continues to incorporate parental ideas about good and bad and firms up the evolving superego. Parents continue to be a primary object choice, but this is also the period in which the child seeks a superparent or hero.

Latency Stage. From about ages five to twelve, the child is in the **latency stage**. No new physical zones take on significance, and the energy associated with seeking physical pleasure is rechanneled into learning new skills and forming peer friendships.

Late Genital Stage. During adolescence, the last or **late genital stage**, the genital area is again experienced as especially pleasure-related, and there is movement toward adult heterosexuality. The heterosexual love object takes on special significance.

Fixation. It should be stressed that the age boundaries given for each developmental stage are not really boundaries, but flexible conceptual divisions that allow for the overlapping of stage-related behaviors. Frequently, however, the individual gets stuck or **fixated** at a certain level of psychosexual development. His or her behavior, object choices and symbol production reflect this fixation. In this case, an excess of libido will be directed toward trying to meet needs at a specific level, and the individual will not successfully move on to the next stage. The result will be an immature and/or restricted manner of dealing with the self, others and things.

For example, an adult fixated at the oral stage will select objects and activities (perhaps symbolic) that reflect an over-reliance on oral pleasure (e.g., eating). In relationships the person may want to be parented, rather than engage in a mature adult-adult relationship. Or, the person might be overly anal in object relationships. He or she might deal with objects or media in an overly messy, or in an overly controlled manner. The person might be unable to give and take comfortably in a love relationship, rather, seeing the relationship as a continual struggle for control. A failure to be clear about one's sexual identity and sexual roles might be a reflection of an inability to deal effectively with the tasks of the early genital stage.

Psychosexual Development and Occupational Therapy

Being fixated at any given psychosexual stage of development tends to limit the range of need-satisfying objects and ways of dealing with the environment. Being cognizant of norms of psychosexual development, the occupational therapist could look at a patient's object choices, ways of handling media, and manner of relating and begin to determine if too much energy was being "spent" to accommodate immature psychosexual development. Table 3.1 outlines briefly Freud's stages of psychosexual development and suggests some

implication for working with adults in occupational therapy.

Exploring the Unconscious

Believing that the unconscious portion of the psyche exerted a prowerful influence over behavior, Freud attempted to determine thoughts that were held in the unconscious. One approach he took was to look in depth at the individual's symbol production through free word association and "slips of the tongue" and by exploring with a person his or her dreams.

In reading *The Interpretation of Dreams*, one can discover that Freud interpreted symbols on a case by case basis, and a great many dream symbols were not interpreted sexually. However, when Freud did summarize his beliefs regarding symbols (see especially pages 242–258, *The Interpretation of Dreams*),[27] there

TABLE 3.1

NORMAL PSYCHOSEXUAL DEVELOPMENT

Age	Zone of Special Sensitivity	Pleasurable Activities	Object Choice	Therapy Implications
Birth - 2	Oral Stage (a) early oral (b) late oral	(a) Sucking, encorporating, swallowing; (b) Biting, destroying	Self; Oral object Maternal Figure	Characteristics of adult fixated at this stage: May be clingy; overdepenent or unrealistically independent; enjoys talking, finds comfort in food, smoking, etc.; unable to form close relationships.
1-3	Anal Stage (a) early anal (b) late anal	(a) Excreting, touching excrement, being messy (b) Controlling, retaining, holding on to excrement; being very neat	Parent Figure; Anal object	Early: Might be overly messy; enjoys paints, clay etc. Late: Finds being messy repugnant; enjoys being the organizer, the collector. Generates conflicts over who is in charge.
3-5	Early Genital Stage (phallic)	Touching or exploring genitals; learning about own and genitals of opposite sex	Parent; superparent (hero)	May have difficulty accepting appropriate roles, manner of dressing, etc., or may have exaggerated sex role behavior. May be most comfortable with same sex relationships or fear them due to homosexual concerns. May appear to be without conscience or remorse for antisocial behavior.
5-12	Latency (no new zone)	Sublimation of energy into learning new skills	Companion of same sex	
12-18	Late Genital Stage (adolescence)	Touching, investigating, fantasizing about own genitals and genitals of opposite sex	Self; Emergence of love for companion of opposite sex	Struggles with issues of independence versus dependence. May appear especially concerned regarding own physical appearance; may be preoccupied with matters of genital sexuality. May experiment with homosexual and heterosexual activity.

was a strong focus on the sexual dimension of dream symbols.

For example he suggests, "elongated objects, sticks, tree-trunks, umbrellas . . . all sharp and elongated weapons, knives, daggers, pikes represent the male member . . . Small boxes, chests, cupboards, and ovens correspond to the female organ; also cavities, ships, and all kinds of vessels . . . Steep inclines, ladders, and stairs and going up or down them, are symbolic representations of the sexual act."[27]

Personal Context of the Symbol

A further listing will not be given here; rather, the interested reader is encouraged to read Freud's work. Too often, the listing of Freudian symbols suggests that a therapist need only compare a patient's symbol production to such a list and come to some valid conclusions. A symbol *cannot* be taken from the personal context in that manner, but must be related in a meaningful way to the individual's personal experiencing.

Motivation and Anxiety

The person wants to satisfy himself or herself on the one hand (the so-called **pleasure principle**), whereas reality often requires that gratification be postponed or even abandoned. The pull of pleasurable objects versus the reality of a situation in which it is difficult to reach desired goals creates a tension that motivates the person to act.

At times this tension is felt as anxiety, especially when needs cannot be met or when the individual feares that he or she will commit an act that would be harmful or guilt-inducing. This action would be especially likely to occur when ego strength was diminished or when demands on the ego were increased. The ego might try to manage anxiety by trying to "deny, falsify or distort reality" via special constellations Freud termed **defense mechanisms**.[37]

Defense Mechanisms

Defense mechanisms are summarized in Appendix E. Although we all use some defenses

and defenses can be adaptive, over-reliance on them, Freud said, limits one's perceptions of realistic object choices. Given the influence of psychosexual development, a person was believed to form characteristic ways of trying to meet personal needs, overcome obstacles and deal with anxiety. Together, these are reflected as **personality**.

The Therapy Process

Although Freud thought that some thoughts about the self and the environment could be kept **repressed** (out of current awareness), use of any defense mechanism took libidinal energy. The process of therapy would seek to free up libidinal energy, allowing it to be voluntarily invested in a variety of socially acceptable, need-satisfying object relationships. Freud called this process **psychoanalysis**.

He saw his role as neutral in which he could allow the patient to play out on the "therapist-screen" the unresolved conflicts and unconscious dramas that needed to be remediated. The major activity of psychoanalysis was interpretation, especially interpretation of the patient's behavior and affect during therapy sessions with the analyst, plus interpretation of dreams recounted by the patient. This interpretation was designed to increase insight and understanding. Although the past was inevitably recounted in the psychoanalytical process it was the patient's memory of the past, "the world of reconstructed subjective experiences," that was considered important; the accuracy of such memory was not a primary concern.[61]

It is interesting to note that Freud viewed personality as tending to stabilize as one reaches maturity (in the early twenties) and as more and more libido is tied up. As a result, the older adult (age 50 or older) was not believed to be a good candidate for change nor for psychoanalytical treatment.[74]

Traditional Psychoanalysis

Traditional psychoanalysis was typically carried out by medical doctors who then gained specialized training in psychiatry or psycho-analysis. The traditional or Freudian occupational therapist, under the close direction and supervision of the physician, used activities as a means to assess personality structure, learn more about unconscious content, provide opportunity for the ego to learn more about the self, and provide opportunity for the ego to improve its problem-solving ability. Because Freud believed that left unresolved old conflicts would dictate current behavior, much emphasis was placed on understanding the patient's history, especially those significant events that were being held by the unconscious and tying up an undo amount of libido. In accounting for behavior by looking at past events, Freud's theories are referred to as **causality**.

Projective Activities and Ego Adaptation

The occupational therapist used activities in which the patient could **project** aspects of the unconscious into the visible therapeutic milieu. Patients were encouraged to use unstructured media such as paints, clay and collage because they tended to facilitate symbol production, especially personal, unconscious symbols that could be then seen and integrated into consciousness. Activities were also selected to help determine the ability of the ego to organize and problem solve and eventually to provide an opportunity for the ego to better adapt to the environment.

Parent Child Relationship

Perceiving the therapist-patient relationship as implicitly reminiscent of the parent-child relationship, the occupational therapist followed the physician's cue in allowing patients to **transfer**, or put onto the therapist, their feelings (often unconscious) about their parents. The therapist then helped the patients to understand and potentially reexperience aspects of this parent-child relationship. The occupational therapist believed that people are influ-

enced by the past, but that they had will and ability to choose.

Influence of Jung

Mosey included ideas attributable to Carl Jung as part of her proposed object relations frame of reference.[63] It is difficult to assess how this man, who was a contemporary of Freud's and a groundbreaker in the field of psychology, influenced beginning object relations practice. It is not within the scope of this text to discuss Jungs' constructs in depth, and the reader is referred again to the bibliography. However, several concepts in current practice owe their inception to Jung and are discussed here.

Jung was a psychoanalyst who, like Freud, believed in the existence of an unconscious. He too identified tensions within the individual. Jung saw behavior as motivated by past events (causality) as well as future aims (**teology**). That is, Jung saw in the person a constant, internal striving for creativity, a search for wholeness, and a yearning for the development of the self.[44,45,46]

Polarities in the Self

Jung was himself well versed in and influenced by Eastern philosophy. The image of the individual as struggling to balance many opposing forces, as is conceptualized in the Eastern image of the yin-yang, is key in Jungian thinking. Agreeing with Freud that much memory and thought is unconscious, Jung thought that the predominant tension in the unconscious was created by the pull of opposite forces that exist in the self.[14]

Some opposing forces identified by him included 1) the tendency of the self to be **introverted** (focused on the self) versus **extroverted** (focused on others), 2) the tendency of the individual to gain information through tangible seeing versus the tendency to favor gaining information through intuition, 3) a striving in the self for material comfort versus a striving for spirituality, and 4) the existence in a man of latent or unexpressed feminine qualities and in a female of latent masculine qualities.

Jung thought that all these polarities in the psyche needed to be developed and be given expression in a person's life. He called this process **individuation**. Further, he conceived of a governing structure that would strive to bring all these polarities into balance and work toward the goal of wholeness. This force he called the **transcendent function** and the process, the ultimate goal of personhood, he termed **transcendence**.

The dualities discussed by Jung also correspond to the dualities suggested by split-brain studies. In the right-handed person, the left or dominant hemisphere corresponds to feelings of "light" and to a sense of masculinity, as well as the verbal-intellectual function, as was mentioned earlier. The right, nondominant hemisphere corresponds to a sense of "dark" or night, to feelings of femininity, as well as the acausal-intuitive function of perceiving and problem-solving. Ornstein[67] makes the observation that various occupations tend to depend more on the function of one or the other hemisphere: "Many different occupations and disciplines involve one of the major modes of consciousness. Science and law are highly involved in linearity, duration and verbal logic. Crafts, the "mystical" disciplines and music are more present-centered, aconceptual and intuitive."

Jung introduced concepts that have found a great deal of contemporary acceptance among a generation who is concerned about achieving a personal balance and inner harmony and who has now turned to the field of psychology, not just for advice about illness but also assistance with personal growth.

Changes in the Second Half of Life

Whereas Freud's concept of psychosocial development tends to stop with the advent of a person's adulthood and sexual maturity, Jung addressed the changes that occurred in self-perception, values and social roles throughout the life process until death. In conjunction with his belief that both men and women carry within themselves latent qualities of the opposite gender, Jung felt that in middle age, after relative success in meeting societal role expectations, persons of either sex could allow themselves to give expression to some of these qualities.

For example, a rather passive mother of 40 may become more assertive in her relationships and may seek a significant role in the business community. In contrast, the 40-year-old man who had been a bit ruthless in his business pursuits may start to feel that perhaps business is not so important and may want to spend more time in nurturing his children. Both men and women at middle age would, said Jung, tend to turn from materialistic concerns to spiritual concerns.

As indicated by Hall and Nordby,[38] Jung is one of the few psychologists until recently who has tried to understand the psychology of the middle years. In an evocative passage Jung states, "A human being would certainly not grow to be seventy or eighty years old if this longevity had no meaning for the species. The afternoon of human life must also have significance of its own and cannot be merely a pitiful appendage to life's morning."[45]

Jung felt that "middle age" extended well into the fifties, sixties and even seventies—old age implying senility or a return to the unconscious. He predicted that the older person would achieve real wisdom and wholeness. Implicit is the premise that Jung valued the roles and accomplishments of the older person, in contrast to Freud's inference that older age brings rigidity and little growth.

With so much of our population now in middle or older years, it is not surprising that a very widely read, lay psychology book popular in the late 1970s, *Passages*[75] by Gail Sheehy, was a restatement and popularization of Jungian philosophy.

Collective Unconscious

Perhaps the greatest stir in the analytical community was raised by Jung's conception of a **collective unconscious**. Jung conceived of the psyche as being conscious and unconscious in content, as did Freud. He went further, however, in suggesting that the unconscious held not only thoughts and reflections of personal experience, but images and ideas and a predisposition to seek certain experiences in a way that our ancestors had experienced them. These universal images and predispositions, thought to be racially inherited, were called collective and said to be stored in the collective unconscious. Pointing to similar themes and content in mythology, religion and cross-cultural art, and finding these same themes in the symbolic expression of his patients, he looked at symbols in a much broader vein than did Freud. *Man and His Symbols*[46] (we suggest the hardcover edition) is an excellent introduction for understanding symbols as is the writing of Joseph Campbell.[13,15–17]

Jung and the Use of Art

As his ideas about the unconscious developed, Jung began to encourage his patients to make drawings of their dreams and daydreams (or fantasy material). Although the drawings were usually not made during a therapy session, they were shared between patient and therapist.[22] The purpose of such drawing appeared to be to help the individual understand and integrate what was depicted therein. As Jung writes, "It is true, I must add, that the mere execution of the pictures is not all that is required. It is necessary besides to have an intellectual and emotional understanding of them; they must be consciously integrated, made intelligible, and morally assimilated."[22,44]

Jung does not in his writing specify techniques for involving patients in drawing; however, many contemporary therapists who specialize in the use of art as an expressive and integrative medium refer to Jungian theory as their base.[22,81] The occupational therapist who is well acquainted with cross-cultural themes

in mythology, art and religion has the opportunity to help the patient look at his or her own life and struggles in terms of broad themes.

Ego Psychology

Although Freud regarded the ego as the decision maker in the personality, he continued to view it as subservient to the whims of the id, trying to reduce tensions and resolve conflicts. Many of those who followed in psychiatry (a medical discipline) and psychology (nonmedical) thought that the ego had a broader, more autonomous role. Writing mainly in the 1950s and 1960s, these persons came to be referred to as ego psychologists. Heinz Hartmann and R.W. White are two ego psychologists often referred to in the occupational literature. Hartmann wrote that the ego does not develop "out of" the id, but on its own at birth. He said that although some ego-energy is used to meet instinctual id needs and to reduce tension, the rest is used to help the person adapt and prosper within the environment in ways that are not conflict-ridden. The person not only adapts to his or her environment, but helps to create that environment.[41] This theory is echoed in the writing of White who stressed that the ego (the person) gains great satisfaction from exploring and accomplishing within his or her world.[82,83]

Hartmann refers to his own ideas as differing in emphasis from Freud's ideas, not as a major break from them. However, the difference in emphasis was one that occupational therapists would increasingly point to in the literature because it helped to explain why "doing" (occupational therapy's key tool) was a natural part of a healthy state of being and was satisfying in and of itself.

Input from Existential-Humanism

With its roots in the writing of such articulate philosophers as Sartre, Camus, Tillich, Kafka and Heidegger and in the neo-Freudian therapies of Horney, Sullivan, Klein, Adler, Rank, Fromm, and Erikson, existential-humanism has evolved over the past 40 years into a significant influence in philosophy, psychology and education. Generally included as part of the existential-humanistic movement are those theories or therapies referred to as Gestalt or field theory organismic theory, phenomenology, Rogers' client-centered therapy, Frankl's logotherapy, plus a broad range of psychologies referred to as "existential" and "humanistic." We focus here on the elements common to existential-humanism, as they have contributed to the object relations framework for occupational therapy.

The existential-humanistic approach to psychology was elaborated in the literature in the 1960s and early 1970s (see especially Rogers,[72,73] May,[56-58] Maslow,[54,55] Jourard,[43] Perls,[69] and Moustakas,[64,65]) even now, one can discern the continued influence of existential-humanism across a broad range of theoretical frameworks and across many disciplines.

Existential-humanism has focused on the issues of what is the essence of the human condition and how one individual might best help another. With science now able to extend or maintain life, questions of life, death and quality of life push us to reexamine our beliefs in this regard.

Appreciation of Subjectivity

Believing as Freud, that the therapist must understand and appreciate the subjective experiencing of the individual, the existential-humanist professes a much different concept of what constitutes an optimum therapeutic relationship. In this unique conceptualization of the therapeutic relationship, existential-humanism has been especially evident in the field of occupational therapy. Existential-humanism conceived of a much different human nature than that identified by Freud, a view quite consistent with the generally positive posture taken by occupational therapists.

Existential-humanism has also been a part of the movement across our society encouraging the individual to be "true to yourself," and to act with integrity rather than blind con-

formity. One result, evident in the practice of many contemporary occupational therapists, has been the reevaluation of age and sex stereotypes, especially as regards role behavior and object choice.

Nature of the Therapist-Patient Relationship

Originally schooled in Freudian ideology, existential-humanists challenged Freud's premise that a therapist must be passive and impersonal, and that he or she must facilitate a reenactment of the parent-child relationship or the doctor-patient relationship. As Rogers stated, "I was asking the question, 'How can I treat, or cure, or change this person?' Now I would phrase the question in this way: 'How can I provide a relationship that this person may use for his own personal growth?' "[73] The humanists suggested that the therapist and individual were each responsible for their own behavior and the ultimate outcome of therapy.

Freedom to Choose

Existential-humanists stressed that the individual has the ability for self-awareness and, with it, freedom to choose his or her actions and determine a personal destiny.[20] With this freedom of choice comes the responsibility for ones own behavior, a responsibility that includes a need to acknowledge one's effect on and relatedness to others. The aim of existentia-humanistically oriented therapy is to assist the individual to become more aware of personal needs, feelings, options and goals; to understand realistically the needs and feelings of others, and to facilitate the acceptance of personal responsibility for one's life.

Unconditional Positive Regard

Existential-humanists believed that to assist the individual in meeting personal goals, the therapist needed to understand the subjective-experiencing or **phenomenal world** of the individual. They suggested that the individual was most able to be honest with the therapist and honest with oneself in the context of an authentic relationship. In this relationship the therapist openly expresses concern for the individual, shares his or her attitudes and feelings, and conveys a message (verbal or nonverbal) of acceptance. The therapist communicates that he or she would not reject the patient upon really "knowing" the person.[72,73] Rogers coined the terms **unconditional positive regard** to describe the therapist's position.[72,73] Unconditional positive regard did not mean that the therapist necessarily agreed with or liked everything the individual did, but he or she continued to value the individual and respect his or her right to feel differently from the therapist.

The Person as a Whole

Existential-humanists focused on the wholeness of the individual, in contrast to what they perceived as a psychoanalytical tendency to compartmentalize the person. In addition to seeing the individual as functioning as a holistic unit, they conceived of the individual as needing always to perceive "wholeness" (or to discern meaning from fragments, ambiguity or nonmeaning). This need for wholeness operates from the most elemental perceptual level to the most complex cognitive or emotional level.†

Existential-humanists also expressed the belief that in each person certain issues, called by Perls "unfinished business," (often emotional in nature) will be most pressing and need to be dealt with accordingly. Failure to do so or failure in closure on old business prevents the individual from attending fully to new experiences.[69] Therefore, the therapist attempts to ascertain with the individual those experiences that are his or her priorities in therapy.

---

²The foundation for such holism may be found in the early works of the Gestalt psychologists Wertheimer, Koffka and Kohler, whose studies were focused on the study of visual perception and learning, and on the organismic theory of Kurt Goldstein.[31,32] This work is not to be confused with the writing of Perls and his Gestalt therapy.[69]

The Here and Now

Existential-humanists placed emphasis on the here and now of an individual's life, rather than the past, but they do not discount the past. Rogers, for example, saw in early childhood experiences the basis for many distortions in the individual's self-awareness. The youngster, seeking parental approval, may behave according to parent wishes and mimic the feelings that parents communicate are valid. If this behavior continues into maturity, the individual loses touch with personal values and perceptions. Parental hopes for the patient become the patient's hopes for himself or herself. Frequently, adult life is spent seeking an external approval that is never forthcoming, or that never seems quite sufficient.

Self-Approval

Moving away from the parent-child model, the therapist sought to help the individual realize that the locus of approval was in the self. The therapist did not see the individual as there to make the therapist feel important, to follow his or her advice, or to model the therapist's expectations. One important function of the therapist was to relate to the individual perspectives and options that she perceived in the "here and now" and that the individual had blocked from self-awareness. This approach did not mean that the individual necessarily chose these options; but with more information about tools, paths, and activities, the range of potential opportunities became greater.

Existential Anxiety

Anxiety is viewed by existential-humanists as a significant concern in therapy and is conceived as deriving from one or more of four essential conditions: 1) the individual recognizes the need for a significant change in life or is in the midst of change; 2) the individual recognizes his or her failure to live authentically, that is, consistently and in accordance with personal beliefs and values; 3) the individual can find no real meaning or purpose in his or her life; and 4) the individual recognizes that he or she has not developed unique skills and has failed to be "all he can be."[20]

The therapist realizes that the individual might be out of touch or unaware of personal values and skills, due to prior concern for acting as he or she believed others wanted. The occupational therapist supports the individual's attempts to risk change, to try new roles and to experience the self in new ways. The therapist understands that such change may feel very scary to the patient.

Motivation

Whereas Freud conceptualized a tension-reduction model of behavior, and ego psychologists and Jung saw both tension-reduction and fulfillment as motivating behavior, existential-humanists conceived one driving force: the innate striving in each individual to be all he or she can be. They termed the life-long striving toward this ultimate goal of **self-actualization**.

Self-actualization can include the kind of biologically rooted drives described by Freud, but goes much further. As discussed by Rogers self-actualization is "... the urge which is evident in all organic and human life—to expand, extend, become autonomous, develop, mature—the tendency to express and activate all the capacities of the organism...."[73] One is reminded of Jung's conceptualization of transcendence—a state perhaps achieved by only a few—where all aspects of the individual find expression during the course of his life.

If there appears to be a loftiness or esoteric quality to this goal of self-actualization, a humbleness and integrity inherent in existential-humanism should not go unnoticed. This ideology holds the basic belief that all individuals have wisdom and worth, that one person's path to knowledge and purpose is no more or less valuable than another, provided that each is using his or her abilities as best each can, and living according to one's personal beliefs.

Therefore, a simple task or basic skill has as much essential worth as great intellect.

Parallels Between Existential Humanism and Occupational Therapy

The reader will discern many themes in existential-humanism that are parallel to basic tenets of occupational therapy: the belief that individuals need to feel valuable and purposeful in their lives, the belief that the therapist must understand an individual's goal for therapy in terms of the patient's priorities and in accordance with his or her perceptions, and the belief that the individual has inner motivation to explore and to master. These tenets have been recounted in occupational therapy literature from the beginning of the profession to the present day.[3,30,85,86]

It may be useful, however, to remind ourselves of some of these tenets. Not too long ago, occupational therapists believed that their professional obligation to patients was to decide, without collaboration, what was best for them. They sought to instill confidence through behavior that was designed to accentuate their difference from patients rather than their relatedness to them.

Therapist's Humanistic Approach

The therapist comfortable with existential-humanistic ideology within the object relations framework tries to understand the patient's subjective experience and then may share his or her personal view of the patient's perceptions and feelings. The therapist trusts that, even in anxiety or confusion, the individual has much wisdom and information about what contributes to well-being. The therapist strives to encourage patient responsiveness to inner-directed motives, rather than overconcern for the approval of others. He or she realizes that personal growth occurs in the context of relatedness to others and tries to help the individual gain a realistic understanding of how his or her behavior is received by others.

Activities

Activities that have their origin in existential-humanistic ideology include values clarification activities, body awareness experiences, gestalt art experiences, and "new" less competitive games.[25,71] However, the therapist realizes that all activities have the potential to be meaningful and facilitate growth.

Freudian Psychotherapy and Ideology Today

Mental health treatment and object relations practice continue to be affected by Freudian ideology, albeit with modification. Whether or not it is accurate to refer to most contemporary Freudian treatment as "Freudian" at all is probably a valid question, as it has moved far from Frued's original model. Nevertheless, today's psychosocial occupational therapist will likely be directly or indirectly influenced by this ideology in contemporary practice, especially when this practice interacts with a traditional medical or medical-model setting.

Current trends in psychotherapy and psychoanalysis (Freud's method) are not duplicated in object relations occupational therapy, but parallels that can be discerned. In the broader perspective, these trends parallel many of the concerns of contemporary society as a whole. One cannot be certain where the mental health treatment community has led and where it has followed or reacted in the response to these concerns.

The following brief overview is designed to assist the reader in recognizing significant changes in Freudian-based mental health treatment as they influence object relations practice in occupational therapy.

Altered View of the Role of Past History

Whereas Freud stood firmly by his belief that events in the past (through their retention in conscious and unconscious memory) caused events in the present and that therapy should attempt to understand these causes, current

Freudian thinking operates under a newer model. Today, childhood experiences are not conceived as necessarily causing events to occur in adult life, and therapy is believed to be most productive when it focuses on the here-and-now interaction between the therapist and the patient.[35,53,61]

Although focusing on the here-and-now of the patient-therapist relationship may be reminiscent of the existential-humanistic mandates, the nature of the here-and-now interaction in the psychoanalytical process is quite different than that in the humanistic interaction. The psychoanalytical exchange is not the give and take, mutual sharing and disclosure by therapist and patient, but rather a unidirectional interpretation by the analyst of the patient's behavior.

New Conceptualization of the Development of Gender Identity

Altered View of Femininity. Freud's perspective on women has been especially criticized as patriarchal, biased and totally inadequate.[5,6,23,50,62,66,70] It was a view based on the belief that psychology was rooted in biology; that women wished (unconsciously) to be men; that appropriate female behavior was dependent, passive, and masochistic; and that the proper feminine role was associated with nurturing and child-bearing. It was an interpretation (or perhaps an absence of one) that was based on the belief that female and male gender was not established until about age four, with the advent of the early genital phase. Undoubtedly, it represents Freud's own observations of the women of his times, and as such, represents his incorporation of the cultural bias and values of his day.

Gender Identity. Today's Freudian therapist is knowledgeable about the information gained in the area of child development and as regards the importance of cultural shaping in gender identity. **Gender identity** is "the knowledge and awareness, conscious or unconscious that one belongs to one sex and not the other."[66,80] The child is now understood to be establishing gender identity upon birth (and quite possibly before birth). Countless studies and simple observation have shown that males and females begin to diverge in interests, mannerisms and conduct by one to one and one-half years.[34,36,59,62,66,70,80]

The understanding of gender identity is one of many areas in which today's therapist views Freud's original premises as too rooted in biology, and as placing too much emphasis in the phallic period. Differences in gender role are now attributed to many antecedents including biological differences, social learning, scripting and cultural myths.[34,36,70]

Changing Roles of Men and Women. The women's movement has challenged the Freudian bias that women needed to be passive and dependent to be "feminine" (and psychologically healthy). Cultural changes, the emerging role of women in positions of power and authority, the increasingly diversified models for child-rearing and family role-taking have all affected the societal norms regarding appropriate female and male conduct. Today's therapist, looking beyond anatomy, has a much broader view of masculinity and femininity.[34,35,36,53,59]

Gender Stereotypes. Gender stereotypes have special implication for the occupational therapist working to facilitate meaningful object-involvement for patients, both male and female. Even if the therapist has incorporated a liberalized perspective on appropriate gender activity, he or she may encounter in practice individuals who still grapple with sexual stereotypes about themselves and others. The occupational therapist needs to be aware that both in terms of the activities and media made available to patients, and in terms of his or her role of therapist (possibly a female in a position

of authority), the therapist may precipitate patient's conflictual feelings about gender role.

Challenging the Supremacy of Biological Determination. The change in views regarding appropriate male and female behavior reflects a contemporary ability to see behavior as determined by more than anatomy. Freud is described as never having been able to adequately resolve the conflict between cultural injunction and individual psychology.[70]

Today, object relations theory attempts to understand the significance of all aspects of the external world (environment and culture) as experienced by the individual and giving unique meaning to his existence. Even sexual objects (e.g., those related to genital sexuality) are considered in light of their cultural-societal association, not merely as appendages to an instinctive, biologic drive.

Prephallic Experiencing

For a long time, the Freudian and neo-Freudian therapist thought the therapist-patient relationship was, at an affective level, a reexperiencing of the child-parent relationship of the early genital period; in other words, the therapist was the longed-for Oedipal parent.[23]

Today the Freudian psychotherapist is aware of the special relationship of infant to mother, which is critical in terms of mother's physical and emotional nurturance. As the ego develops, the child is increasingly able to go off alone, thus beginning the process of separation-individuation. Successful separation-individuation depends on the ability of the child to experience mother as consistent and nurturing, to retain her in memory and to trust that she will be there when he or she returns.

With much more emphasis being given to early (prephallic) development, it is not surprising that current psychotherapists also perceive the development of superego as beginning much earlier than conceived by Freud.[8] This view would be more consistent with the work of such developmentalists as Piaget and Kohlberg.

Geriatric Psychiatry

With the increased longevity of the average American, public priorities about the elderly are changing. Whereas Freud thought that change was not likely to occur in the older individual, therapists have become increasingly involved (within their professional organizations and as reflected in their practice) in better understanding the special problems of the elderly and making treatment available to them.[35,12]

In an associated shift in priorities, those individuals with cognitive impairment (e.g., the organically impaired, those with senile and presenile dementias, and the traumatically assaulted) have, according to Sloane, been "rediscovered by American psychiatry in the last decade."[34,77] The medical community's renewed interest in the function and chemistry of the brain is reflected in its extensive coverage in recent literature. Whether the contemporary Freudian therapist can retain an allegiance to Freudian constructs while accommodating the special problems posed by neuropsychological dysfunction remains to be determined. If this change is not possible, neuropsychiatry will emerge as a unique specialty, divested from the traditional constructs of conscious-unconscious, id-ego-superego, defense mechanisms, and the like.

Supportive Treatment

The final trend that has emerged in literature and practice is the acknowledgment of a need for shortened psychotherapeutic treatment. (This trend does not extend to the traditional process of psychoanalysis, but certainly helps dictate whether or not psychoanalysis is a viable alternative.)

Shortened treatment duration is in some cases a reflection of changing therapeutic directives. For example, more treatment programs are directed toward crisis intervention and prevention. Intervention that is not expected to bring about personality change nor change in ego function but is designed to bolster existing ego strengths is referred to as **supportive**. Shortened supportive treatment

must be also viewed as a response to the increasing need to contain medical costs.

Current Practice in Occupational Therapy

Person and Behavior

The object relations frame of reference as described by Mosey and as practiced to date brings together many constructs that seem the antithesis of each other.[63] It is not possible to be strictly Freudian, neo-Freudian, Jungian and humanistic-existential at the same time. However, the occupational therapist who wishes to understand and explore with the patient the feeling side of personal experience will find in object relations ideologies the necessary permission and guides (if diverse). The following discussion is a generalized statement regarding the object relations view of the person.

Dynamic Energy System

A person is a dynamic energy system, composed of parts known to the self (conscious) and parts of which one is unaware. The individual is composed of an id, ego and superego, each with its own role in maintaining selfhood and continuous experiencing, but each a psychological construct not to be confused with selfhood itself. The individual knows the self better than anyone else can.

Object Choices and Relationships

Early experiences tend to determine object choices and ways of relating to human and nonhuman objects, but objects have no meaning in and of themselves. Individuals give meaning to them through their unique perceptions and experiences. Understanding his or her own behavior and being given the opportunity to do so, a person may make deliberate choices to change the manner in which he or she relates to objects. A person needs to feel safe in the environment and to love and feel loved and accepted. He or she needs to be true to the self and strives to recognize personal assets, limits and potential. Thus, he or she strives toward self-actualization.

Process of Self-Actualization

Although the person may fear change or resist seeing the self in a new way, each person has an innate striving to grow, mature, and be all he or she can be. When mature, the individual accepts responsibility for his or her own actions, is congruent, and changes personal perceptions according to real data and values of self and of others.[73]

Only the person can develop his or her opportunities. No one can do it for another. **Self-actualization** is a process more than an outcome. A person moves toward self-actualization when he or she uses thoughts, feelings, senses and perceptions to increase self-awareness and develop personal talents while respecting one's limitations and the rights and boundaries of others.

Psychological Dysfunction

Whereas Freudian ideology contributed to a system of labeling patient behavior according to psychodynamics (psychiatric diagnoses), humanistic-existential proponents have challenged this system of labeling, seeing it as presumptive, unnecessary, and even demeaning. However, with insight as a goal in all of the interpretations of object relations theory discussed, the need remains for the patient to be reality-oriented (for all but the most supportive goals).

Dysfunction is based on the individual's subjective experience. That is, the patient states whether he or she is in distress, and how that distress is experienced.

Implications for Research

Freud based his conclusions on the careful observation of his own patients. He frequently wrote about these in individual case studies (e.g., "Little Hans," the "Wolf Man"). The single case study as applied by Freud was a qual-

itative research design in which the therapist or researcher carefully described the patient's account of his or her experience, the patient/therapist interaction, and how these changed during the course of treatment. The bottom line in qualitative research is the individual's experience of his or her world. This approach has also been referred to as the "insider perspective," and is consistent with the object relations framework's concern regarding the patient's subjective experience.[7]

Role of the Occupational Therapist

The occupational therapist serves as a knowledgeable, empathetic guide who develops a collaborative relationship with the patient and maintains the framework of treatment. The therapist is not an authority who passively participates in evaluation and treatment as was the case in the classical psychoanalytical approach. Nor does the therapist foster a parent-child relationship. The occupational therapist takes a more neo-Freudian, humanistic approach in which he or she provides unconditional positive regard and a framework of concern and interaction.

Mutual Responsibility

In this **collaborative relationship**, the occupational therapist acknowledges that the patient has a will and responsibility for making decisions and choices. Patient and therapist mutually assume responsibility for evaluation, identification of treatment goals and development of a treatment plan. They work together cooperatively during the treatment process. When the occupational therapist has an attitude of unconditional positive regard, he or she sees the patient as equal and accepts the individual's thoughts, feeling and behavior without attaching a value to them.[4] When therapy occurs in a group context, the occupational therapist has a key role in establishing group norms that facilitate exploration and positive social interaction. This role as a group leader is discussed later in the chapter.

Behavior Awareness Through Activity

The framework for interaction and decision-making defines the expectations for participation in occupational therapy and identifies the activities and resources available in occupational therapy from which the patient can choose. Within this framework, the patient makes choices and shares his or her thoughts about the outcome and personal significance of activities. To help the person understand personal symbols and to help the patient achieve a dynamic understanding of behavior and problems as presented during the activity process, the occupational therapist uses his or her knowledge of personality, group process and normal growth and development.

Participant-Observer

Most often the therapist functions as a **participant-observer**. As an observer, the therapist may reflect his or her observations to the patient and check their validity. It is important to remember that the therapist is not there to tell patients what their behavior "means," but rather, to facilitate their own discovery of meaning. The therapist has a responsibility, along with the patient, to maintain the momentum of therapy, that is, to reassess as needed, the goals that have been established for treatment and to redefine them as patients broaden their perceptions and become aware of more choices.

Function of Activities

As each therapist looks at activities in relation to each patient, the following will be at the very core: What activity can best provide this individual with an opportunity to learn more about the self and experience the self in a broader, more successful way? Closely akin to this question: What are this person's most pressing needs now? These are the questions that the patient and therapist consider, from the beginning to the end of therapy. The answers may be difficult to tease out, or they may be quite apparent. The activities may run the gamut, from trying on make-up to preparing a meal, from coping with an unbalanced checkbook to expressing oneself in art, or from learning to give to learning to receive. Patients are viewed as always changing, and the process of growth is more important than the tangible end product.

Appropriate Expression of Feeling

If patients are feeling confused, describing themselves perhaps as "out of touch with feelings," as "sad" but "not knowing why," or "anxious" but uncertain of what, then the therapist might suggest expressive media, such as art, poetry, clay, drama, dance and expressive movement. When art is used in this way it may serve as what Frye and Gannon[29] refer to as a "safe alternative to violence." Strong aggressive id impulses or unchanneled anger can be released acceptably through expressive media. Then, when some of the energy behind the anger has been released, the patient can be helped to identify the source of this anger. This process depends on the patient's knowing that he or she will not be permitted to get out of control.

Activity Process

In this case the activity process is the primary focus of treatment. As Mosey states, "The therapist tells the patient that the 'purpose of using art media is to help him discover unknown aspects of the self, not to develop his skill as an artist.' "[63]

Further, the activity may serve as a catalyst in facilitating interaction between the patient and therapist, or among patients, and can be used to help the patient relate present experience to a past or future situations. Whatever activity or media is chosen, when the patient is given some choices within the activity as to color, design or other personal preference, one expects to see some projection of the patient into the activity. In many cases, this projection is far from mysterious.

We recall a woman who came to an outpatient facility because of feelings of depression. When she was asked to draw herself, she depicted a small, female stick figure hanging up the laundry. It was not difficult for her to verbalize her belief that not only did she have a housekeeping role, this role encompassed all that she was. With children gone to college and less housekeeping to do, her identity was severely assaulted. The kind of expressive activities suggested here tend to stimulate fantasizing, an id activity, and to tap into unconscious content.

Regaining a Sense of Control

In some persons, the most urgent need may be to regain or strengthen a sense of mastery and control. Hence, the occupational therapist is equally concerned about ego function as it is reflected in a patient's ability to problem-solve, to manage frustration, to accomplish a task, to feel confidence in one's ability, and to integrate new insight into awareness and put it into action. The following example illustrates this concept.

A woman in her early thirties came into the occupational therapy facility during her brief hospitalization. She was attractive and articulate and very pleasant as she assured the therapist that there was "nothing" that occupational therapy could do for her. When asked what she might do for herself, the patient laughed and said, "Are you kidding? Everything I touch, I mess up. I'm a walking disaster area." Here, the pressing need was for this woman to experience herself as successful, and it became clear, as she gradually did try some activities, that she was determined to fulfill her prophecies. Through her interaction with very structured media and tangible results, she was able to learn about her own need to "mess up" and could gradually make some choices that were far more positive.

Improving Ego Function

To assess and ultimately improve ego function, the occupational therapist might offer the patient a selection of activities that are more structured. In other words, the activity should be performed in logical steps and that there may be a plan or design to follow. The patient will be required to organize and plan ahead in anticipation of each new step, and gratification may not be immediate, or it may be achieved in increments as each step in the activity process is completed.

Offering a Choice

Think for a moment about the requisite demands in following a sewing pattern, building a birdhouse, repairing a broken clock or baking a cake. By offering the patient a choice, perhaps from a selection of structured activities, the therapist communicates his or her belief that the patient is a competent human being, capable of making decisions, and ultimately responsible for the outcome of his or her actions.

Even where freedom of choice results in a less-than-perfect outcome, looking at one's own errors in a atmosphere of tolerance, acceptance and patience can turn a "disaster" into an education and need not be an assault on one's self-concept. By seeing his or her successes and limitations, the patient can move toward an improved yet realistic self-confidence.

Sometimes, when given free choice, a patient feeling emotionally empty may try to substitute nonhuman objects for persons and may verbalize the wish to complete as many projects as possible in order to take home many tangible goods. It was not uncommon for many of the adolescent patients at a community mental health center who were, not incidentally, having a great deal of family problems, to attempt to carry literally armfuls of material from the clinic, plants from the greenhouse, and cookies from the kitchen to fill the vacancies they experienced in people relationships.

Seeing Oneself in a New Way

For others, occupational therapy activities may be a vehicle to explore untapped skills and see themselves in new roles. We might think for a moment of what is probably a classic situation: A male patient, about age 55, is brought to the occupational therapy setting for the first time. He looks around and sees what appears to be a great deal of art and craft material, or perhaps a greenhouse, or even a woodshop. Red flags figuratively flash before him and he announces in his own fashion something like, "Get me out of here!" With appreciation of the roles and values this patient brings into the occupational therapy setting, this man can be helped to look at the ideas he has about himself and the kind of tolerance he has for others. Perhaps he has never allowed himself to enjoy play, a hobby or time for quiet thinking. The choices may be reaffirmed or disavowed. It will always be up to him to decide.

When occupational therapy offers group activities, patients may learn about themselves and their concerns in a group. The have an opportunity to learn more about how others view them, and may have a chance to test out their ideas about others. The patients have a vehicle for developing trust and for trying out dependence or independence. They may have the chance to compete or to try noncompetitive play. They may learn more about their feelings about sharing, about losing and about winning. They may try out a new role as a leader or as a follower.

Processing the Activity

Whatever the media and the activity, any activity may be explored dynamically. When looking at the **dynamics** of the activity, the patient and the therapist together look at the end product, form, content and process that occurred. Patients are encouraged to talk about the significance of the activity: How did it feel to have so many others compliment you on your work? Is this (product) for you or a gift for someone else? How was it to win or lose? What did you learn about yourself? What did you learn about the others?

In their book, *Occupational Therapy: A Communication Process in Psychiatry*, Fidler and Fidler[24] have a substantive discussion on the use of activities. As they state, the "extent to which a patient is encouraged to talk about feelings associated with the activity process..." will depend partially on ... "the patient's readiness or ability to communicate certain associations verbally."[24]

One could add to these views, that the degree to which a patient is encouraged to talk about an activity will depend equally on the therapist's comfort in instigating and following through with such a dialogue. This framework asks, if we are not comfortable with ourselves, how can we expect our patients to be comfortable with themselves? Frequently, students and beginning therapists do not want to analyze or delve too much. If one can provide "permission" for a patient to explore his or her own activities and ultimately, his or her world rather than make demands that the person do so, it is suggested that most of us have a healthy curiosity to know more about ourselves; one may well find a patient who is disappointed to have the discussion end.

Summary of Activity Functions

In summary, occupational therapy activities in the object relations frame of reference and the discussion around them are seen as serving one or more of the following functions:

1. To provide an avenue for appropriate expression of feeling;
2. To provide an opportunity to improve ego function;
3. To provide a means to establish or reestablish a sense of self and control;
4. To provide a vehicle for learning new skills, improving skills or gaining confidence in skills already held;
5. To provide an opportunity for trying out new roles or gaining confidence with already established roles;
6. To provide a vehicle for learning more about one's self and one's relationship to others;
7. To provide a means toward increased self-acceptance;
8. To facilitate movement toward flexibility in approaching life tasks.

Theoretical Assumptions

Before embarking on the discussions of the evaluation and treatment processes in occupational therapy, the basic theoretical assumptions that provide a framework for practice based on the principles of object relations theory are outlined.

1. A patient is a valuable, unique individual.
2. A patient's perceptions of his or her reality and experience are more valid than any diagnosis.
3. A patient capable of logical thinking is capable of developing increased understanding of self and other, cause and effect, and the interplay of past, present and future referred to as insight.
4. A patient's most pressing needs will naturally emerge and need to be dealt with first.
5. The id-ego-superego are useful constructs if they are understood to represent portions of the self, each serving to enhance the experiencing of the self while helping the self to respond and accommodate to the real needs of others. When the wholeness and integrity of the self is lost in focusing on these parts, these have ceased to be useful constructs.
6. A therapist who is comfortable with oneself, able to communicate concern, and able to see personal responsibilities in the therapy process is most able to foster a helpful relationship and positive movement in therapy.
7. A patient is not likely to be open to increased insight when his or her sense of self is threatened.
8. Objects have no meaning in and of themselves. Persons give them meaning.
9. Objects and object relationships can stand for more than themselves and thus serve as symbols.
10. A patient can be assisted to understand the self in a new way when he or she can learn to understand the significance of personal symbols, as they may be produced during an occupational therapy session.
11. The patient who can be more self-accepting and have less need to keep "secrets" from personal awareness has more energy to put toward establishing an abundance of satisfying object relationships.
12. A patient who can try out a new experience, as in the occupational therapy setting, has an opportunity to integrate verbalization, insight and action, which verbalization and hypothesizing alone can not provide.

Evaluation

The purpose of the occupational therapy evaluation is to gather information that will increase the mutual understanding of the patient's difficulties, which will help in clarifying the thoughts, feelings and experiences that are influencing behavior, which will identify the areas in which the patient wishes to grow and to identify the means and resources available for achieving that growth. To gather this data, the occupational therapist uses projective tests and an interview that allows for open-ended responses.† The intent is to gain insight into the patient's view of experience. Structured activities may be used to help determine the effectiveness of the patient's ego in adaptive problem-solving. Interview questions and assessment activities are designed to gain an understanding of the following:

1. Does the patient have a well-established sense of self?
   What are his or her thoughts and feelings about his or her physical image?
   What is his or her level of self-esteem?
   What are his or her social roles and responsibilities?
   Can the patient identify personal strengths

---

³The term **projective** was coined by Lawrence Frank[26] who wanted indirect methods for eliciting patterns of internal organization. Projective tests are based on the Freudian belief that the most influential aspects of personality are not in the person's conscious awareness, but are suppressed by the ego. Projective tests are designed as a means to sidestep the ego and superego and reveal data believed to represent underlying personality and conflicts.

and weaknesses? Does he or she accept them?

What does he or she perceive as available resources?

2. Does the patient have the ability to trust? Does he or she trust oneself? Can he or she trust others? Does he or she feel free to share personal thoughts and feelings with the therapist?

3. Is the patient's primary mode of communication verbal or nonverbal? Feeling oriented or intellectual? Spontaneous or controlled?

4. What is the patient's affect? Is behavior consistent and congruent with his or her verbalization?

5. Does the patient have significant relationships? Family? Friends? Peers? Colleagues? Community ties? Can he or she establish and maintain these relationships? What are his or her relationships with patients and staff?

6. Can the patient identify and meet personal needs? How are safety, physical, love, belonging, self-esteem, and self-actualization needs being met?

7. How does the patient respond to change?

8. How does the patient invest and use energy?

9. What does the patient value?

10. Does the patient want to participate in the evaluation and treatment process?

11. What does the patient hope to achieve in treatment? In occupational therapy?

12. Can the patient cope with the anxiety of self-discovery and change?[24,63]

Assessment Instruments

The Azima test battery was one of the first occupational therapy evaluation instruments to be well documented. It consists of four tasks: 1) draw a picture using a pencil, 2) draw a whole person and draw a person of the opposite sex, 3) make an object out of clay, and 4) make a finger painting. The purposes of the test battery were to uncover the psychodynamics of behavior and to determine the level of psychosexual development.

After the development of the Azima battery, Fidler modified the battery and expanded the evaluation process through the identification of five general areas to be assessed. The modified battery has three activities: 1) draw a person, 2) make a finger painting, and 3) make an object from clay. As a result of the activities, the occupational therapist assesses the patient's concept of self, concept of others, ego organization, unconscious conflicts and nature and manner of communication.

Fidler and Fidler[24] outline the method of interpreting patient behavior by considering the patient-therapist, patient-group and patient-activity relationship. They also provide an outline for activity analysis, which can be used with any activity as an assessment instrument. These outlines by the Fidlers continue to influence the use of projective activities as assessment tools.

The test battery that Mosey suggests in the area of object relations is a modification of the ones developed by Azima and Fidler. The patient completes three tasks: 1) a drawing with colored pencils, 2) a finger painting, and 3) a clay object.[63]

Although not identified with a particular frame of reference, recent literature gives an extensive list and description of projective instruments that includes the following: 1) The Azima Battery; 2) The Shoemyen Battery: 3) The Goodman Battery; 4) The BH (Barbara Hemphill) Battery; 5) The Lerner Magazine Picture Collage; 6) The Ehrenberg Comprehensive Assessment Process: A Group Evaluation; 7) The King Person Symbol As An Assessment Tool; and 8) The Activity Laboratory: A Structure for Observing and Assessing Perceptual, Integrative and Behavioral Strategies.[42]

Because projective media and approaches are identified with the object relations frame of reference, they are listed and summarized here. For a thorough discussion of the evaluation process and protocol for each of the evaluation summarized, refer to Hemphill, *The*

Evaluative Process in Psychiatric Occupational Therapy[42] or the original sources cited.

Azima Battery. The battery consists of three media that facilitate free association and exploration of personality dynamics. The patient is asked to complete the following tasks: draw anything using a paper and pencil; draw a whole person, then draw a person of the opposite sex; make anything out of a clay ball; make a finger painting. The therapist then makes interpretations based on the following: 1) organization of mood, 2) organization of drives, 3) organization of the ego and 4) organization of object relations.[2,42]

Shoemyen Battery. The therapist evaluates one to four patients at a time and requests the patients to complete four projects: 1) construct a mosaic tile trivet, 2) using three primary colors, paint whatever finger painting you want, 3) carve an object from a 4-inch vermiculite-plaster cube and 4) model a human figure from clay. The therapist then completes a data form that summarizes the patient's responses to the task, media and the discussion between therapist and patient.[42,76]

Goodman Battery. The battery consists of four tasks that begin with the most structured and become progressively less structured. First, the patient copies a mosaic tile design to reproduce a tile trivet. The second task is a spontaneous drawing; then the patient does a figure drawing, and finally he or she is asked to make an object from clay. The therapist then rates the patient's behavior, using a seven-point scale.[42]

Barbara Hemphill (BH) Battery. The BH battery consists of a mosaic tile trivet and a finger painting. The therapist evaluates the patient's approach to the media, the manner in which he or she uses space, and the patient's verbal responses. A rating form is used.[42]

Lerner Magazine Picture Collage. The patient is given colored construction paper and magazines and is asked to construct a collage.

The therapist assesses cognitive-perceptual skills; the nature and quality of defenses; and the patient's affect, sense of self, and the quality of object relations. A scoring sheet is used to objectify results.[48,49]

Ehrenberg Comprehensive Assessment Process: A Group Evaluation. During three, one-hour group sessions, patients are asked to complete a tile trivet, choose one of three projects, (a collage, group drawing or a problem-solving task) and then complete one of the three chosen activities. The therapist evaluates general appearance, interaction skills, work skills and activities of daily living skills. The assessment defines behaviors that need to be assessed.[42]

King Person Symbol as an Assessment Tool. The patient is given a pencil and paper and asked to draw a person. There is no discussion of the drawing with the patient. The therapist uses the Goodenough-Harris Scale to interpret the drawing.[42]

Other Person-Symbol Assessments. Therapists have used several other versions of a draw-a-person test to assess body image in adults. Many of these were initially designed as assessment tools for children, including the draw-a-man test,[33] later revised to the Goodenough-Harris draw-a-person test;[40] the house-tree-person;[9] and kinetic family drawings.[10,11] Guidelines for the interpretation and use of these assessments are in the citations noted, but should be understood as informal, at best, if applied to adults.

Fidler: Activity Laboratory, A Structure for Observing and Assessing Perceptual Integrative and Behavioral Strategies. Fidler states that this assessment is used to establish a tentative behavioral profile. Five activities are used: 1) the patient traces one of two pictures and cuts it out, 2) a finger painting, 3) a collage, 4) the patient performs through an obstacle course, and 5) a ball tag game. The patient then completes a questionnaire.[42]

Broad Interpretation of Projective Terminology

All of these assessments have been categorized as projective assessments. This categorization is based on a broad interpretation of projective testing, perhaps somewhat broader than that used by the psychology community. Do activities of daily living, ball games and obstacle courses provide stimuli that are open to interpretation? Might these also be "amorphous, somewhat unstructured situations" onto which the patient projects his or her needs?[47]

Guides for Evaluation

Interview. During the evaluation interview, the therapist allows time to establish **rapport** with the patient. Rapport is enhanced by the therapist's attitude of warmth, openness, and regard, as discussed previously. In addition, confidentiality may be discussed and the therapist is open in stating the reasons the patient is asked to engage in the specified evaluation activities.

Instructions. When giving instructions for evaluation tasks, the therapist gives clear, specific instructions but does not give suggestions for methods of task accomplishment. As the patient works, the therapist observes and notes verbal and nonverbal behaviors. The patient completes each task and then the therapist discusses the activity process and behaviors that were observed. Discussion during the activity may be too distracting for the patient and can affect patient performance.

Atmosphere. The atmosphere during the evaluation should be one of mutual sharing and learning, not interrogation. The patient gains personal awareness and the therapist learns about the patient's thoughts, feelings, and concerns as well as his or her manner of approaching certain tasks. In this frame of reference, the therapist is often open in sharing his or her views with the patient. During the interview the therapist may orient the patient to occupational therapy, its purposes, and how

the patient might benefit from the activities available.

The Figure Drawing as an Evaluation Task

Increasing Self-awareness. The projective assessments previously summarized stimulate the reflection of unconscious content and, as such, are quite traditionally analytical in their assumptions. Additionally, these batteries provide a means to assess the ability of the person for (ego-directed) problem-solving. With the moderating input of human-existential theory into the object relations frame, the object relations therapist would be not so much wishing to analyze patient productions but rather focusing on using the evaluation activities as a springboard for helping the patient become more aware of his or her approach to activity; personal strengths and limitations; and feelings about self, interests, and relationship to others.

Because the person drawing is used in several of the aforementioned batteries, as well as in assessments to be discussed in other frames of reference that follow in this text, we will illustrate how a person drawing might be presented and followed up as part of the evaluation process.

Draw a Person Versus Draw Yourself. When using the classical, projective presentation of the person drawing the therapist requests the patient to draw a "person." After noting the gender in the drawing the therapist then asks for a second drawing depicting the opposite gender. Most often, the individual will draw first a figure that is the same sex as himself or herself; projectively speaking, both drawings relate to aspects of the self.[39] Another option is to request one self-drawing, which can then be discussed directly as a reflection of the self. The method that follows is not cut-and-dry, but provides an example. The use of other evaluation media such as collage, structured tasks, and clay could be presented and discussed in much the same way.

Adapted Person Drawings. The request for a person drawing might be as part of a given projective battery, singly with an interview or as part of other structured assessments. The drawing requested might be of a person, the self, or the self engaged in an activity; of the self doing something with the family; of the self in the future; or of the idealized self.

Person Drawing Protocol. The therapist has available several pieces of white paper (at least 8-1/2×11 inches; larger pieces can produce more expressive results), two or more pencils and functioning erasers, crayons or colored marking pens or pencils (if the therapist wishes to allow color to be an aspect of the drawing and increase the opportunity for expression).

The patient is typically seated with the therapist and asked "Please draw a picture of yourself" (or "yourself with your family"). Patients may express the concern that they "can't draw" or "can't do this." The therapist will communicate his or her understanding, and give assurance that artistic ability is not the concern and that he or she would like the patient to try. The therapist can also assure the patient that when the drawing is finished, they will look at it together. This approach lets the patient know that the drawing will not be interpreted, but rather, the patient will have the opportunity to look and see what he or she thinks. This attitude of valuing the patient's opinion frequently lessens the resistance to what can be a very anxiety-laden task. If possible there is no limitation on the time allowed for the drawing. Individuals frequently feel a strong need to get the drawing right. When there is a time limit, however, the patient is told about it in advance.

Guide for Activity Processing and Feedback. The therapist pays attention to the following: 1) the manner in which the patient selects and uses the media; 2) comments made while engaged in the task; 3) the parts or aspects of the body or drawing, which are given special time or care, or which are ignored or glossed over; 4) the patient's general affect while doing the drawing; 5) peripheral drawings or scribbles on the page and when, in the process, they were made; and 6) the person figure itself. After the drawing is completed, one might ask the patient to pause, look at the drawing and then give it a title.

In this example, when the drawing is made as part of a battery of evaluation tasks, the drawing is the last task presented in the sequence. This task sequence also allows time for the therapist to establish rapport with the patient and for the person to get comfortable with the evaluation process while completing the other tasks. As a consequence, there is usually less resistance when it comes time to draw.

After completing the drawing, the therapist communicates a wish to look at the drawing with the patient so that they might both learn more about the patient. The process might be started with a statement such as, "I am hoping that together we can look at this drawing and learn more about you and get a better understanding of what you want to accomplish for yourself while you are here in treatment. What can you tell me about the person in this drawing?" or "Please tell me about the person in this drawing."

When a patient is reluctant or unable to respond to an initial request to tell about the drawing, the therapist might facilitate the process by making an observation about the drawing, or the manner in which it was approached, always with a note of tentativeness in his or her voice, so that the patient feels invited to expand on or correct the therapist's observation. For example, the therapist might say, "I noticed that you drew a very light figure, almost as if it wasn't supposed to be seen. How do you feel looking at it?" or, "I noticed that you erased your drawing several times, and I wondered how you felt while doing the drawing?"

Using Observation and Discussion Questions. Some patients are unable to talk about their figure drawing even with support and assistance, and their limitations must be respected. Occasionally, these patients are able to structure their thoughts in writing, and the therapist might ask them to respond to one or more issues this way.†

Some questions that might be posed about the figure drawing include:

- What is the figure doing?
- Is the figure male or female (if that is not evident)?
- What does the figure in the drawing like about himself/herself?
- What would he/she like to change?
- What are his/her roles? And to whom is he/she responsible?
- If engaged in a task, why was this task chosen?
- If the patient makes a family drawing, to whom is he or she placed nearby?
- Who is close to whom in the family? Who is isolated?
- What is the significance of the title (if one was requested)?
- What is the person in the drawing thinking about?
- What is the person in the drawing feeling?
- What does the patient feel while looking at the drawing?
- What has he/she learned about himself/herself from doing the drawing?
- If a physical change or disability is reflected, what does the person feel about it? Are physical changes accurately depicted?

Although several manuals are available for the projective interpretation of person drawings,[19,52] the therapist is encouraged to respond to the feeling tone of the drawing and to the organization of the task as well as the approach as a whole. For example:

---

†The manner in which a person-drawing is handled is a reflection of both the integrity of the concept of self, as well as, more broadly, the development and integration of a person concept as applied to all persons. The ability to depict visually as well as talk about a "person" advances predictably in a developmental sequence. The reader is referred to *Person Perception in Childhood and Adolescence* by Livesley and Bromley.[51]

1. Small, lightly drawn and frequently erased drawings tend to appear apologetic; they do not communicate confidence or comfort.
2. Large, bright drawings may exude confidence and a sense of importance; however, one needs to ask how this fits with the fact that the patient is in treatment.
3. Body parts may be missing or covered, scribbled and erased when there is discomfort with their function.
4. Drawings tend to appear masculine, feminine, or asexual or bisexual. What does the drawing communicate about the individual's comfort with his or her sexuality?
5. A figure's expression, posture and use of color communicate an affect or feeling-tone. Is it sorrow, confusion, "flatness" (lack of affect), joy, anger, other?
6. A loss of integration in the figure (e.g., body parts disconnected, distorted, or missing) or the use of excessive symbolism often reflects a loss of integration in the individual.
7. Inability to complete the task or a highly symbolic rendering may reflect an inability to deal with the self as a real and meaningful entity.
8. Background objects placed with the figure in the drawing may provide emotional support or help define the individual's roles.
9. Drawings may be internally congruent or incongruent. For example, the title of the drawing is "I'm Me and I'm OK" but the figure in the drawing is frowning. The drawing may also be congruent or incongruent in relation to the patient doing the drawing. For example, the patient may appear sad and state that he or she is in treatment due to depression, but the figure in the drawing is smiling.
10. The amount of time and energy spent on the figure drawing and on specific figure parts may relate to their importance to the individual.

Figures F1 through F18 in Appendix F are self-drawings completed by patients with whom we have worked. Some pertinent biographical data are included. They illustrate the manner in which figure drawings can reflect vividly an individual's sense of self and related concerns.

Sample Interview Dialogue. For Figure 3.1, we have included the beginning patient-therapist dialogue, to further illustrate how communication around a task can be developed. This figure was drawn by a 19-year-old white woman. She sought outpatient treatment because of feelings of depression, but was then hospitalized because of her physician's concern about her suicide potential. Her parents are recently divorced. In the interview she appears a bit heavy, wears a very short dress, and is well groomed. When asked to "please draw a picture of yourself," she uses the pencil to draw a figure about 6.5 inches tall in the middle of a 12×16-inch piece of paper, and titles it "Little Girl." When the task is completed the therapist initiates the following interview:

Therapist: What can you tell me about this drawing?

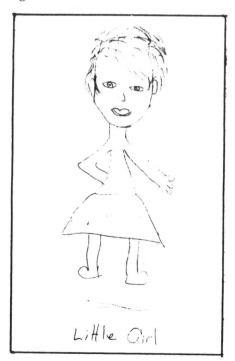

FIGURE 3.1. Self-drawing of a 19 year old female.

Patient: I like my eyes, I think they're my best feature.

Therapist: And the rest of you . . .?

Patient: I'm too fat (pause). I don't like my body.

Therapist: I'm struck by the title that you gave this picture. Can you tell me how you came to this title?

Patient: Sometimes I feel like a little girl (pause). I wish I were a little girl again. It was so much easier.

Therapist: Easier than being a woman?

Patient: I know my parents don't approve of me, especially my father. They don't like the way I dress . . . or the guys I date. I'm dating a guy right now, "R." Sometimes he calls me at 11 o'clock and wants me to come over (pause, looking down). You know what I mean. He doesn't even ask me out on regular dates. When I come home, I feel really crummy.

Therapist: It sounds like you disapprove of yourself as much as your parents do.

Patient: That's right—I really hate myself. I wish I could be little again; then my parents would love me, and they'd be together and I wouldn't have to feel so crummy. I don't even know what I want to be and I have a crummy a job as a . . . I'm a big flop . . . Do you know what I mean?

Therapist: Well, I think I'm starting to understand why being little again could seem so appealing.

Summary of Evaluation Process

The evaluation process is designed to help clarify both the problem or pressing need(s) as perceived by the patient and to help identify the patient's strengths and available resources. The person drawing was discussed to illustrate the development of an evaluation task in the evaluation process. Both structured and unstructured evaluation tasks as well as patient-therapist dialogue are used to help identify the patient's personal perceptions, goals for treatment, and the ways in which these goals might be accomplished. During the evaluation, the patient is helped to focus on and identify specific details about goals for treatment and for occupational therapy. A patient unfamiliar with occupational therapy may need assistance from the therapist in understanding what resources are available and how these might be used. Once the initial evaluation has been completed, the therapist turns the process to goal setting and program planning. The evaluation process is really an ongoing process of reassessing patient participation and change and helping to identify new areas in which growth is desired.

Treatment

Goals

In the early history of psychiatric occupational therapy, an analytically oriented approach was used under the close supervision of the physician who prescribed treatment. Knowledge of psychodynamics and activities were used to identify personality structures, object relationships, defenses and conscious and unconscious meanings of behavior. The occupational therapist used projective activities to develop object relationships, ego function and defenses and to increase the conscious awareness of the dynamic reason for symptoms.[24]

Therapist Responsibility

The philosophy of treatment based on object relations and the communication process has come to expect the occupational therapist to function more independently in evaluation and treatment planning and to assume more responsibility for decision-making. The physician or primary therapist refers the patient to occupational therapy and expects the therapist to evaluate the patient and design a treatment program that effectively responds to the patient's needs. Setting treatment goals encompasses 1) stating what the patient would like

to accomplish and 2) planning a program that will provide the patient a means to this goal.

The occupational therapist may continue to use projective or expressive media to achieve traditional analytical goals. In addition the therapist strives to increase the patient's ability to identify and satisfy personal needs, achieve greater insight, and to be able to use this insight to interact more effectively within the environment. Within the broad goals of increasing self-awareness, developing insight and improving problem-solving, the occupational therapist sets specific, individualized treatment goals for each patient.

Specific Treatment Objectives

Ten years ago, one might find occupational therapy treatment goals to be lofty but vague. Such goals might state that the therapist aimed to "increase self-esteem" or "decrease depression" or "improve problem-solving." The contemporary occupational therapist writes more specific objectives which are easily understood and are stated in terms of patient outcome. Usually the goals are behaviorally identified and agreed on by the patient and treatment team. They may be used by third-party payers when making reimbursement decisions.

Sample treatment goals include the following:

1. The patient will describe feelings of inadequacy and identify sources of these feelings.
2. The patient will increase self-esteem through the completion of a (specified) occupational therapy activity.
3. The patient will identify and explore through occupational therapy media feelings of loss and grief.
4. The patient will identify personal strengths and weaknesses within the context of the occupational therapy activity.

The treatment goals are discussed jointly by the patient and the therapist and a treatment plan is developed. Treatment goals are then reevaluated periodically, typically weekly or bimonthly, and modified as needed.

Treatment Process

The application of the object relations frame of reference in the treatment process occurs in individual and group situations in occupational therapy with patients who are reality oriented and capable of logical thinking. To facilitate a dynamic understanding of behavior and problems, the occupational therapist uses creative media or semistructured experiences to help the patient project personal thoughts, feelings, needs, fantasies, desires and frustrations onto the end product (activity), or uses structured activities to assist the patient to increase organizational and problem-solving skills.

Creating a Climate. Individual treatment sessions usually last 40 to 60 minutes and group sessions are 1 to 1.5 hours long. Optimum group size is from five to eight patients. During the treatment sessions the therapist is an observer and participant-observer. The therapist participates in the activity when processing the activity or trying to influence the treatment outcome. Therapist participation can also ease patient anxiety or the initial resistance due to the threat posed by the activity. When participating in treatment groups, the patient can influence the focus of the group.

For example, when a patient refuses to experiment with drawing media, the occupational therapist might suggest that they experiment with colors, or each do "scribbles" and then share their view of the identifiable images in the scribbles. Sharing in this manner can help establish rapport. Or, perhaps the occupational therapist is aware of much anger in the patient group and senses that the group is threatened by the expression of this feeling. The therapist could request that each patient pantomime a feeling, and then have the group discuss what they saw. During this process, the therapist might mime anger and depict how he or she handles anger. This is one way of **role-modeling** and gives the group permission to express angry feelings. If the group resists this permission, however, the therapist should be sensitive to this resistance and would not try to force anyone to go beyond

his or her present need or capacity. The process of change may be both inviting and threatening, and thus, tends to occur slowly.

Increasing Self-knowledge. As an observer during the treatment process, the occupational therapist notes significant behaviors that occur during the activity process. These behaviors, as well as the significance or symbolic meaning of the activity, are discussed when the activity is completed. During the discussion, the occupational therapist tries to do the following:

1. Help patients explore the thoughts, feelings, and memories aroused by the activity;
2. Help patients make conscious association between the activity experience and past, present and future experiences and difficulties;
3. Using conscious associations, help the patients increase their self-understanding and broaden their perspective on current behavior and problems and possible solutions;
4. Help the patient interpret the meaning of symbols and integrate this new knowledge.[63]

When an activity, process or medium is believed to hold special symbolic content, the occupational therapist might try to help the patient understand the latent as well as obvious significance therein. It is believed that symbols are expressed not only in art form but in all our actions and interactions. For example, when I jog, I may do so because I really enjoy jogging or perhaps because it symbolizes to me health and well-being, prosperity or independence. When I draw myself jogging, I may be symbolizing my quest for health or prosperity, or I may wear jogging shoes as a symbol of having attained prosperity.

When interpreting symbols, the occupational therapist focuses on the function of the symbol. When looking with a patient at a person drawing, he or she does not ask the patient to defend specific symbols. For example, he or she does *not* ask, "Why did you draw this person wearing jogging shoes?" Rather, "I wonder how this person feels jogging?"

Validating Patient's Interpretation. The therapist may give a personal view of the meaning of a symbol, but it must always be validated by the patient. The ultimate purpose of looking at symbols is to help patients understand for themselves the unique purpose of their symbols. Even when Freudian and Jungian symbolism is of special interest to the therapist, it is felt to be a great disservice to overgeneralize these interpretations if doing so loses the unique personal context.

A brief example from practice illustrates the preceding point: It is not uncommon for patients working with clay to rather absent mindedly make snakelike coils. On one occasion, a young man did this, then presented this "snake" to the therapist. He smiled and asked, "How do you like your present?" The therapist asked, "Is this a snake?" He responded, "Yes," and again asked, "Do you like it?" The therapist then asked, "How do you expect me to react?" He smiled, and explained, "When I was a lot younger I brought home a small garter snake. My mom freaked out! You should have seen her. It was so fun to scare her."

Neither the Freudian tendency to see snakes as a phallic symbol, nor the Jungian tendency to see the snake as a symbol of power (as in the physician's caduceus) is discounted in this example; but the personal experience of the young man with his mother gives this symbol its personal meaning.

Guidelines for Exploring Symbols

The therapist wishing to explore symbol production is referred to the guidelines suggested by Mosey in *Three Frames of Reference in Mental Health,*[63] which are summarized here:

1. Symbols have no fixed meaning.
2. Symbols have individual significance.
3. Symbols are given reality through reproduction such as artwork, speech and behavior.
4. Explore the content of symbols—their size, shape, form, placement on the page, the method of production and the use of materials.
5. Identify themes or commonalities that relate to the past, present and future life situations.
6. Relate in the here and now.
7. Note the process of symbol production.
8. Use interpretations sparingly. Too many interpretations are confusing and may be difficult to integrate.[63]

It cannot be overemphasized that in looking at symbol production, the therapist does not simply look to a list of Freudian, Jungian or other symbol discussions and apply them to the patient's symbols. The **symbol** is a nonverbal expression of something personal. When the patient has the ability for insight and can talk about his or her own symbol production, he or she may learn about the self.

Impact of Group Process in Treatment

As stated, occupational therapy in the object relations framework frequently is carried out in a group context. The therapist needs to consider special characteristics of group influence and group process when this situation occurs.

Patient Expectations. Patients new to treatment are usually quite uncertain about what is expected of them in a patient group. They may be frightened that the patient group will see them as sick, or a "mental case," and they may be equally concerned about the pathology they see in other patients. The therapist needs to respect these concerns, while setting a tone of mutual regard. The therapist also needs to be certain that the patients are introduced to each other, and that they are given a chance to become more comfortable before numerous demands for interaction are made of them.

Varied Forms of Interaction. Depending on the format within a clinical setting and on the therapist's goals, the following degrees of interaction may be in evidence, and are reminiscent of the development of play interaction among children.

1. Individuals are working by themselves on their own projects, with little interaction, but in the same work space as other patients.
2. Several patients are sitting together, sharing materials and talking, but each is working on an individual activity.
3. Several patients, or the entire group, are working together, cooperating on accomplishing an agreed upon task; interaction and sharing, which are high as well as personal feelings, occur around the task.

Leader as Gatekeeper.   Even when the level of patient interaction is minimal, the therapist has a **gatekeeping** responsibility. In this role he or she sees that safety needs (physical and emotional) are met, disruptions (subgrouping, scapegoating, abusive behavior) are responded to, materials and equipment are shared and used appropriately, and patient and clinic scheduling needs are met.

When the therapist wishes individuals to function cooperatively as a group, the concerns become much broader. Materials and seating may be arranged to facilitate sharing and interaction. Group tasks, activities or games my be introduced that will depend for their vitality on patients' interdependence.

Example: A Cooking Group.   One community health center outpatient group experienced frequent change in patient population, with the average length of patient treatment being one month. To encourage interaction and build specific skills, the occupational therapist had the patient group, which varied in size from five to ten, plan and carry out the preparation of a noon or evening meal. Patients purchased all supplies, prepared food and cleaned up. The occupational therapist was a resource person only. On some occasions, the patient group would vote to invite one guest each to share their meal. It was useful for the group to look at their own feelings about having guests. When the group had achieved a strong sense of unity and each patient felt accepted by the group, the issue of having guests was not volatile. When there was less ease and cohesion, the prospect of having guests made many patients anxious. When potential guests included persons not in psychiatric treatment, many patients had to confront the personal struggle they were experiencing about being in treatment.

This group had many tasks and subtasks that required good organization and problem-solving. Equally significant, patients had the opportunity to experience themselves in a social setting that was quite similar to an everyday social situation.

This cooking group was a popular patient activity. It should be noted that food and feeding play important symbolic functions in our culture. In breaking bread together, patients could give to themselves and to each other in a significant way.

Example: An Art Group.   To provide another perspective on the therapeutic use of group, we cite an art therapy group described in the literature.[18] The group consists of four to six psychiatric inpatients, with one or two new patients at any given session. The group meets two hours a week. During each group session the group engages in an activity such as those listed.

1. Each patient is asked to draw a lifelike portrait of each parent or a significant other. Afterward, each patient holds up the drawing(s) and describes the persons depicted in the group. A male and female in the group are selected to role play the parents, and each patient is encouraged to tell that "parent" what they had always wanted to tell them.
2. Each patient is given some clay and told to imagine that they are lost in the forest and to make tools with which they will survive. A group discussion follows.[18]

Group as a Social Microcosm.   It has been suggested that whenever people get together in this way, a **social microcosm** is formed. An individual tends to replicate, in each group of which he or she is a member, the patterns or ways of behaving that typify everyday social interactions. Thus the occupational therapy group experience is a vehicle for learning about and possibly enhancing social skills. When the group provides a chance for intimacy and mature interaction (that may be lacking or minimal in everyday life), the patient in the group has an opportunity for what Alexander called a **corrective emotional experience**.[1,68]

Feedback. If the group is open in its verbal sharing, the patient can be given **feedback** about behavior (i.e., the person is told how he or she is perceived by others), not just from the therapist, but the entire group. Yalom[84] suggests that in a group context, the patient may gain insight at several levels. Those most applicable to an occupational therapy group are the following:

1. Insight as to how I am perceived by others: Am I tense? Warm? Aloof?
2. Insight as to how I interact with others: Do I tend to exploit them? Reject them? Overdepend? Do I behave differently toward men than toward women?
3. Insight about why I behave the way I do: How does my behavior make me feel?[84]

By receiving this kind of feedback, the patient can engage in **consensual validation**; that is, he or she can compare thoughts and viewpoints with the statements that others make and can reassess these views when he or she becomes aware of discrepancies. Studies suggest that whether the patient receives so-called "superficial" or "deep" insight appears to not influence the degree to which the patient finds feedback to be helpful. Any accurate feedback is considered useful.[84]

With dynamics similar to those of the therapeutic one-to-one relationship, if group feedback is to be openly received by a patient, he or she must perceive the group as accepting and supportive. Otherwise, the patient feels too strong a need to defend against perceived assaults on his or her self-esteem.

Establishing Behavior Norms. To ensure that the group is one in which patients feel a

sense of acceptance and trust and one in which feedback is given effectively, the therapist must be cognizant of the important role he or she has in helping set the norms of behavior. These norms would include free interaction among members; nonjudgmental acceptance; respect for individual boundaries; honest expression of affection, displeasure and other feelings; and confidentiality.[84]

One way for a therapist to help establish norms is to be a model-setting participant, as we have discussed. However, therapists cannot get so involved as a participant that they lose their perspective and ability to stand back and process the group interaction. Therapist openness has its place, but the therapist is not in the group to solve personal problems.

Processing the Activity Group. Group activity sessions may be viewed in much the same way as individual activities, with the added dimension of group interaction. The occupational therapist continues to focus on the process of the activity rather than the end product. The therapist notes the following:

1. The choice of the activity and how this choice is made;
2. The individual skills demonstrated when manipulating material: motor coordination, workmanship, ability to follow instruction;
3. The satisfaction of each group member with the end product or the activity outcome;
4. The attitude of the group members toward each other and toward the therapist;
5. How each patient evaluates the activity and the group experience;
6. The role that each group member assumes;
7. The feelings of each group member about the group;
8. How the group members respond to feelings or situations that arise during the activity process;
9. The type, quality and system of communication that occurs during the group;

10. Overt behavior of the individual or the group during the activity.[24,63]

The ultimate aim is to assist patients to better understand their social and task behavior and thereby allow them to make conscious efforts to change or expand the manner in which each relates interpersonally and approaches activities. Further, when patients have the chance to try out new more successful behaviors within the group, they may have the added advantage of having the group express their approval and appreciation of this new manner of relating. Patients thereby increase self-esteem and this confidence is carried into future situations.

Summary

"Physical concepts are free creations of the human mind, and not, however it may seem, uniquely determined by the external world. In our endeavor to understand reality we are somewhat like a man trying to understand the mechanism of a closed watch. He sees the face and the moving hands, even hears its ticking, but has no way of opening the case. If he is ingenious he may form some picture of the mechanism which could be responsible for all the things he observes, but he may never be quite sure his picture is the only one which could explain his observations. He will never be able to compare his picture with the real mechanism and he cannot even imagine the possibility of the meaning of such a comparison."—Albert Einstein[87]

Regard for Subjectivity

The object relations framework for understanding a person and his or her endeavors depends on the therapist's belief in the integrity of subjective experiencing. Although the framework draws its philosophical base from a diversity of sources—Freud, Jung, contem-

porary Freudians, the humanist-existentialists—these beliefs are key:

1. That as a person sees his or her world, so is the world;
2. That a person's feelings and perceptions about personal endeavors have a significant impact on his or her actions;
3. That persons are interested in learning more about the obvious as well as hidden parts of themselves;
4. That the more a person is aware of personal needs, beliefs, and values and feelings, the more real freedom he or she has in making choices;
5. That understanding a patient's personal and social history can assist the therapist to understand the patient's current approach to life;
6. That the patient-therapist relationship significantly affects the therapeutic process and its outcome;
7. That each individual has an internal drive to love and be loved, to use unique skills, and to feel purposeful and significant, and that this is achieved through active interrelatedness with persons and nonhuman objects;
8. That human endeavor is influenced by conscious and unconscious intent;
9. That the person who is more self-accepting has more means available to interact positively with others and to develop his or her potential.

Although consideration is given to the social context and the quality and function of activity, the locus for looking at activity is from the view of the individual. Although not specifically addressed in this text as a developmental theory, the object relations approach is, in fact, developmental in its ascribing to the person a sequential development in self-perception, relatedness to others, relatedness to objects, and ability to successfully engage in activity. Before considering the contributions and limitations of the object relations framework for occupational therapy, we need make some precursory comments.

Disenchantment with Freud

First, there is a growing tendency in occupational therapy literature and in the field of psychology to discard Freudian ideology. Because object relations theory has much basis in Freudian theory, therapists need to evaluate their stance regarding the incorporation of Freudian concepts. As the scientific community and helping community look with hindsight on Freudian theory, there are obvious limitations, limitations acknowledged by Freud himself. As Corey[20] comments, it is easier to discern the need for change and reach out to build new theories when one "stands on the giant's shoulders."

Freud was a product of his times and own biases, much as we are of ours. In each frame of reference in this text and in each discipline, we encounter leaders whose ideas have at one time been accepted with authority, ideas that eventually have succumbed to selection and adaptation. If one chooses to discard, nonselectively, all constructs that are Freudian in origin, one may discard constructs that address aspects of human thought and activity not as thoroughly or adeptly handled by other theoretical frameworks. The final judgment lies with each reader.

Occupational Therapy, Not Psychoanalysis

The occupational therapist who is knowledgeable in object relations theory and applies it appropriately in practice is not undertaking psychoanalysis; the method suggested by Freud is not that of the occupational therapist, nor is the goal of extensive reworking of unconscious content and major personality change. It should be added that most contemporary psychotherapists are not engaged in psychoanalysis. Moreover, the occupational therapist can work from Freudian constructs without actually using psychotherapy.

Contemporary object relations theory speaks to the function of activity in the development of personhood, and one can accept certain aspects of Freudian ideology and approach and use this understanding to enrich one's practice. Occupational therapy provides a living laboratory for active engagement and verbal exchange.

Second, for a long time, subjectivity was held with great disdain by the scientific community and occupational therapy has been pressed to objectify its data, along with other health professionals. As a profession whose personnel have been historically better at considering feelings than clarifying fact, the need to objectify may seem clear and unquestionable. Before we become overly zealous in discarding subjective data, however, we need to recognize that we can never really separate ourselves from our own goals and interests in our research, and we must realize that our science can only discover what its tools and tests accommodate. If we choose, we can determine that thoughts and feelings are irrelevant as indices of change. Then with this decision, will we increase or decrease our understanding of the human condition and the therapeutic process?

Contributions and Limitations of the Object Relations Frame of Reference

Contributions

As has been stated, the object relations framework provides a vocabulary and hypothetical constructs for talking about and understanding feelings or the subjective self, and proponents of this framework emphasize that subjective experience is a valid and integral part of the human condition. It may be that patients who have the opportunity to express their feelings and trust that they are understood can more easily turn their attention to objective tasks. Further, patients who have both a limited and a broad range of ability for insight have demonstrated an interest in increasing their understanding of why events within and outside of themselves occur. Although we cannot all gain insight to the same degree, the desire to understand "why" is evident in most of us.

The object relations frame provides a context for approaching and understanding an individual's history or previous experience. This characteristic has been considered by many to be a detriment, rather than a contribution, to the extent that traditional Freudian ideology is judged by some as having placed too much emphasis on patient history. However, patients are given an opportunity to reflect on and better understand their past experience while being encouraged to recognize that it is today that offers the opportunity for change.

We might each pause to reflect on our own feelings about our personal past. How often do we, upon making new friends, wish to share with them information about where we come from, our family upbringing, meaningful events and relationships in our lives? How often do our children ask us to tell them about ourselves when we were children? Understanding and reflecting on our roots need not keep a person forever looking back.

The therapist conceptualizing life as a process of continuing development (much as Jung and humanist-existentialists do) would be encouraged to explore the recent work in the study of the adult life span as a developmental, task-related process. This process is discussed in more detail in Chapter 5.

The humanistic-existential influence has moderated the deterministic analytical view of the person, providing a positive posture about the individual and his or her potential for change. It is an optimistic posture that emphasizes the possibilities not fallibilities of the individual.

Humanistic-existential input emphasizes the importance of the human element and the therapeutic relationship in treatment. It encourages the therapist to be more conscious of the role and responsibilities in the therapeutic relationship, requiring active participation, not passive neutrality. For those new therapists who may be especially concerned that they will harm a patient by saying or doing the wrong thing, the emphasis on listening to the patient and respecting his or her pace and choices might lessen therapist anxiety.

In encouraging patients to be independent and emphasizing their responsibility for their welfare, the object relations framework strives to facilitate carryover of treatment benefits to home when the patient is no longer in treatment. In addition, by looking to internal, naturally evolving rewards, rather than rewards designed by staff members, behavioral change is viewed as more stable.

An important contribution of humanistic-existential and contemporary Freudian input into object relations theory is that it encourages the therapist to consider each person as unique. Thus, there is no one best approach or technique, and the therapist would profit by being aware of a diversity of philosophical and treatment principles.

Limitations

When subjective reality forms a basis for treatment, the veracity of one's conclusions about therapy and the efficacy of treatment intervention must be demonstrated through research and verifiable outcomes. Both the Freudian use of case studies to exemplify the outcomes of treatment and the humanistic reliance on feeling barometers have been criticized as too subjective. Freudian, Jungian, and existential-humanistic constructs (e.g., libido, ego, unconscious, collective unconscious, and unconditional positive regard) have been described as picturesque but not useful for scientific inquiry.

Further, no comprehensive research in occupational therapy (beyond descriptive case studies) support an object relations treatment approach. In contrast, cognitive theorists (discussed later in the text) have attempted to objectify thoughts and demonstrate the outcome of therapeutic intervention using behavioral indicators. Eventually, the theorist and practitioner within this framework must ask, "Does feeling-oriented therapeutic intervention improve the quality of individuals' lives? If so, how can this improvement be demonstrated?'' Indeed, are both the objective and subjective worlds of experience available for scientific inquiry?

The contemporary Freudian, humanistic-existential and Jungian understanding of the development of object relationships in early childhood, although much more concerned with social and cultural influences on early personality development, has not rejected much traditional Freudian conceptualization of early object choice. As a result, the object relations framework can be accused of placing too much emphasis on the role of anatomy and the significance of the parent-child relationship in the development of behavior.

As with any body of knowledge, there is a danger in knowing just enough to be conversant and believing that one knows all that he or she needs. We have been acquainted with students and longtime therapists who became quite fascinated with their encounter with elements of the unconscious. However, haphazard dabbling with unconscious constructs and misguided efforts to analyze symbols and the like lend themselves to a great deal of useless interpretation and much misinterpretation and little in the way of helpful intervention. Further, therapists may think that they somehow know more about patients than patients know about themselves.

When humanistic principles are applied, there can be a tendency to view therapy as overly simplistic. Being warm and concerned about patients is important, but does not mean that therapy has occurred. Unconditional positive regard is not viewed as desirable by all therapists and may be one of the most difficult postures to achieve; yet it may appear simple. Finding one's own place within this construct depends on experience and a maturing into the therapist role. Phony acceptance by the therapist of behaviors that he or she finds unacceptable confuses the patient and confounds the relationship.

The object relations use of interpretation and insight is most successful with patients who have a good functioning ego and capacity for logical thinking. One must remember, however, that even patients who present as more confused often are at times quite lucid, and they may well have more ability for insight than treatment staff acknowledge. Further, when insight is not the goal, the therapist's ability to conceptually understand the behavior may make the behavior more meaningful and manageable and thereby facilitate a constructive response. Attempts at empathic understanding and the communication of positive regard are believed to be important with all patients.

The object relations framework as presented is an eclectic framework. Therefore, it is open to criticism on a variety of grounds. As Patterson[68] notes, eclecticism has been considered undesirable for its lack of direction, the inevitable inconsistencies in practice, and the difficulties in its examination through research. If one accepts that no one current theory or technique best fits each individual treated or each situation, however, then one can try to synthesize common, compatible and workable constructs from a range of therapy approaches. Patterson cites the definition of **eclecticism** given by English and English in *A Comprehensive Dictionary of Psychological and Psychoanalytic Terms*:

''Eclecticism . . . in theoretical system building, the selection and orderly combination of compatible features from diverse sources, sometimes from incompatible theories and systems; the effort to find valid elements in all doctrines or theories and to combine them into a harmonious whole. The resulting system is open to constant revision even in its major outlines . . . Eclecticism is to be distinguished from unsystematic and uncritical combination, for which the name is syncretism. The eclectic seeks as much consistency as is currently possible but he is unwilling to sacrifice conceptualizations that put meaning into a wide range of facts for the sake of what he is apt to think of as an unworkable overall systematization. The formalist finds the eclectic's position too loose and uncritical. For his part the eclectic finds formalism and schools too dogmatic and rigid, too much inclined to reject if not facts, at least helpful conceptualizations of facts."[68]

The object relations framework for understanding a person and his or her activity is an attempt at the kind of integration of which English and English speak. As we leave this model and move to the next, we are confronted again and again with trends toward eclecticism in other theoretical frameworks. The reader is encouraged to be open-minded and journey with us.

References

1. Alexander F: *Fundamentals of Psychoanalysis.* New York, Norton, 1963.
2. Azima H, Azima F: Outline of a dynamic theory of occupational therapy. *Am J Occup Ther* 8(5): 215, 1959.
3. Baum C: Occupational therapists put care in the health system. *Am J Occup Ther* 34(8):505–516, 1980.
4. Benjamin A: *The Helping Interview.* Boston, Houghton Mifflin, 1969, p. 42.
5. Bernstein D: The female superego. *Int J Psyhcoanalysis* 64(2): 187–201, 1983.
6. Blum H: Masochism, the ego ideal and the psychoanalysis of women. *J Am Psychoanalytic Assoc* 24:157–191, 1976.
7. Borg B, Bruce MA: Assessing psychological performance factors. In Christiansen C, Baum C (Eds): *Occupational Therapy: Overcoming Human Performance Deficits.* Thorofare, NJ, SLACK Inc., 1991, pp. 539–586.
8. Brickman A: Pre-oedipal development of the supergo. *Int J Psychoanal* 64:83–91, 1983.
9. Buck J, Jolles I: *House-Tree-Person Projective Technique.* Los Angeles, Western Psychological Services, 1972.
10. Burns R, Kaufman S: *Actions Syles and Symbols in Kinetic Family Drawings: An Interpretive Manual.* New York, Brunner/Mazel, 1972.
11. Burns R, Kaufman S: *Kinetic Family Drawings.* New York, Brunner/Mazel, 1970.
12. Busse E: Introduction to part II, geriatric psychiatry. *Psychiatry Update: The American Psychiatric Association Annual Review, Vol. II.* Washington, DC, American Psychiatry Press, 1983, pp. 83–87.
13. Campbell J: *Creative Mythology.* New York, Viking Press, 1968.
14. Campbell J (Ed): *The Portable Jung.* New York, Viking Press, 1971.
15. Campbell J: *The Masks of God.* Harmondsworth, England and New York, Penguin Books, 1976.
16. Campbell J: *The Mythic Image.* Princeton, NJ, Princeton University Press, 1981.
17. Campbell J: *Transformations of Myth Through Time.* New York, Harper and Row Perennial Library, 1990.
18. Chapman L: The art of therapy in a psychiatric OT program. *Occupational Therapy Forum,* 1(15), 1986, pp. 1–3.
19. Cohn R: *The Person Symbol in Clinical Medicine.* Springfield, IL, Charles C Thomas, 1960.
20. Corey G: *Theory and Practice of Counseling and Psychotherapy.* Ed 2. Monterey, CA, Brooks/Cole, 1982, pp. 34, 30.
21. Dowling C: *The Cinderella Complex.* New York, Simon and Schuster, 1981.
22. Edwards M: Jungian analytic art therapy. In Rubin J (Ed): *Approaches to Art Therapy.* New York, Brunner/Mazel, 1987, pp. 92–113.
23. Eichenbaum L, Orbach S: *Understanding Women—A Feminine Psychoanalytic Approach.* New York, Basic Books, 1983, p.71.
24. Fidler G, Fidler J: *Occupational Therapy—A Communication Process in Psychiatry.* New York, MacMillan, 1963, p. 82.
25. Fluegelman A (Ed): *The New Games Book.* New York, Dolphin Books/Doubleday and Co., 1976.
26. Frank L: Projective methods for the study of personality. *Journal Psychology* 8:389–413, 1939.
27. Freud S: *Interpretation of Dreams* (1900). (Translated by Brill AA) New York, Random House, 1950, pp. 465, 242–243.
28. Freud S: Three essays on sexuality(1905). In *Standard Edition of the Complete Psychological Works of Sigmund Freud, Vol. XII.* (Translated under the general editorship of J. Strachey, in collaboration with Anna Freud, assisted by Starchey A, Tyson A). London, The Hogart Press, 1953, pp. 135–243.
29. Frye B, Gannon L: The use, misuse, and abuse of art with dissociative/multiple personality disorder patients. *Occup Ther Forum* 5(24):3, 1990.
30. Gilfoyle E: Caring: A philosophy for practice. *Am J Occup Ther* 34(8):517–521, 1980.
31. Goldstein K: *The Organism.* New York, American Book Co., 1939.
32. Goldstein K: *Human Nature in the Light of Psychopathology.* Cambridge, Harvard University Press, 1940.
33. Goodenough F: *Measurement of Intelligence by Drawings.* New York, Harcourt, Brace, 1926.
34. Grinspoon L (Ed): *Psychiatry Update: The American Psychiatric Association Annual Review, Vol.III.* Washington, DC, American Psychiatric Press, 1984.
35. Gruenbaum H, Glick I: The basics of family treatment. In Grinspoon L (Ed): *Psychiatry Update: The American Psychiatric Association Annual Review, Vol. II.*

Washington, DC, American Psychiatric Press, 1983, pp. 185–203.

36. Hales R, Frances A (Eds): *Psychiatry Update: The American Psychiatric Association Annual Review, Vol. IV.* Washington, DC, American Psychiatry Press, 1985.

37. Hall CS: *Primer of Freudian Psychology.* New York, New American Library, 1954, pp. 29, 35, 85.

38. Hall CS, Nordby V: *Primer of Jungian Psychology.* New York, New American Library, 1973, p. 93.

39. Hammer E: The clinical application of projective drawings. In Rabin A: *Projective Technique in Personality Assessment.* New York, Springer Publishing Co., 1968.

40. Harris D: *Children's Drawings as Measures of Intellectual Maturity.* New York, Harcourt/Brace, 1963.

41. Hartmann H: *Ego Psychology and the Problem of Adaptation.* New York, International Universities Press, 1958, p. 31.

42. Hemphill B: *The Evaluative Process in Psychiatric Occupational Therapy.* Thorofare, NJ, SLACK Inc., 1982.

43. Jourard S: *The Transparent Self.* Rev ed. New York, Van Nostrand Reinhold, 1971.

44. Jung C: *The Practice of Psychotherapy: Collected Works, Vol. 16.* Princeton, NJ, Princeton University Press, 1966.

45. Jung C: *The Portable Jung.* Campbell J (Ed), New York, Penguin Books, 1971, p.17.

46. Jung C (Ed): *Man and His Symbols.* Garden City, NY, Doubleday and Co., 1979.

47. Kaplan H, Sadock B: *Modern Synopsis of Psychiatry III.* Baltimore, Williams & Wilkins, 1981, p. 209.

48. Lerner C: The magazine picture collage: Its clinical use and validity as an assessment device. *Am J Occup Ther* 33:500–504, 1979.

49. Lerner C, Ross G: The magazine picture collage: The development of a scoring system. *Am J Occup Ther* 31(3):156–161, 1977.

50. Lerner H: Female dependency in context. *Am J Orthopsychiatry* 53(4):697–705, 1983.

51. Livesley W, Bromley DB: *Person Perception in Childhood and Adolescence.* London, John Wiley and Sons, Ltd., 1973.

52. Machover K: *Personality Projection in the Drawing of the Human Figure.* Springfield, IL, Charles C Thomas, 1949.

53. Malone C: Family therapy and childhood disorders. In Grinspoon L (Ed): *Psychiatry Update: The American Psychiatric Association Annual Review, Vol. II.* Washington, DC, American Psychiatric Press, 1983, pp. 228–241.

54. Maslow A: *Toward a Psychology of Being.* Rev ed. New York, Van Nostrand, 1968.

55. Maslow A: *The Farther Reaches of Human Nature.* New York, Viking Press Inc., 1971.

56. May R: *The Meaning of Anxiety.* New York, Ronald Press, 1950.

57. May R: *Man's Search for Himself.* New York, Norton, 1953 (Also New York, American Library, 1967).

58. May R: *Love and Will.* New York, Norton, 1969. (Also New York, Delta Books, 1973)

59. McFarlane W.: New developments in the family treatment of psychotic disorders. In Grinspoon L (Ed): *Psychiatry Update: The American Psychiatric Association Annual Review, Vol. II.* Washington, DC, American Psychiatric Press, 1983, pp. 242–256.

60. Menninger K: *The Vital Balance: The Life Process in Mental Health and Illness.* New York, Viking Press, 1963.

61. Michels R: Contemporary psychoanalytic views of interpretation. In Grinspoon L: *Psychiatry Update: The American Psychiatric Association Annual Review, Vol. II.* Washington, DC, 1983, pp. 61, 69.

62. Money J, Ehrhardt A: *Man and Woman, Boy and Girl.* Baltimore, John Hopkins University Press, 1972.

63. Mosey AC: *Three Frames of Reference in Mental Health.* Thorofare, NJ, SLACK Inc., 1970, pp. 71–81.

64. Moustakas C: *The Self: Exploration in Personal Growth.* New York, Harper, 1956.

65. Moustakas C: *Loneliness.* Englewood Cliffs, NJ, Prentice Hall, 1961.

66. Notman M, Nadelson C (Eds): *The Woman Patient: Aggression, Adaptations and Psychotherapy, Vol. 3.* New York, Plenum Press, 1982, p. 5.

67. Ornstein R: *Psychology of Consciousness.* New York, Penguin Books, 1973, p. 83.

68. Patterson, CH: *Relationship Counseling and Psychotherapy.* New York, Harper and Row Publishers, 1974, pp. 270–271, 459–460.

69. Perls F: *Gestalt Therapy Verbatum.* Moab, UT, Real People Press, 1969.

70. Person E: The influence of values in psychoanalysis: The case of female psychology. In Grinspoon L (Ed): *Psychiatry Update, Vol. II.* Washington, DC, American Psychiatric Press, Inc., 1983, pp. 36–50.

71. Rhyne J: *The Gestalt Art Experience.* Monterey, CA, Brooks/Cole, 1973.

72. Rogers C: *Client-Centered Therapy.* Boston, Houghton-Mifflin, 1951.

73. Rogers C: *On Becoming a Person.* Boston: Houghton-Mifflin, 1961, pp. 32, 35–36.

74. Sadler A: Psychoanalysis in later life: Problems in the psychoanalysis of an aging narcissistic patient. *J Geriatr Psychiatry* 11(1):5, 1978.

75. Sheehy G: *Passages: Predictable Crises of Adult Life.* New York, E.P. Dutton and Co., 1976.

76. Shoemyen C: Occupational therapy orientation and evaluation. *Am J Occup Ther* 24: 276–279, 1970.

77. Sloane R: Organic mental disorders. In Grinspoon L (Ed): *Psychiatry Update: The American Psychiatric Association Annual Review, Vol.II.* Washington, DC, American Psychiatric Press, 1983, p. 106.

78. Springer S, Deutsch D: *Left Brain, Right Brain*. San Francisco, W.H. Freeman and Co., 1981.

79. Stafford-Clark D: *What Freud Really Said*. Excerpt from Freud S: *An Outline of Psychoanalysis, Vol. 23*, (1939). New York, Schocken Books, 1966, p. 134.

80. Stoller R: *Sex and Gender*. New York, Science House, 1968.

81. Uecker E: Tarot thematic projective technique: A structured exercise for facilitation of self-awareness and problem solving. *Occupational Therapy Forum*. 1(14):1, 1986.

82. White RW: Motivation reconsidered: The concept of competence. *Psychological Review* 66: 297–333, 1959.

83. White RW: The urge toward competence. *Am J Occup Ther* 25:271–274, 1971.

84. Yalom I: *The Theory and Practice of Group Psychotherapy*. Ed 2. New York, Basic Books, 1975, pp. 32–33, 84.

85. Yerxa E: Authentic occupational therapy. *Am J Occup Ther* 21(1):1–9, 1967.

86. Yerxa E: The philosophical base of occupational therapy. In *Occupational Therapy: 2001 AD*. Rockville, MD, American Occupational Therapy Association, 1978.

87. Zukav G: *The Dancing WuLi Masters: An Overview of the New Physics*. New York, Bantam Books, 1980, p. 8.

Chapter 4

THE BEHAVIORAL FRAME OF REFERENCE

Focus Questions

1. How are function and dysfunction identified in this framework?
2. Cite an example of a conditioned behavior that you exhibited today.
3. What is the difference between primary and secondary reinforcement? Give several examples of each.
4. How is behavior extinguished? Why is it difficult to extinguish most behaviors?
5. Why is it so important to be specific when targeting behavior for change?
6. What characterizes the behavioral assessment?
7. Describe three or more means by which new behaviors can be learned.
8. What are the benefits and drawbacks of a token economy?
9. Support the view that behavioral treatment is a humanizing influence in mental health treatment. Support the opposite view.

Introduction

The behavioral frame of reference is built on experimental inquiry and principles of cognitive, social and conditioned learning theories. Within the context of a therapeutic relationship, these principles are systematically applied to develop behavioral techniques and procedures that bring about behavior change and build functional skills necessary for the individual to function successfully in the environment.

Occupational therapists identify building functional skills as their professional commitment, regardless of frame of reference.[19,44] Identifying psychiatric illness in terms of ability to function, the mental health community has also placed increasing emphasis on behaviorally identified outcomes in treatment.[58] Viewed in this light, the behavioral frame of reference can be described as both a theoretical and treatment approach that stands on its own, but that also affects much, if not most, contemporary psychiatric care.

Definition

Therapy within the behavioral frame of reference is concerned with identifying and eliminating problem behaviors and building necessary functional skills. It is not primarily concerned with feelings, past history or the development of insight. Human maladjustment is viewed as the result of faulty learning; no disease process is implied. Behavioral techniques and procedures use action-oriented experiences to teach, shape and reinforce adaptive behavior. The therapist and patient actively participate in a learning process designed to develop skills needed for activities of daily living, work and leisure. These skills consist of overt behaviors that can be observed and measured in occupational therapy and in the patient's expected environment.

Theoretical Development

Since the 1960s, occupational therapists have documented the efficacy of the behavioral approach to treat patients exhibiting psychosocial behavior problems.[11,22,23,27,42,53,54,57] Professionals have also described the theoretical basis for behavioral treatment within occupational therapy.[17,37,39,40,46,52,55,56]

Originally, the approaches used in occupational therapy were derived from principles of conditioned learning. Today the behavioral approach in occupational therapy incorporates cognitive, social and operant learning theory, although cognitive behaviorists tend to view themselves as being in a different camp from traditional behaviorists and are discussed in Chapter 8 in this text.

Additionally, many psychologists, counselors and behavioral scientists have contributed to the theory and development of behavior therapy. Those most often cited in the occupational therapy literature include Hilgard, Bower, Clayton, Tolman, Bandura, Skinner, Wolpe, Dollard and Miller, Goldfried and Davidson, Lieberman and Spiegler, Azigan, Bakker, and Armstrong. Although each behaviorist may give a different explanation for learning and the application of learning theory to therapy, the reader should view these differences as being mainly in emphasis. In addition to the countless numbers of texts describing behavioral treatment, more recent works may refer to *functional* treatment or *functional* approaches in their titles, also suggesting a behavioral focus.

How Learning Occurs

All behavior—both adaptive and maladaptive—not attributable to physical maturation or accident is learned, and behavioral therapy rests on the assumptions of learning theory.† When an organism learns, certain factors interact: the organism (for our discussion, we use the word person), his or her capacity, intelligence, and bodily functions; the drive or motives that impel the person to act; the thoughts, perceptions and feelings of the person; the situation or setting in which he or she is interacting; and the response or behavior that is present, as well as behavior that is desired. Of these factors, much is internal and must be inferred; (e.g., intelligence, motives, feelings, thoughts and tolerance of change); even when they can be described or verbalized, they are not external and measurable.

The setting and the existent and desired behavior or response(s) can be seen and measured; these factors define learning.† Although a setting typically consists of many sights, smells and other stimuli, here setting is referred to in its most basic unit, as a single **stimulus**. Similarly, most behavior is very complex, but is described here as the simplest behavior, a single **response**. When a new stimulus brings about or elicits an already demonstrated response, or when a given stimulus brings about a new response, **learning** is said to occur.

For example, yesterday a child could climb only the stairs from the family basement. Today the toddler was able to climb the stairs to the attic. Or, yesterday confronted with any of the stairs in his or her home, the child could only crawl up them. Today, confronted with

---

[1]The term **learning theory** as used here refers to behavioral learning theory. In addition, a wealth of theory addresses the question, "How does the individual learn?" from the perspective of psychoanalytical, developmental, humanistic-existential, cognitive, neurological, and other frameworks[7].

[2]Although coined in slightly different terms, the process of imitation and modeling, as described by Bandura, is quite similar to the process of identification and the development of superego as conceived by Freud[8].

these stairs, he or she walked up them for the first time. In both cases, learning took place. When a given stimulus consistently brings about a given response, one says that an **association** has been made between them. In every day behavior, such an asssociation may also be termed a **habit**.

Beginning with the Tolman's pioneer work *Purposive Behavior in Animals and Man* (1932), behaviorists began to grapple with the possibility that internal processes, as mediated by the central nervous system, also need to be considered when looking at behavior. Tolman conceived of a "cognitive map," or internal integration of data by the organism. He suggested that the individual, rather than responding in an automatic stimulus-response habit, is capable of holding a cognitive awareness of several means to achieve a desired goal. Tolman theorized that in the development of these cognitive maps, the organism is learning not just movement patterns but also meaning.[26] The attention given to cognitive processes was to be especially significant in the work of behaviorists who were interested in the development of language and has ultimately led to a division between traditional behaviorists and cognitive behaviorists.

Classical Conditioning

According to behavioral inquiry, learning occurs in several ways. In **classical conditioning** (also called respondent conditioning) a new stimulus becomes capable of evoking a given response because the new stimulus is presented together with a stimulus that already evokes the response. For example, eating a bit of lemon will cause a person's mouth to pucker. This puckering is a natural autonomic bodily response and does not need to be learned. Most often, a person tasting a lemon will also be seeing the lemon, and in very

short time, just the sight of a lemon, without any necessity for tasting, will elicit the puckering response. For this kind of learning to occur, the two stimuli (taste of lemon, sight of lemon) need to be presented at virtually the same time, or in what is termed **close temporal contiguity**. If the lemon were shown over an extended time, but not tasted, the tendency of the sight of the lemon to elicit puckering would diminish until it had become eliminated or extinguished through a process called **spontaneous recovery**.

Stimulus Generalization

Classical conditioning most often has been carried out in relationship to autonomic functions. As such, its application to therapy might seem limited; however, dimensions of classical conditioning have important implications in learning. Learning occurs in classical conditioning and in operant conditioning, which will be discussed, in part because of stimulus and response generalization. For example, if the sight of an actual lemon makes your mouth pucker, a photograph of a lemon, or perhaps a plastic facsimile evoke the same response as a result of **stimulus generalization**.

Stimuli that seem alike become capable of eliciting the same response. For instance, most newborn and young infants attach emotionally to their mothers and experience a positive response such as body relaxation when their mother holds them. It is quite typical for young infants to respond more positively to other women than to men because women are more like the mother. This response is due to a series of stimulus generalizations. Similarly, a patient may respond to a female therapist or very nurturing man much as he or she does to Mom because of stimulus generalization.

Response Generalization

In **response generalization**, two or more responses are evoked by the same stimulus because these responses occur in close temporal contiguity, or because the two responses are perceived as similar. For example, we may learn to say "thank you " upon being given a present; or we may, upon receiving a gift, shorten our response to "thanks." Or, as may occur in treatment, when an individual builds certain social skills in the clinic setting (learning to say "please," waiting to take his or her turn), frequently other, nontargeted social skills also improve. Response generalization is often complex and therefore difficult to specify; yet it plays a significant role in everyday learning.[33]

Importance of Learning Generalization

Stimulus and response generalizations are most likely to occur when the stimuli look or act similarly and when the responses are similar or occur in close temporal contiguity. Through an infinite number of response and stimulus generalizations, the stimuli that become capable of evoking a given response may become very different, and the repertoire of responses that may be elicited by a given stimulus may become vast. Because of this generalization in learning, we do not need to relearn how to drive a car every time we purchase a new automobile. Nor, do we have to relearn how to button our clothes every time we change our shirts.

The ability to generalize learning depends on the ability of the person to recognize and respond to the similarities in a variety of situations and behaviors. The occupational therapist uses this principle when he or she plans learning experiences. The more similarities between two or more environments, the more likely it becomes that the individual can perceive and respond to these similarities, and the more vivid the similarities, the greater the likelihood of generalization. Therefore, the therapist often creates a learning structure that uses multisensory stimuli and amplifies similarities between the learning and natural environment.

Operant Conditioning

B.F. Skinner focused his attention on the role of reward or **reinforcement** in learning and described the process known as **operant (also called instrumental) conditioning.**[47–50] Skinner looked first at the behavior or response that was in evidence. When the response was desirable, it was rewarded or reinforced.

Discriminating Stimulus

When the response was reinforced in the presence of one stimulus but not in the presence of another, the response tended to occur in the presence of the former and not the latter. The former stimulus, called a **discriminating stimulus**, was said to act as a **cue**, telling the person when to emit the response. If the stimulus and response were paired repeatedly, but without the reward, the response ceased and **extinction** was said to have occurred.

To illustrate, a patient might have difficulty in asking for help and making his or her needs known to others. As a goal of treatment, the patient might agree to come to your desk and ask for assistance when needed. You would wait for the patient to come and ask for help; when he or she succeeded, you might smile and say, "I'll be glad to help you" (reinforcement). If the patient approached you while you were away from your desk helping someone else in the clinic, you would ignore his or her evocation (no reinforcement). Seeing you at your desk is the cue that he or she should come and ask for help.

Discriminatory Behavior

In the preceding example, the cue has two parts—you are alone and you are at your desk—and two responses are desired—approaching you and asking for help. Being able to perceive the difference between your being at your desk and your being elsewhere in the clinic is the basis for **discrimination**. Discriminatory behavior is the opposite of generalization. It depends on being able to see the differences between situations or settings, thereby enabling the individual to determine when a behavior is appropriate and when it is not. It is because of many stimulus and response discriminations that we know to act differently in a movie theater than during a church prayer.

It is easier to discriminate between gross or obvious differences in stimuli than between subtle differences. For example, the junctions of most busy streets use discriminating stimuli designed to be noticed; these are the red and green traffic signals that cue our traffic behaviors. However, discriminating among subtle differences in stimuli makes possible the execution of more skilled motor and social acts. For instance, if an individual is adept at perceiving slight changes in the voice or nonverbal behaviors of his or her peers and can respond accordingly, one might tend to say this individual is sensitive or gracious. If he or she fails to take notice of such changes, he or she might be considered to be insensitive, "crude," or a bore. Or, one might say that the individual needs to be "hit over the head before getting the message."

In the object relations framework, the power of discrimination would be considered an ego function. From the behavioral stance, in order for effective and adaptive discrimination to be learned, there must be appropriate giving and withholding of reinforcement according to the situation, and the individual must be able to perceive differences in stimuli and cues.

Facilitating Discrimination in Therapy

The occupational therapist would be aware of his or her role in the therapeutic milieu in relation to 1) seeing that only properly discriminated behavior is supported and 2) making certain that the individual perceives the differences between given stimuli. Regarding this second aim, the therapist might direct the patient's attention to the discriminating features of a setting or amplify the differences between settings.

Reinforcement

Skinner defined **reinforcement** as anything that increased the likelihood that a behavior

would recur. For our discussion in this chapter, we speak primarily of positive reinforcement, although some behavior therapists use also what they refer to as negative reinforcement. A significant role for the therapist planning to use operant conditioning is to identify what in the environment serves to reinforce, and therefore maintain, specific patient behaviors, both adaptive and maladaptive.

Negative reinforcement, the use of **adverse stimuli**, when removed, increases the tendency for the desired behavior to occur. The behavior acts on the environment so as to remove the adverse stimuli or to remove or keep the individual from the situation. Adverse stimuli cause escape or avoidance behavior. For instance, in the winter we put on a coat to avoid getting cold; the cold weather outside negatively reinforces the behavior of putting on a coat. One might also consider that getting warmer is a rewarding result of putting on a coat. Thus, as some suggest, negative reinforcement may be a somewhat misleading term for adverse stimuli.

Types of Reinforcement

Although one tends to hear of certain types of reinforcers quite frequently (e.g., attention, hugs, tokens and material goods), Martin[33] suggests five categories that seem especially helpful to consider in planning a behavioral occupational therapy program. We combined these into three broad categories: consumable reinforcers, social reinforcers and activity reinforcers.

Consumable reinforcers are those such as candy, cigarettes, fruit, snacks and coffee. **Social reinforcers** include any signs of attention, hugs, smiles, pats on the back, verbal praise, etc. **Activity reinforcers** cover a broad range, and may require some diligence on the part of the therapist and patient to identify. These include the opportunity to engage in a favored activity (e.g., to tinker with one's car, to ride a bike, to read a book, to spend time alone, to work with art or crafts, or to go shopping). Activity reinforcers may also include the opportunity to wear one's favorite shirt, to hold a favored toy, or to sit in one's favorite chair. Martin[33] refers to these last three activities as **possessional reinforcers**.

Schedules of Reinforcement

In day-to-day living, environmental goods and opportunities are reinforcing to the individual, in part, because they are not constantly available. For instance, food is rewarding because we do not eat constantly and we get hungry. Reading a book may be reinforcing because it represents a diversion from a more exacting, or work-related task. We function in a world where although we are not flooded with reinforcement, we are reinforced often enough to encourage given behaviors.

Continuous Versus Fixed Reinforcement. In therapy, reinforcement is supplied according to what is termed a **schedule of reinforcement**. If behavior is reinforced every time it occurs, **continuous reinforcement** occurs. If it occurs after a given number of correct responses (e.g., every third or fourth time the behavior is exhibited), a **fixed ratio** of reinforcement occurs. If behavior is reinforced at a consistent interval of time (as every 10 minutes) a **fixed interval** of reinforcement occurs. There are also variable or unpredictable ratios and intervals of reinforcement and complex combinations of ratio and intervals. When a new behavior is being learned, the individual may need continuous reinforcement. This situation occurs in occupational therapy when the therapist acknowledges the patient's achievement by giving verbal praise or attention, candy or tokens every time a desired behavior is exhibited.

Intermittent Reinforcement. Over a period of time in therapy the patient is usually weaned to less frequent reinforcement. In **intermittent reinforcement**, behavior is reinforced only occasionally. Behavior that is maintained by reinforcement that is both intermittent and unpredictable is the most difficult to extinguish and, therefore, most stable. This effect is illustrated, for example, by the behavior some may exhibit when hoping for a phone call from a new romantic interest. If we expect a call from our would-be date, we may stay near the phone for many nights, hoping for a call. If he or she calls only once during the week, that may be enough to keep us at home waiting for many more days, because there is the chance that this person will call again. If no such call has ever been received (no reinforcement), however, we would typically stop waiting around for the call within a relatively short time.

Determining Reinforcement. It is difficult to determine how often an individual will need to be rewarded in order for a specified desired behavior to occur. For instance, one employee may require a great deal of recognition and many pats on the back from his or her employer to maintain a high level of output; another might find only a yearly brief, "Thanks for a good job," adequate reinforcement. The extent to which each of us needs external and predictable reinforcement from outside sources is related to the extent that we achieve self-satisfaction from our own behavior.

Guide for Implementing Operant Conditioning

In addition to what has already been discussed, behavioral scientists have learned the following characteristics about reinforcement, which may be especially useful to the therapist planning to use operant conditioning:

1. An agent or event will be particularly reinforcing if one has been deprived of it, as least briefly. Therefore, food will be more rewarding in the clinic setting if the patient has not just finished lunch; being able to work on a

fine-motor craft will be more satisfying if the patient has not been working a similar task before occupational therapy. Even smiles and praise, when available in excess, tend to lose their capacity to be rewarding. When an agent or activity is no longer experienced as reinforcing because the patient has had enough, **satiation** occurs, and an alternative reinforcement must be used.

2. An individual should be reinforced immediately after a desired behavior in order for the correct response-reinforcement association to be made.

3. By providing verbalization along with the reinforcement, one can, through the principle of stimulus generalization, make the verbalization alone a reinforcement. For instance, when a patient is on time for therapy five days in succession, he or she may earn the right to take a walk to a local shopping mall unattended. If, when informing the person of the reward, the therapist adds enthusiastically, "I'm really proud of you, and I'll bet you feel good too!," therapist praise has been coupled with the earned walk. If this association is repeated many times, therapist praise alone may eventually be adequate reinforcement for the patient to maintain promptness.

4. The thoughts or internal statements that an individual tells himself or herself may act as stimuli for action, as cues telling him or her when to act, as drives impelling actions, as responses and as reinforcement.

5. Behavior that depends solely on external reward for its maintenance is precarious behavior, for reinforcement may be removed by others without recourse by the individual. The most stable behavior is that in which personal satisfaction (e.g., living up to one's standards) is the most important reinforcement.

Reinforcement is the term used most typically to describe the positive consequences that follow a given behavior. When an individual consistently demonstrates a behavior as a consequence of a specified reinforcement, re-gardless of whether it is behavior the person has consciously thought about, learning is said to have occurred.

Punishment

Behavior may also be followed by a consequence that is not positive. One instance of this negative consequence is referred to as punishment. **Punishment** occurs when a given behavior is followed by an adverse stimulus that can not be escaped or avoided. Punishment has been shown to suppress behavior but not to extinguish it; there is no change in learning. For example, if the therapist criticizes a patient for interrupting conversation, the patient may stop talking, but no new response has been associated with the situation; instead a behavioral vacuum is created. Behavior stopped in this fashion is likely to recur. Further, the therapist has to deal with the possibility that he or she has fostered negative feelings from the patient about the therapy setting or the therapist. On the other hand, an undesirable response is ignored (neither positive nor negative reinforcement follows) and positive reinforcement is withheld until the desired response occurs, a pattern of desired behavior is more likely to be achieved.

To cite an example from the literature, time-out-on-the-spot (TOOTS) is used as a way to neither reward nor punish inappropriate behavior. The therapist responds to a behavior (e.g., patient demanding a third or fourth dessert at lunch) either by walking away for a brief period (20 seconds or so) or by continuing to pay attention to the patient but ignoring the behavior and talking with the person about something else.[22]

Punishment may be useful in so far as it interrupts an undesirable behavior, thereby providing an opportunity for some alternative, desirable behavior to be exhibited. The key is to not only suppress undesirable behavior but to replace it with an adaptive behavior that is rewarded. In the example of interrupting a conversation, the patient may be taught to jot down his thoughts and express them when there is a lull in the conversation.

Both reinforcement and punishment are used when an individual has shown that he or she is capable of a specified behavior. When a desired, adaptive response appears not to be in the patient's behavior repertoire, other behavioral techniques may be used. These techniques include shaping, building chains of behavior and modeling.

Shaping

If the desired behavior of asking for the therapist's assistance is not demonstrated, then shaping techniques could be used. In **shaping**, any action that is similar to or preliminary to the desired behavior is reinforced, as are successive actions that more closely approximate or lead to the desired response. For example, if the patient in the earlier example did not succeed initially in approaching your desk and asking for help, you might watch to see if he or she arose from his or her seat, or, even just looked your way. Then you might choose to reinforce this anticipatory behavior and continue to reinforce subsequent behavior (e.g., with smiles) that brought the person closer to you. While using the principle of shaping, the therapist would also be careful not to reinforce any maladaptive responses.

Identifying Approximate Steps

When using shaping as part of a behavior program, the therapist must begin with a behavior that the patient can complete and be prepared to reinforce rather small steps toward the final, desired goal. Martin[33] suggests that the therapist begin by making a list of the approximate steps that will lead from the beginning to the final behavior. It should be understood that each step in the sequence might have to be repeated and reinforced many times before the therapist can expect the next step in the sequence to be exhibited. In other instances, however, several steps might follow in quick succession.

Building Chains of Behavior

Skinner believed that most complex behavior can be understood as chains of stimulus-response connections, links in which a completed response acts as a stimulus signaling that it is time for the next in the series of responses. One might consider the steps in planting a flower garden. We see the seedlings at the store, which signals us that it is time for a planting, which cues us to collect our tools and other paraphernalia, which leads us to select a potential site for planting, which when chosen cues us to begin digging a hole, and so on. In fact, each of these primary steps in itself consists of even smaller, discrete stimulus-response links.

Backward Chaining

When we think about learning, we tend to conceive of developing learning chains in a forward order. Frequently in therapy, however, **backward chaining** is used. The term backward chaining might seem to imply that the individual is taught to do a procedure backwards, but that is not the case. The example of planting a seedling illustrates backward chaining and its potential advantage.

Suppose for a moment that you are teaching a young child or adult who has a short attention span the procedures just indicated. By the time you help the child select tools, choose a planting site, and dig a hole, he or she may have lost interest in completing the process. For most, the most rewarding part of planting is seeing the young plant standing upright firmly in the ground. If we prepare the ground and call the child over to put the plant in the hole, or just ask him or her to cover the roots of the plant with dirt, the child begins with the final step and immediately gains the reward of seeing the plant in the ground.

After helping us with several plants in this manner, the child may express the wish to help dig the holes. In that case, we might start the hole for the child so that not too much digging is needed, then let him or her finish the digging, insert the plant, and cover its roots with soil. As the child becomes more interested and better able to persevere, we continue to add steps in a backward chain, always allowing the child to move from the chosen step through the subsequent steps he or she has already learned, to the last step and the reinforcement. In this way, the final reward comes to sustain a long series of stimulus-response links.

As with shaping, the therapist may find it useful to make a list of the approximate steps taken from start to finish in a given process. The therapist then starts with the last step and upon its completion, provides a suitable reinforcement. Then, the therapist proceeds backward down the chain, giving the patient ample opportunity to practice each step or series of steps, as needed, before trying to add a new behavior link.

Modeling

One hears a great deal about the significance of the therapist as a role model. In terms of learning theory, modeling has been better understood largely due to the investigation of Albert Bandura.[3-5] Along with such others as Mischel[35,36] and Rotter,[45] Bandura has proposed a social learning theory that attempts to incorporate not only the traditional reinforcement and contiguity elements of behavioral theory, but also to add to these the significance of imitation in learning. Bandura and his associates believe that when a person observes the actions of another, he or she can learn vicariously a new behavior that later can be demonstrated through imitation. Much learning appears to be accomplished more easily by imitation than through the development of stimulus response chains or the shaping of behavior.

For example, when an individual wishes to learn to swing a golf club correctly, he or she often imitates his or her teacher. Learning new words, learning to drive a car, learning to play baseball—all these can be viewed as highly imitative forms of learning. Nothing in this concept is new to most occupational therapists who have long known the value of demonstration and imitation when trying to teach new skills. However, modeling needs to be understood as being quite different conceptually from other applications of learning theory, for the **modeled behavior** is conceived as having been learned internally and vicariously before any actual response has been demonstrated or rewarded.

Guides for Using Modeling

Bandura highlights significant dimensions of modeling that can be considered by the occupational therapist who wishes to be more aware of the impact he or she may have as a model:

1. A person is more likely to be imitated if he or she is perceived as having high status; consequently a therapist, typically viewed by patients as having status, has a potentially significant impact as a social model.
2. A person is more likely to be imitated if the observer can see the similarities between self and the model.
3. An individual will more likely imitate behavior perceived as leading to reward (e.g., when the person sees the model receiving a reward). In addition, he or she is more likely to inhibit a response perceived as leading to punishment, as when the model is observed being punished.
4. Hostility, aggression and moral behavior have all been shown to be highly accessible in learning through modeling.
5. To be successfully imitated, the model behavior must be well attended to. Distraction in the learning setting can be expected to decrease imitative learning.
6. Many skilled acts, especially those involving fine motor coordination, can be learned only in part through modeling; participation and practice are necessary adjuncts to learning.
7. When the individual can give verbal labels or descriptions to the behavior observed, that behavior is more successfully remembered and imitated.[25,26]

Bandura and other social learning proponents differ from traditional behaviorists with their inclusion of concepts such as vicarious learning, symbolic representation, imagery and cognitive problem-solving. Social learning has become an increasingly significant part of behavioral theory and, along with cognitive-behaviorism, appears to represent the direction of much recent behavioral inquiry. More of Bandura's theory and cognitive-behavioral approaches are discussed in Chapter 8.

Token Economies

Token economies are systems of operant conditioning designed to alter behavior with several or more individuals, especially where internal or intangible reinforcements (e.g., social approval) have not proven effective. Tokens, which can be metal washers, plastic discs, credit cards that can be punched, and the like, are tangible rewards, given for appropriate designated behavior. They can be exchanged for privileges, cigarettes, candy, involvement in desired activities and other desired outcomes.

For example, if a hospitalized patient makes his or her bed, he or she might receive three tokens; if the individual completes an occupational therapy project, the reward is five tokens. A candy bar might cost three tokens; a pass home might cost 20 tokens. Whereas some token economies use only positive reinforcement, others use negative procedures as well; for example, fines (tokens given back) are assessed when a patient fails to meet a requirement. As noted by Corey,[16] tokens can have several advantages:

1. Tokens reduce the delay between appropriate behavior and its reward.
2. Tokens can be used as a concrete measure of motivation.
3. Tokens involve an element of choice in that the person has an opportunity to decide how he or she wishes to spend them.

Concern for Patients' Rights

During the 1960s and 1970s there was a proliferation of token economies, especially in programs for patients with long-term or chronic problems, the person with developmental delay and those in a forensic setting. Some major and positive outcomes were seen in the ability to affect behavior, teach new skills to those who up until then had seemed unteachable, and to manage large populations more effectively. As journals cited cases in which bizarre behavior was improved dramatically, token economies and the concomitant strict observance of operant behaviorism were touted as breakthroughs in mental health care.[42,43]

More recently, however, token economies have been criticized. Overbaugh, Bradley and Bucher[43] describe a male patient who had been in treatment for 45 years, yet continued to respond with little in the way of appropriate behavior. The decision was made by the treatment team to apply a rigorous token system. As the authors state:

"Throughout the therapy, the patient was on a deprivation schedule. He received no breakfast at any time during the study and received cigarettes only from the therapist. Receipt of tokens redeemable for the noon and evening meals was contingent on meeting each day's global performance criterion (quality and quantity)."

The authors go on to say that in a short time the patient exhibited markedly improved behavior and was more manageable within the institution.

The ethics of depriving an individual of such a basic need as food is at issue—even for what is described as a "short period" and for positive intent.

In 1962, President Kennedy outlined a Consumer's Bill of Rights, which provided for the consumer's right to safety, right to be informed, right to choose, and right to be heard. Since then, patients and clients have been viewed increasingly as consumers and these rights also extend to them. However, persons in institutions, especially those involuntarily committed, often have not received treatment sensitive to patients' rights.

In 1972, the court decision of *Wyatt vs. Stickney* represented a significant move toward increased specificity regarding patient rights. As part of the resolution of this case, the court assisted by the American Civil Liberties Union, the American Orthopsychiatric Association, the American Psychological Association and the American Association of Mental Deficiency specified in detail rights for those individuals who were under involuntary commitment. These rights include the right to privacy, the right to wear one's own clothes, the right to have personal possessions, the right to regular physical exercise, the right to be outdoors from time to time, the right to nutritionally adequate meals, and to the "least restrictive conditions necessary to achieve the purposes of treatment."[21] These are absolute rights and cannot be made contingent on a token economy or other treatment system. One can certainly operate a token economy without depriving individuals of their basic rights, but the kind of things spelled out in the *Wyatt* decision tended to be in the areas where reinforcement was identified in many of the token systems until that time.

Effectiveness of Token Economies

Contemporary therapists are sensitive to these legal rights and take care to use tokens as part of programs designed to foster patients' dignity. Finding effective reinforcements for very regressed and uncommunicative or uncooperative patients can be difficult. This problem has been addressed by Lorna Jean King,[30] who noted that many institutionalized patients suffered from anhedonia, or the inability to experience pleasure from the kind of everyday events most of us find pleasurable.

Other questions have been raised by token economies. There is no clear evidence that the gains made within a token system are sustained once the individual returns home or to a nontreatment setting. To sustain behavior, internal or other external reward must reinforce behavior that had been maintained by tokens. For instance, self-satisfaction or a spouse's approval must be sufficiently rewarding at home; this is not always the case. Although token economies do seem capable of managing behavior within an institution, they are not the panacea for behavior change that they were once conceived to be.[34]

Desensitization

Since the late 1950s, **systematic desensitization** has been used as a behavioral strategy to reduce anxiety. Although the reasons for the success of this technique are not entirely understood, persons with test anxiety, speech anxiety, interpersonal-social anxiety, stuttering and phobias have been successfully treated by desensitization.[15] After identifying the source of fear or anxiety, the patient participates in experiences that help him or her to gradually get comfortable with the situation. The anxiety-provoking stimuli is presented in a series of graded experiences that proceed from low to high intensity. The graded experience may incorporate imagery, role playing, simulated activities, homework, or real situations inside or outside the treatment setting that stimulate fear and anxiety.[15]

Biofeedback and Stress Management

Biofeedback emerged from behavior and learning theory as applied in a controlled environment to shape behavior and from advances in technology that promoted the use of electronic equipment during the evaluation and treatment process. **Biofeedback** is "a process of using equipment (usually electronic) to reveal to human beings some of their internal physiological events, normal and abnormal, in the form of visual and auditory signals to teach them to influence these otherwise involuntary or unfelt events by manipulating the displayed signals."[1] The signals that the patient receives may act as stimuli or cues to act and as reinforcement.

Physical Medicine and Mental Health Settings

Biofeedback has been applied by occupational therapists and other professionals in physical medicine and mental health treatment settings. In rehabilitation settings, biofeedback can be used for physical reconditioning, muscle reeducation, increasing motor control and coordination, and strengthening muscles. It is also used in physical medicine settings to monitor heart rate, visceral activities, blood pressure and skin temperature. It has been used in pain management programs and with psychosomatic conditions such as tension and migraine headaches and fecal incontinence.[1]

In mental health practice biofeedback more frequently is applied to promote relaxation and manage stress. It has also been successful in helping patients manage symptoms that are an outcome of neurotic disorders, phobic reactions, depression, drug addiction, schizophrenia and character disorder.[1,53]

Biofeedback in Occupational Therapy

In occupational therapy, biofeedback is used in conjunction with activities and is integrated with the application of other major theoretical treatment approaches such as biomechanical, neurodevelopmental, rehabilitation, psychodynamic or sensory integrative approaches. During evaluation and treatment, biofeedback is given to identify the effects of the occupational therapy activity on the individual. Patients have been monitored during group projects, home activities, social experiences, work projects and community outings. This feedback is used to teach the patient self-control, to change intervention strategies and to document progress.[1]

Difference in Approaches

Before proceeding, we pause to illustrate the difference between a feeling-oriented approach and a behavioral approach to understanding and treating psychosocial difficulties.

Psychodynamic Response to Depression

One can take as an example the common difficulty of sadness or depression. The psychodynamically oriented therapist might note that the individual who identifies himself or herself as depressed has poor self-esteem; that he or she feels helpless; that the individual has poor social relationships, lacks confidence in tasks, and feels that others do not approve of him or her; and that the person does not approve of himself or herself.

The feeling-oriented therapist might try to understand and help the person recognize when these feelings began and how they were experienced. The therapist might help the patient become aware of the ways in which significant relationships influenced personal feelings about self and others.

The therapist would provide a relationship in which the patient felt warmly and positively regarded, without condition, and he or she would try to understand the internal experiences of this patient. The therapist would want the patient to know that he or she could express sadness without reprisal, and the expression of sadness would frequently be encouraged, based on the belief that such expression was a pressing need and would result in therapeutic gain.

The therapist would try to make available experiences in which the person could try out a variety of new ways of relating, without fear of failure. The patient would be encouraged to understand and explore his or her own interests, beliefs and values, and to behave in a manner that was not only socially acceptable, but in which the person was consistent, "real," and in tune with his or her inner voice.

Behavioral Response to Depression

The behavioral therapist would not be primarily concerned with how the depression began historically, but might elicit history related to positive and negative reinforcers and environmental cues. Further, the therapist would identify behaviors that were associated with this depression: the inability to carry out everyday tasks; a reduction in social interaction; crying and fatigue; concerns expressed regarding health; self-deprecating statements; and changes in grooming, eating, sleeping, and other kinds of self-care.

The therapist would try to identify forces in the environment that tended to sustain the sad behaviors (e.g., attention from a concerned spouse or other patients). The therapist might note that the more depressed the patient became, the more his or her behavior(s) tended to reaffirm the negative feelings (e.g., the more the patient withdrew from social contact, the fewer positive interactions he or she had with others, thereby affirming the belief that "no one likes me"). The therapist would try to reverse this process. He or she would be concerned about encouraging expressions of sadness because the attention to sadness would be a positive reinforcement for an undesired behavior. Instead, the therapist would try to help the patient identify some activity that he or she enjoyed and that evoked positive personal feelings. Concurrently, the therapist would identify what in the environment reinforced positive behaviors. He or she would try to elicit from the patient a commitment to engage in a specified activity in which the patient could learn new skills that would ultimately bring success.

For example, the therapist might involve the person in a patient group in which he or she would be positively reinforced for assertive behaviors. Or, the therapist might try to engage the patient in an activity that he or she found pleasurable. To help ensure a successful outcome, the therapist would, when necessary, break the activity into discrete, achievable units in which success was discernible, and that would lead to accomplishment of the larger goal. When the patient's depression tended to cause him or her to withdraw or be minimally communicative, the therapist would attend to and reinforce any behavior, however slight, that represented a step toward appropriate involvement while simultaneously ensuring that withdrawal behavior was not reinforced. Achievement of treatment goals would be measured by the increase in patient participation, in the reduction of depressive behaviors, and in the increase in behaviors identified as pleasurable, socially acceptable, and behaviors indicative of increased competency.

Current Practice in Occupational Therapy

Person and Behavior

From 1940 through the 1960s, the deterministic view of behavior predominated. This view was "radical" because it viewed people as limited in the ability to actively choose and learn.[16] The early behaviorists, operating on Skinner's behavioral theory, believed that virtually all behavior was determined and, therefore, controlled by the introduction and maintenance of reinforcement.[50] Persons who controlled reinforcement were identified as those in charge, and the concept of free will was challenged. Since the late 1960s, the behavioral position has incorporated cognitive and social learning theories, which consider the individual to be both the product and producer of the environment.

Man's essence is neither good nor bad. Whether behavior is considered adaptive or maladaptive depends on the degree to which it conforms to societal norms.

Motivation

People are believed to be motivated by basic biological drives (e.g., the need for food, sex, and the avoidance of pain) as well as the secondary needs for love, approval, and other social needs. In this regard, motivation may relate to the drive to reach external rewards or to satisfy internal needs. Behavioral therapists do not deny the existence and importance of internal motivators, but because these motivators are intangible and unquantifiable, behaviorists identify them in terms of the behaviors that these internal drives elicit. For example, the need for self-satisfaction might be exhibited as diligence at a task.

Fear and anxiety are considered important learned motivators. Thoughts, words and memories are believed to become associated with and, therefore, to mediate between motive, stimulus and response and may act as cues, helping to define where, when and how behavior should occur. Thoughts and words may also become associated with and act as rewards or reinforcement.[18]

Function as Adaptation

The person is an active and choosing agent who interacts with and acts on his or her environment. The environment responds to the individual and selectively reinforces behavior. Those behaviors that are reinforced will most likely recur. As a result of environmental interaction and selective reinforcement, the individual becomes socialized and develops a repertoire of behaviors that are used for adaptation through work, activities of daily living and leisure.

All behavior may be broken down into observable, measurable actions or discrete skills. These discrete skills plus the larger behavior of which they are a part will be viewed as adaptive if they enable the individual to satisfy personal needs, live according to his or her values, achieve independence, achieve pleasure, and live in harmony with others in the society.

Dysfunction

An important influence of behavioral therapy has been to challenge the supposition that deviant behavior is illness. Deviant or maladaptive behaviors are considered the result of faulty learning or previous learning in which undesirable behavior has been intentionally or inadvertently reinforced.

Role of the Occupational Therapist

The behavioral frame of reference identifies the occupational therapist as a motivator, a re-

inforcing agent, a teacher, a social role model and a consultant. The therapist assumes one or more of these roles in the therapeutic learning environment, which is where he or she and the patient work in collaboration to identify and accomplish specific goals through identified learning experiences. Contrary to common belief, the occupational therapist is not an expert who assumes total responsibility and authority for treatment. Rather, the therapist recognizes the patient's ability to contribute to the therapeutic process and the benefits of the patients' assuming mutual responsibility for the treatment outcome.

Therapist as Motivator and Reinforcing Agent

Therapy may involve motivating the patient to try new behaviors that are anxiety-producing. Techniques for motivating include giving explanations to the patient about his or her condition, providing explanations and assurance regarding the function of activities, and offering support and affirmation that the patient can succeed.

Treatment teams including the occupational therapist frequently award privileges as a motivator for participation in therapy. The patient who refuses to participate in occupational therapy or other therapy programs in the therapeutic milieu may be refused passes home, free time away from the nursing unit, passes for community visits or time free of staff supervision.

Rapport between patient and therapist allows therapist attention and approval to serve as an effective reinforcement. The patient who might otherwise avoid participation in an occupational therapy activity may participate to gain this approval, or the patient who enjoys occupational therapy may be given extra time in the clinic as a reward for appropriate participation in other therapeutic activities. How and when this interdependent relationship is presented to the patient and how it is enforced determine whether motivation, reinforcement or punishment is occurring.

Therapist as Teacher

In the role of teacher, the occupational therapist provides new learning or relearning experiences.[38] When teaching new skills the therapist uses activities that help the patient learn to cook, apply for a job or use community resources. These skills are most frequently taught to the patient with a history of chronic problems who has had limited life experiences or to the younger patient who needs these experiences as a part of the process of normal development.

New Learning. The patient who has come through a trauma or one of life's natural changes that occur in the process of normal development may also need to learn new adaptive responses. For example, when children leave home or a spouse is lost through death or divorce, the patient must adjust to a new life-style. Part of this adjustment may be facilitated in occupational therapy through the process of learning to be more independent in home management, financial planning, and socialization, to name just a few areas. During treatment sessions, the occupational therapist targets skills needed for independence and does not focus on the feelings that the patient experiences due to the loss and changes that have occurred. It is assumed that if the patient's skill level improves, then his or her feelings will also change, even though feelings are not the primary focus.

Relearning. Another form of teaching occurs when relearning is required. For example, the patient may have the basic knowledge and skills, but for some reason is not using them to function independently. The patient knows how to cook, has had a job, and has gone to the store, library, or bank but has failed to do so for an extended time. Perhaps the patient has not had the opportunity to assume these responsibilities, is depressed, or needs support to gain the confidence needed for independent functioning in activities of daily living, work or leisure. The reasons that skills have not been exercised is not the concern. Eliciting and

reinforcing the desired skill or behavior is the aim of the treatment learning experience.

Corrective Learning. In the psychiatric learning setting, the occupational therapist may also provide corrective learning experiences through social skills groups in which the patient can acquire verbal and behavioral skills that will enhance his or her ability to function within the social network. For example, children who are abused by a parent often reenact these abusive behaviors with their own children when they become adults. The therapist may teach the patient to recognize internal signals that he or she is losing control and then educate the patient in alternative means of handling feelings, or the therapist may choose to build parent effectiveness by teaching the individual specific child-rearing skills.

Regardless of the learning focus, it is assumed that as a teacher the therapist has specific skills and expertise, which are shared with the patient during learning activities. These activities are chosen to reflect the patient's interests and goals and are selected for their ability to develop the skills needed for adaptation and independent functioning in the patient's natural environment.

Therapist as Role Model

As a social role model, the therapist exhibits behaviors from which the patient can learn. Here the learning process occurs as the patient identifies with and imitates the therapist.† The patient can learn verbal behavior as well as other specific skills, particularly social skills. This knowledge may occur quite naturally as the patient observes the therapist in a variety of interactions about the clinic. The identification process in interactions is also apparent as we see one patient teach another the activity process, imitating what the therapist does.

---

†When the behavioral model is applied in a medical setting or when reimbursement is sought from the government or an insurance carrier, it may be required that the patient be given a medical, psychiatric diagnosis[9].

Behavioral Rehearsal. The occupational therapist may use activities that incorporate role playing (also called **behavioral rehearsal**). During role plays, the therapist demonstrates desirable verbal and nonverbal behaviors, which can later be mimicked by the patient when he or she role plays a specific situation. Individual and group role play experiences are used to teach new behaviors or to provide support to patients in allowing them to explore multiple responses to problem situations.

Role Reversals. Role playing can involve practicing an expected social role, as well as learning more about the roles of others through role reversals. The authors recall situations in psychodrama sessions in which patients and staff were asked to reverse roles. The modeling and identification process was readily apparent. Both patients and staff benefited from the humor as well as the serious implications of the role play situation. These role plays frequently resulted in meaningful discussions between the two groups, eased the tensions in the patient unit and facilitated the resolution of ward problems. (These sessions were lead by a trained psychodramatist.)

Problem-solving Through Role Play. Role playing is frequently used in occupational therapy to practice skills such as applying for a job, asking for a date, saying "no" to a friend or spouse, or talking with parents about a concern. These scenarios allow the patient to experiment with introducing himself or herself to a potential employer or new acquaintance and to decide how he or she will respond to the situations encountered. For example, patients often worry, "What will I do if someone knows I've been in a psychiatric hospital? What should I say or do? Should I lie?" The occupational therapist can help the patient group experiment with different verbal and nonverbal behaviors and help patients become aware of their options and their likely consequences in addition to gaining confidence in the options chosen.

Therapist as Consultant

In the consultant role, the occupational therapist designs the behavior program that best responds to the patient's goals and problems and may train an aide to work cooperatively with the patient or with the family or staff to implement the intervention plan. The occupational therapist teaches methods of providing reinforcement and documenting behavior change.

Whatever his or her role, the occupational therapist is always aware that therapist interest, approval and disapproval have an important influence as reinforcers of behavior and that through reinforcement, he or she facilitates the learning of specific skills that lead to an adaptive or maladaptive response.

Function of Activities

Building Skills

The behavioral occupational therapist uses activities to teach situation specific skills, to provide simulated learning experiences, and to serve as a reinforcement. The therapist breaks down activities into their component parts and is aware of the level of challenge presented to the patient and skills required of the patient when completing each activity component. Activities are graded from simple to complex and used in evaluation and treatment. Activities are selected according to their interest to the patient and to the degree which they are consonant with sociocultural expectations. When operant conditioning is used, the activity must begin at the level of behavior that the patient is currently capable of emitting. When modeling and imitative behavior are incorporated, activities may be selected that begin with novel, not previously emittted, behavior.

Frequently during evaluation, the therapist observes the patient performing tasks in simulated experiences in the occupational therapy clinic or in the patient's natural (post-treatment) environment to determine the extent of adaptive and maladaptive behavior.

Treatment activities are the concrete specific tasks that the occupational therapist uses to develop specific skills for independence in activities of daily living, work and leisure. Activities are identified that are consistent with the interests and expectations of the adult patient. These activities are broken down into specific tasks and skill components, some of which may be called splinter skills.

Splinter Skills

A **splinter skill** is "a specific motor or mental skill that is performed only under specific circumstances and not integrated into a person's total behavior."[6,7] A splinter skill is nonstage specific and may be performed without the development of subskills or enabling skills, which are acquired in a chronological developmental sequence. Splinter skills are needed in the present situation; they may be lost if not practiced continually and usually are not generalized.[41]

For example, a child can memorize the alphabet song without understanding the concept and function of letters. He or she will forget the alphabet if the song isn't practiced frequently. Therefore, treatment activities often include teaching both situation-specific skills plus strategies that the patient can use in a variety of situations. For example, the patient preparing to live independently might be taught how to scramble an egg at home on a gas range. Additionally, if the person didn't already have the information, he or she would be taught safety procedures to be used with any gas oven.

Activities are graded, and specific tasks are presented to provide progressively more difficult learning challenges, which develop skills and strategies and shape adaptive behavior needed for the patient to fulfill his or her roles and responsibilities. Some skills will have to be practiced repeatedly to be maintained.

Activity Components

Activities can be broken down into almost endless behavioral components. A simplified example is provided here.

Meal planning and preparation require knowledge of nutrition and knowledge of and skills in budgeting, food purchase, meal preparation, serving and clean-up. These major components can then be further delineated and used to form behavioral objectives for the intervention program. Food purchasing can be broken down into the following skill components: 1) Make a shopping list that would include items from the major food groups and that would be sufficient in quantity to feed a given number of persons; 2) use public transportation to get to the supermarket; 3) use interpersonal skills that enable appropriate discourse in the community setting; and 4) use financial skills necessary for purchasing the food (e.g., making change).

End Product

Activities frequently used when applying this frame of reference include craft activities, task groups, prevocational or work experiences, relaxation experiences, assertiveness groups, social skills training, desensitization experiences and activities related to the use of token economies. The therapist uses activities to achieve an end, that is, to produce an end product and not to give primary attention to the activity process that occurs during the activity. The focus is on the outcome, as one asks, "Can the patient initiate a conversation? Can the patient cook a meal? Can the patient go to the bank and set up a new account? Did the group finish the task and accomplish its goal?" The focus is not on, "What does it feel like to be in this group? What did you learn about yourself from this experience?" These feelings and process concerns are the primary emphasis in the object relations frame of reference.

Activity as a Reinforcer

Activities can also reinforce behavior. For many, but not everyone, mastery of activities and one's environment becomes an internal reinforcer. Although not directing the discussion to how the patient feels about a task experience, the occupational therapist recognizes that successful task experience and the sense of accomplishment that comes from the task completion can be a source of reinforcement. He or she can further reinforce the patient's behavior by commenting on the quality of the end product and give strokes, saying, "I like your breadboard; you did a good job sanding and smoothing the surface" or "I know that you have worked hard to finish this project and carry through with your choice." The therapist may also ask the patient to confirm his or her accomplishment by asking the individual to identify the skills that were acquired during the activity process. The therapist might say, for example, "Tell me what you learned about yourself, about how to work with others, about how to approach a work problem."

Theoretical Assumptions

When applying the behavioral frame of reference in occupational therapy, the therapist bases evaluation and treatment on the following assumptions, which have been derived from behavioral theory and are summarized here.

1. Behavior is predictable, measurable and objective.
2. A person's verbalization and self-descriptions are behaviors.
3. The patient has a repertoire of behaviors, adaptive and maladaptive, that have been learned through selective reinforcement within the environment. The therapist is concerned both with extinguishing maladaptive behaviors and with establishing adaptive behavior.
4. The patient's repertoire of behavior determines the ability to function in activities of daily living, work and leisure.
5. Through positive and differential reinforcement and the systematic application of learning techniques, the patient can learn to modify and control his or her behavior.
6. Only behavior that is demonstrated can be reinforced.

7. New behavior may be established through the use of continuous or frequent and predictable reinforcement; however, the most stable behavior and the most difficult to extinguish is that maintained by intermittent reinforcement.
8. If maladaptive behavior is only occasionally reinforced, it is strengthened.
9. The strength of the patient's response is influenced by bodily conditions such as those related to emotions, drives and the use of drugs.
10. In occupational therapy the patient can learn new skills or refine present skills, or learn to manipulate the environment to problem solve and improve his or her functioning in the community.
11. The skills for adaptive functioning in the natural environment are independent and nonstage-specific.
12. In occupational therapy, the therapist seeks to increase the patient's ability to transfer (or generalize) the behaviors learned during treatment to a broad range of appropriate situations.
13. Clear, concrete goals increase the patient's understanding of the focus of treatment, which in turn expedites the treatment process and facilitates the evaluation of the treatment outcome.

Evaluation

The behavioral assessment elicits objective, measurable data that can be used to 1) identify problems and target behaviors to be extinguished and skills to be learned, 2) help identify viable intervention strategies and 3) act as a basis against which progress can be measured. It is recognized that skills are situation-specific.[2,44,51,58] For example, certain skills or repertoires of behavior are needed by a mother to care for her three year old at home in the playroom; different skills will be called for if the same child is being supervised on a train ride.

Because of this situation specificity and because there are practical limitations on what can be learned during treatment, the assessment must identify precisely characteristics of the environment in which the learned behavior is to be used, and the exact behaviors required for function in this setting. With this information, the therapist and patient together identify areas of concern, specific to the patient's expected environment.

Database Guide

In each area of concern, the therapist and patient will typically identify the following factors:

1. Existing behaviors that contribute to adaptive function;
2. Behaviors that interfere with adaptive function;
3. Behaviors necessary for adequate function in the patient's natural environment;
4. Frequency of specific adaptive and maladaptive behaviors;
5. Which stimuli are acting as cues;
6. Reinforcers for specific behaviors and where appropriate, who supplies reinforcement;
7. Sources of motivation for the patient's behavior;
8. Patient's ability to discriminate among stimuli and to generalize learning effectively.

From the preceding information, the occupational therapist often establishes a database, or baseline, sometimes depicted in a chart or graph, in which he or she notes the frequency and strength of specified responses during a limited time.

A characteristic of the behavioral evaluation is the specificity sought in designating the strength of behavior. For example, rather than making a general evaluative statement indicating that the patient "fails to ask for assistance in the clinic, as needed" or "tends not to clean up his work area," the therapist may indicate as part of the database that (the patient) "asked for assistance one time during a 50 minute session" and (the patient) "cleaned his work area one time during a five-session week."

Method of Assessment

The method of assessment is typically a combination of observation and rating of task performance along with an interview. Behavioral observation guides are often used in the assessment of task behavior and to structure the interview. Structuring is believed to help objectify the data gathered, increase the likelihood that necessary information is not overlooked, and help to minimize the impact of therapist-observer bias on the assessment process. This method contrasts with the traditional psychodynamic interview in which the patient responds to open-ended questions or is assessed using nonstructured media.

Behavioral therapists tend to emphasize that knowing what one wants to do or should do does not necessarily translate into the ability to take the desired action. Similarly, seeing where one has made a mistake in the past does not necessarily prevent one from repeating similar mistakes in the future.

The word **insight** is used when the behavioral therapist tries to increase the patient's recognition that a particular behavior has brought about a specific, predictable result.

When an interview is used, the behavioral interview is also different from the psychodynamic interview in that it is not designed to help the patient develop insight. It is not designed to establish a medical diagnosis,† nor is it designed to help the patient understand more about his or her feelings or past history. It does aim to elicit the required information about current targeted problems, and is concerned with history only to the extent that history influences current treatment.

---

‡Although observation in the patient's natural environment may seem ideal, it can also be problematic, such as when behaviors that the therapist had hoped to observe do not occur in the natural setting, or when there are unexpected interruptions in the normal routine[10].

Behavioral Database

One example of behavioral evaluation and goal setting was given by Kaye, Mackie and Hitzing[29] in their article, "Contingency Management in a Workshop Setting: Innovation in Occupational Therapy." In describing their work with eight male chronic patients, they noted that all of the patients exhibited minimal social skills, "bizarre motor and verbal behavior," "tardiness and inattention."[29] The patients participated for an hour each weekday in a workshop occupational therapy setting. During the baseline phase, the patients were observed for several weeks, and then a list of undesired behaviors (at least six per patient) was made up and restated in terms of a posi-tive behavioral objective. For example, the following behavioral goals were among those listed by the authors: "on time; cleaned up assigned work area; told the truth; stayed at the job with no pausing or pacing longer than . . . minutes per session; initiated relevant, appropriate conversation at least . . . times."[29]

The therapist tallied the six behavioral goals for each patient on a survey sheet. The authors included a sample behavioral survey sheet to illustrate the vehicle for weekly tallying (Table 4.1).

The progress of each patient was then made visible by means of a graph (Figure 4.1). This process concluded the establishing of behavior baselines. Baseline data surveys and

TABLE 4.1
TYPICAL BEHAVIORAL OBJECTIVES SURVEY SHEET
OBTAINED DURING BASELINE

NAME Joe Smith   **WEEK OF 5/19-23/69**

BEHAVIOR	M	T	W	TH	F	WEEKLY TOTAL
1. On time: Present before 10:03			X	X	X	3
2. Stayed at job with no pausing or pacing longer than 5 minutes per session		X			X	2
3. Cleaned up assigned area(s)		X		X		2
4. Well-groomed; Shaven, hair combed, clothes properly secured	X		X	X		3
5. Initiated relevant, appropriate conversation 2 times			X			1
6. Smiled (at least 3 times)	X				X	2
TOTALS	2	2	3	3	3	13

Kaye J, Mackie V, Hitzing EW Contingency Management in a Workshop Setting . . . Innovating in Occupational Therapy. AJOT 24(6):415, 1970. Reproduced with permission.

graphs were then displayed prominantly, and the therapist spoke to each patient about the goals of treatment and the responsibility of each for filling out his or her own behavior objectives survey, for being able to verbalize personal behavioral goals from memory, and to cite criteria for appropriate behavior. Reinforcement revolved around the accumulation of token points, as well as social reinforcements such as smiles and pats on the back.

Behavioral Self-Inventory

This example describes an adapted behavior evaluation format that incorporates the use of a behavioral check list and an interview.

During the evaluation interview, the patient is asked to complete a self-inventory. The one from which this excerpt was taken had 50 self-statements. The patient, a 21-year-old woman, came to the interview somewhat carelessly dressed, appeared overweight, and had facial acne. She was asked to rate her perform-

ance as described by each of the 50 statements. The patient assessed her performance by checking one of the following: always (A), frequently (F), sometimes (S), or never (N). The patient was also asked to indicate if she was satisfied with her performance or if she wished to change her behavior. The statements related to the patient's behavior in interpersonal, self-care, task, community and communication activities. The responses on the form were then discussed by the patient and the therapist to target behaviors for change, set treatment goals and discuss the resources that were available for learning experiences in occupational therapy.

It would not be unusual for patients to rate themselves low on may areas of such a checklist and to desire to make multiple changes. This experience can be a huge blow to patients' self-esteem as well as an overwhelming experience. Therefore, the occupational therapist should use questionnaires judiciously and

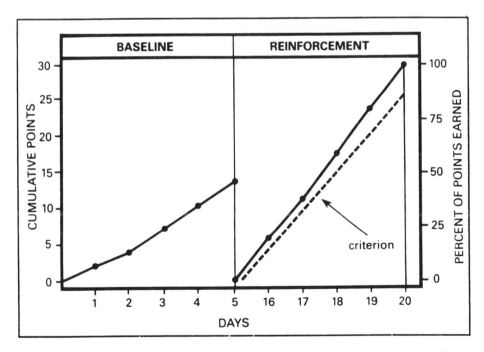

FIGURE 4.1.   Cumulative graph points earned by Patient D during last week of base line and third week of reinforcement. Kaye J, Mackie V, Hetzing EW Contingency Management in a Workshop Setting . . . Innovation in Occupational Therapy *AJOT* 24(6):415, 1970. Reproduced with permission.

help patients organize the information in a manner that helps patients to identify desired changes as well as their own strengths (adaptive behaviors), to establish priorities for the desired changes, and to identify sources that will culminate in a successful learning experience that will enhance the patients' sense of accomplishment.

Discussion of Patient Questionnaire

The following excerpt is taken from the patient-therapist dialogue that took place after the completion of the inventory. The reader will see the contrast between this dialogue and the one in Chapter 3, even when there are similarities in the patients' concerns regarding physical appearance.

OTR: "On your list you have indicated that you'd like to change your appearance and your clothes and improve your physical coordination and skin condition."

Patient: "I'm heavy and clumsy . . . I'd like new clothes . . . I need new makeup."

OTR: "I can't buy you new clothes or makeup, but in occupational therapy I can help you to improve your physical coordination so you're less clumsy, and I can help you plan a weight reduction program. You also can experiment with skin care and make up and clothing selection in occupational therapy." (Pause) "Where would you like to begin?"

Patient: "I can't decide."

OTR: "Let's talk about the first statement that you made about yourself, and I will help you begin. You first mentioned that you're 'heavy.' Are you interested in working toward a weight loss while you're in the hospital?"

Patient: "I've tried. It's hard."

OTR: "Yes, it's difficult . . . and I think we have some supports here that can help you. We could look at both your eating habits and your level of physical activity. Have you spoken to your doctor about your weight concerns? He can order special weight reduction meals for you."

Patient: "No. I don't like many foods. I thrive on junk food."

OTR: "If you decide that you want to work toward losing weight, you will need to speak

---

Table 4.2
EXCERPT FROM COMPLETED QUESTIONNAIRE

Behavioral Statement	Rating*	Satisfaction
I am satisfied with my physical self (Body weight and shape, muscle strength).	N	Want to Change
I can find clothes that fit well and that are attractive and comfortable.	S	Want to Change
I am satisfied with my general appearance (Hair style, skin condition, etc).	S	Want to Change
I am satisfied with my physical coordination (e.g., the way I walk, my ability to use my hands).	S	Want to Change

*N = Never, S = Seldom.

to your doctor when you see him. Perhaps, too, you'll have to work on changing your eating habits."

Patient: "I love the snacks here in the hospital, and my parents always bring me my favorite treat when they come to visit."

OTR: "Do you think that you could ask them not to bring food when they come to visit? You might find it useful to give them a suggestion of something else you'd like since visitors frequently express concern and care for you through a gift."

Patient: "I'll ask for my makeup!"

OTR: "To help you avoid the snacks here in the hospital we could write a contract. A **contract** is a written statement of your goals, such as, 'I want to lose five pounds.' Then you write down how you intend to reach your goal, and what your reward will be for doing it. You might contract to limit your in-between snacks to one or two a day, and reward yourself at the end of the week."

Patient: "I'm not in the mood to write today. I'm tired."

OTR: "I think that we have done enough for today and it is almost time to stop. Tomorrow in occupational therapy we will talk more about your specific goals and work on your contract for occupational therapy."

During this interview the therapist summarized one area of the questionnaire, and worked with the patient to identify specific problems and establish priorities for desired changes rather than pursue the patient's feelings about herself. Although the patient was not ready to complete her contract, the therapist established that there would be an emphasis on action.

Simulated Experiences

Assessment may also occur in the context of simulated experiences in the hospital or occupational therapy setting. Simulated experi-

ences, also called **analogues**, are situations designed by the therapist to replicate the patient's natural environment. Although it may seem ideal to evaluate the patient in the everyday environment, it may be difficult due to the limits imposed by short hospitalizations and lack of funds for home visits. For some information the therapist will more than likely depend on verbal reports from family members or significant others with whom the patient lives. In some hospitals, the living unit or ward is structured as much as possible to simulate an extended family home environment. Therefore, the occupational therapist can gain evaluation data from the informal interaction that occurs between patients and staff, as well as from observation of the patient's room (e.g., organization, neatness) and daily routines that display daily living skills.

Another simulated experience that occurs in occupational therapy evaluation or treatment is in the area of financial management. Financial management includes the ability to make money transactions in the community; make banking transactions; pay one's bills; plan a budget; and identify and use community and personal sources of income. To determine the ability to make banking transactions, the therapists uses bank deposit and withdrawal forms for savings and checking accounts to determine if the patient is capable of managing banking responsibilities that are a part of personal financial management. To complete these forms, the patient also needs to be able to read, write and make mathematical computations.

Situation Specificity

Because much behavior is situation-specific, the therapist does not assume that the patient functioning well in a simulated experience is guaranteed to do equally well when in his or her everyday environment. For example, anxieties might arise in the everyday world that do not arise in the simulated, clinic experience. Nevertheless, simulated experiences are designed in accordance with the principle that although every situation or setting contains a slightly different set of stimuli and cues and calls for a slightly different response, learning is most likely to be generalized when the patient can recognize the similarities between given settings.

Assessment Instruments

The occupational therapy literature identifies the following assessments as behavioral assessments: The Kohlman Evaluation of Living Skills (KELS), The Comprehensive Occupational Therapy Evaluation (COTE), The Bay Area Functional Performance Evaluation (BaFPE), and the Scorable Self-Care Evaluation (SSCE). These evaluations are summarized here. Details and specific protocol are available from the identified sources.

Kohlman Evaluation of Living Skills (KELS). The KELS was developed in an acute psychiatric setting. Interview and tasks are used to determine the patient's ability to function in everyday living situations. Administered in 30 to 45 minutes, this battery identifies 17 living skills that are categorized under the broad headings of self-care, safety and health, money management, transportation and telephone, work, and leisure. Forms and problem-solving tasks are used to identify skills within these broad categories (e.g., reading and writing ability, self-care and appearance, knowledge of danger, use of the telephone, money management, work and leisure interests and abilities). The test manual is available from the American Occupational Therapy Association, Products Division.

Comprehensive Occupational Therapy Evaluation (COTE). The COTE was developed in an acute psychiatric setting to identify behaviors relevant to occupational therapy, to improve communication with staff and to improve the system of data formation and retrieval. It identifies 25 behaviors that can be seen in occupational therapy. They are organized under three major categories: general behavior, interpersonal behavior and task behavior. The behaviors are rated on a 0 to 4 scale. A format

for evaluation and reporting is provided. The assessment is described in detail by Brayman and Kirby.[10,24]

Bay Area Functional Performance Evaluation (BaFPE). The BaFPE has two subtests: the Task Oriented Assessment (TOA) and the Social Interaction Scale (SIS). The TOA consists of five, time-limited tasks that are both structured and nonstructured: sorting shells, completing a money and marketing task, drawing a house floor plan, duplicating a block design and drawing a person. The therapist then rates 9 functional behaviors: 1) the ability to paraphrase instructions, 2) productive decision-making, 3) organization of time and materials, 4) mastery and self-esteem, 5) frustration tolerance, 6) attention span, 7) ability to abstract, 8) verbal or behavioral evidence of thought or mood disorder, and 9) ability to follow instructions leading to correct task completion.

The SIS is a behavior rating scale, not a behavior check list, that depends on the observation of the patient in five specified situations and includes an optional self-report. Developed by Bloomer and Williams,[8] it is used to assess seven categories of social interaction: 1) response to authority figures, 2) verbal communication, 3) psychomotor behavior, 4) dependency vs. independency, 5) socially appropriate behavior, 6) ability to work with peers, and 7) participation in group activities. The test manual and materials are available from Consulting Psychologists Press.

Scorable Self Care Evaluation. A standardized self-care evaluation instrument designed by Nelson Clark and Mary Peters,[14] the evaluation is used to identify baseline performance in basic living skills (personal care, housekeeping, work and leisure, and financial management). The authors provide subtasks for each of the basic living skill areas, a format for administering subtasks, a format for scoring performance during subtasks, reliability studies and standard scores to assist in the interpretation of patient scores and forms for communicating evaluation and progress data. *The*

Scorable Self Care Evaluation is available from SLACK Inc.

Treatment

Treatment Goals

An important contribution of the behavioral frame of reference comes from the guidelines it has established for writing treatment goals. Owing to the desire to establish efficacy of treatment and the requirements of third-party payers, most clinicians have been influenced by the behavioral goal-setting system. In general, goals must be observable and measurable.

Originally, the behavioral occupational therapist identified problems, determined the goals for treatment and designed the intervention plan; this continues to be the role when the patient is believed to be incapable of contributing to the process. More often, however, the patient actively participates in the decision-making process and works cooperatively with the therapist to target the patient's problems and to determine the specific changes that need to occur.

Defining Target Problems. The targeted problems must be defined in observable terms and as measurable outcomes and be individualized for the specific patient. Multiple resources are available to aid the therapist in the goal-setting process.[31] This process is summarized as follows.

After the completion of the evaluation, the therapist and the patient identify the changes that need to occur to improve the patient's functioning within his or her expected environment. These changes may be stated in terms of the patient's feelings, desires, interests, or concerns and are usually general statements.

Next the therapist takes the patient's general statements and works to identify the specific behaviors that would indicate that the patient had learned a new skill or otherwise addressed the changes desired. These behav-ioral statements, which are derived from an analysis of the tasks that relate to the patient's broad concerns, must be understood by the patient and agreed upon as subskills of behaviors to be learned or modified and as indicators that change has occurred.

General Statements Become Observable Goals. After targeting behaviors, observable goals are established. The therapist and patient establish behavioral expectations within a framework that may identify the context, time and place of behavior and the significant persons involved in or affected by the behavior.

Having identified the observable behavioral goal, the patient and therapist then discuss the frequency of behaviors expected and the criteria that indicate success or failure to accomplish the goal. In this way, the observable behaviors become measurable goals.

The Goal-Setting Process. The goal-setting process is exemplified as follows: Let us take a frequent situation that occurs in psychiatric settings with the patient having chronic problems and frequent outbursts of disruptive behavior. A young man's family decides that they can no longer cope with the problematic, childlike adult and inform the patient that he may not return home. The patient's problem and concern are, "Where am I going to live? How am I going to care for myself?" As the patient and therapist discuss the concern, the following issues and adaptive behaviors emerge as issues that need to be addressed. These are described in Figure 4.2.

In the process of determining treatment goals, the patient and therapist will often identify behaviors that are not adaptive and that interfere with goal attainment. Typically, the therapist will take note of these maladaptive behaviors and attempt to remove reinforcement for them. Unless the therapist and the staff have complete control of the patient's environment, eliminating such reinforcement is difficult and at times impossible.

Positive Statements. Goals are most often written in terms of what will be attained, and not what will be eliminated. For example, the "problematic childlike" behavior in our example might include excess time spent by the patient brooding in isolation in his room. Steps taken toward exploring community resources and gaining employment represent adaptive behaviors opposite to brooding and isolative behaviors, and these positive actions can serve as treatment goals.

Patient Priorities.   Usually multiple issues, problems, and behavioral goals are present, as can be easily seen in the previous example.

Concern

Where am I going to live?

Issues

What is important to me about where I live?

How will I pay for the setting (apartment, boarding home, house)?

What are my alternatives and choices?

What supports are available (financial, interpersonal)?

Necessary Skills

Identify alternatives by scanning the classified advertisements and contacting community agencies.

Clarify values and identify personal needs.

Speak to personal and community resources regarding financial support.

Behavioral Goal Statements

Patient will identify two possible settings in which he could live.

Patient will speak to his parents regarding possible financial support.

Patient will participate in values clarification group and identify what type of setting he wants to live in, whom he wishes to live with, and what kind of support group or social network he desires.

Patient will gain employment capable of meeting financial responsibilities.

FIGURE 4.2.   Goal-setting process.

Therefore, the therapist helps the patient to set priorities for treatment in order to set realistic expectations and to avoid overwhelming the patient. Whenever possible the patient will choose where he or she wishes to begin. This process also is indicative of the humanistic influence in behaviorally based occupational therapy.

As treatment progresses, the measurable statements are reviewed frequently to determine progress. Measurable goals and the review process allow the patient to clearly see his or her progress and enable the staff to evaluate the success and limitations of the intervention plan.

Patient Contract.   Sometimes the treatment goals and intervention strategies are written in the form of a contract. A **contract** is a verbal or written agreement between patient and therapist that defines the roles of each during treatment, the behavioral goals, reinforcements and their schedules, the treatment procedures and other related negotiations. If written contracts are signed by both the therapist and patient, the contracts are time-limited and at agreed intervals are reviewed, renegotiated or terminated.

Problem-Oriented Record

Along with the behavioral movement; the increased support for specific, observable, and measurable treatment goals; and the growing interest in data processing came the need for specific formats of documentation. One of these formats was the **problem-oriented record** as described by Weed.[59] This format was not initially designed for occupational therapy or psychiatry. It was first used in general medicine settings, but has influenced documentation in many medical and occupational therapy treatment programs.

Components of the Problem-Oriented Record.   The problem-oriented record has four major components. The **database** includes demographics; medical and social history; medical, laboratory, and psychological test results and related clinical reports; and a statement of the patient's chief complaint. The **subjective data** includes the views expressed by the patient and his or her family. The **objective data** includes staff observations and laboratory reports. Finally, the **problem list** includes past and present psychiatric and medical problems identified from the information in the other three components of the problem-oriented record.

Progress Note Format. For each problem listed by number and title, a diagnostic and a treatment plan are listed. Progress notes are then keyed to a particular numbered problem and are written according to the "SOAP" format. "SOAP" is an acronym for the following: "S," the patient's subjective response to treatment and patient observations; "O," objective data from laboratory studies, diagnostic reports, and treatment; "A," the assessment and analysis of the subjective and objective data; and "P," the diagnostic, therapeutic and patient education plan.[59]

The influence of the problem-oriented record system and its adaptations is evident in the records and documentation in many mental health settings. The problem-oriented record is reflected in goal-oriented treatment in which there is a problem list, specific goals (long- and short-term) and treatment strategies for each problem on the list.

We are also familiar with a system that uses a "NAP" note. NAP is an acronym that stands for "N," a narrative that combines the subjective and objective data; "A," the assessment that identifies the problems and states how they were determined; and "P," the plan, with the goals and intervention strategies that are used to resolve and identify problems.

Treatment Process

Behaviorally based occupational therapy is concerned with building skills that contribute to adaptive function while eliminating those that interfere. The straightforward nature of this statement should not suggest that behavioral treatment is simple or necessarily similar across various treatment programs. Although behavioral therapists hold in common the concern for observable measurable behavior, the techniques used to modify and build specific behaviors vary. We wish to dispel the notion that merely acknowledging a patient's success in occupational therapy (as through smiles or privileges), ignoring maladaptive behaviors, and writing measurable treatment goals suffice as behavioral treatment. The complexity of the human being is such that identifying and isolating the literally thousands of stimulus-response-reinforcement associations that comprise one individual's learning is virtually impossible, at least in the practical sense. The behavioral therapist must be very diligent in the application of behavioral techniques if he or she is to avoid being surprised by the outcome of a treatment experience that failed to take into account the complex interrelationship of stimuli, responses and reinforcements in even the most circumscribed learning setting.

Mapping Out a Plan. The therapist endeavors to collect objective data, and with the patient's cooperation, takes charge of the learning milieu. Together they accomplish the following:

1. Identify and establish priorities for learning needs;
2. State learning needs as specific, observable behaviors;
3. Determine what learning techniques will be used (operant conditioning, modeling, building response chains);
4. Specify one or more individual or group treatment experiences in which learning is likely to occur. An **optimum learning experience** is characterized as follows: a) The learning experience is compatible with the patient's age, interests, values, societal expectations and the expected duration of treatment; b) there will be an opportunity for the desired behavior to be demonstrated (or modeled, shaped, chained); c) there is, when needed, an opportunity for trial and

error problem-solving and sufficient opportunity for repetition of adaptive responses (practice); d) the therapist and designated others can ensure that positive reinforcement be given, per schedule, for adaptive responses, and reinforcement is held in response to maladaptive behavior; e) there is opportunity within the experience to move from continuous or frequent external reinforcement to more everyday (intermittent, patient maintained) kinds of reinforcement; f) the patient can recognize the similarities between the behavior in the therapeutic environment and its enactment in the natural environment (the therapist may amplify salient features of both the therapeutic and natural environment to make these similarities clearer); and g) the patient can perceive the differences between demonstrating the learned behavior in appropriate versus inappropriate settings (the therapist may help the patient identify these differences);

5. Specify criteria for periodic reassessment of treatment.

Behavioral Interaction

Regardless of the activity or techniques used, throughout the treatment process the occupational therapist informs the patient what is expected of him or her, and the goal of each learning experience. The therapist uses a vocabulary and manner of explaining that are understandable to the patient to accomplish this goal. For example, the therapist may state to the patient, "I would like you to work on this leather key case so that you can learn to follow the written instructions. I will be available for assistance if you need help; but I want you to try this on your own first, so that you can become more accustomed to working independently."

Behavior-Consequence Relationship. The therapist uses dialogue with the patient to assist the individual to recognize the relationship of his or her behavior to the consequences that result. The therapist does not attempt to deny or overlook the patient's thoughts and feelings, but she responds to them in terms of the

behavior that ensues. Rather than telling a patient that he or she looks sad, angry, or depressed, for example, the therapist may say, "The way you're throwing that clay around looks angry," or, "You've spent most of the hour sitting by yourself, and it appears that you feel discouraged."

Constructive Feedback. Information that is given back to the patient about his or her behavior is referred to as **feedback**. When relating to the patient, the therapist tries to give positive feedback as well as to makes sure to specify expected behaviors. During a community outing, the therapist may begin by saying, "Please stay with the group when we leave the van and walk to the entrance of the YMCA. Enter the lobby, be seated and wait for the Y program director to join us," rather than just saying "Don't stray from the group."

To cite another example, when a patient in a therapeutic cooking group is using a knife carelessly, the therapist will not only say, "Be careful." He or she will say, "Be careful; your hand is too far down on the knife blade. Here, let me show you." Then, the therapist proceeds to demonstrate the correct procedure. Even when giving criticism, the therapist avoids using blanket remarks that suggest something is bad, wrong, or ugly. Rather, he or she demonstrates how to use a tool or do a process correctly, suggests how a process might be improved, or identifies what characteristics of a task or project have been completed successfully, and which may need work.

The therapist also uses dialogue to help the patient generalize this learning to the natural environment. The occupational therapist encourages the patient to assume responsibility for personal behavior and strives to build a sense of self-control.

Three Behavioral Occupational Therapy Groups

We have selected three examples of behavioral group learning experiences that we feel are representative of the current application of behavioral theory in occupational therapy. Although not all behavioral occupational therapy occurs in a group context, it frequently does occur in adult care; therefore, each of the group experiences discussed here represents or is a composite of behavioral groups that we have observed or that have been part of the fieldwork experience of students we have supervised.

In behavioral group treatment, the therapist must structure the group and learning environment to ensure that specific target behaviors for each group member are facilitated and reinforced. The therapist has the same gatekeeping functions described in the previous chapters. Additionally, he or she must see to it that there is a means to monitor specific behaviors and to supply (or withhold) reinforcement. At times this technique requires having other staff or aides present, all of whom coordinate their efforts.

Group I—Prevocational Activity Group.
One type of behavioral group is typified by the prevocational activity group in which each participant works on an individual project, but the patients have in common a need to learn general task skills that will enable each to ultimately succeed at a job after discharge.

For example, in an in-hospital clinic in a Veterans Administration psychiatric wing, all of the patients are working in the wood shop, which has available both hand and power tools. The number of group members varies from six to eight, and represents a stable group, with an occasional new admission or discharge changing group membership. The group meets twice a day during the week for 90 minute sessions.

The general work behaviors that the therapist tries to promote include the following:

1. The ability to initiate productive work;
2. The ability to pursue a task to completion;
3. The ability to work well alone;
4. The ability to cooperate with others;
5. Social skills related to sharing space and materials;

6. The ability to make timely decisions based on available data;
7. The ability to anticipate consequences;
8. The acquisiton of habits related to punctuality, safety and cleanliness;
9. The ability to identify and use available resources.

> Specialized job task skills are taught by the occupational therapist teacher in vocational rehabilitation centers, sheltered workshops or in simulated work experiences (such as assembly line work) that can occur in an occupational therapy setting. Occupational therapists have been known to contract with local agencies for simple jobs that patients could complete in a short time or to assume responsibility for jobs inside the hospital. Sample jobs include assembling cardboard boxes, packing machine or electronic parts in a container, collating printed materials, stuffing envelopes, folding linen and sorting tasks.

Before coming into the group, each patient has met individually with the therapist and developed a written contract that describes the project, the behaviors that will be learned, the reinforcement and its criteria, and criteria for reassessing goals. The therapist shares with the other staff a copy or the contents of the agreement.

The clinic environment is designed to maximize opportunity for all patients in the group to achieve their personal goals. Such an activity group can accommodate a diversity of individual treatment goals. In some instances, the clinic is structured to encourage sharing and social behavior (e.g., by limiting materials and tools available for use). In other instances, when many of the patients in the group are highly distractable and have difficulty attending to tasks, the work area is structured to minimize socialization.

To maximize the transfer or generalization

of learning, the therapist structures the work setting to closely approximate key aspects of the setting in which the patients will work after therapy. Toward this end, the therapist has included a point system as part of the reinforcement, and each patient in this group has been assigned his or her own work area. Points are given for completing designated steps on the projects, for cleaning work areas at the conclusion of the session, and for promptness. Points are deducted for specified misuse of tools. Socialization is encouraged during a designated coffee break during each work session.

The occupational therapist and often auxiliary staff are primarily responsible for providing reinforcement. The occupational therapist, staff and each patient are involved in determining whether target behaviors have been achieved. In this activity group, the therapist is primarily an observer and not a participant.

Group II—Resocialization Group.   The process of treatment in the resocialization group may begin in much the same way as that of the prevocational activity group. Each patient may meet individually with the therapist to target initial behavioral goals. Or the patients may have been placed in a group to be observed, with significant behaviors targeted and baselined by the therapist. Then, each patient and the therapist mutually set treatment goals. In this case, several patients with similar social learning needs are placed in a resocialization group.

For example, at a local mental health facility, outpatients are periodically selected into FAC (Friday Afternoon Club).

On Wednesday of each week, all group members and the occupational therapist meet. The group typically but not necessarily consists of five to eight younger unmarried adults. Members come and go from the club as their treatment stay dictates. Therefore, the group must constantly respond to changes in its membership. All the patients in the group are unable to initiate or sustain social conversation, lack familiarity with community resources,

have little confidence (especially in situations involving the opposite sex), exhibit poor grooming and dressing habits, and exhibit poor habits as with regard to keeping appointments or arriving on time for appointments.

At the Wednesday meeting, each patient reports to the entire group on his or her progress toward weekly goal achievement. Many weekly goals involve specific social behaviors that each patient is to exhibit while at home. For example, one participant may have agreed to check out a book from the local library, to call a designated friend on the phone, or to obtain a brochure describing extension classes at the community college.

As an additional function of the Wednesday meeting, the group plans a Friday social outing at which the therapist is to be a participant-observer. Arrangements are made to meet at a specified locale (restaurant, skating rink, bowling alley) on Friday afternoon. Each patient is to select one short-term goal for the Friday engagement (e.g., to be on time, to order dinner independently, or to initiate a conversation with a group member or nongroup member). Further, one or two short-term goals to be accomplished at home during the next week are verbalized by each patient and recorded by the therapist.

At the social outing, therapy talk is kept at a minimum. This outing is intended to simulate as much as possible a natural social event. While a participant, the therapist models appropriate social behavior and helps stimulate casual conversation. Group members and the therapist provide reinforcement in the natural sense, responding to the social overtures made by various patients. However, the stringent kind of provision for reward, as might occur in a prevocational activity group, is not present in this group. Because patients have a large responsibility for reinforcing each other, the success of this group depends, in part, on the ability of patients to respond to each other positively.

Once again, the therapist, who is often emulated, plays a key role through modeling in helping the patient group attend to the positive behavior of its members. The therapist notes significant behaviors during the social outing that need to be addressed by the group at the next Wednesday meeting and is responsible for communicating with the other treatment staff on the status of individual patients regarding goal attainment.

Group III—Assertiveness Training Group.
A third type of behavioral group is typified by an assertiveness training group.† As in the FAC group, patients are selected into the group according to similar needs and similar targeted behavioral goals. Patients who might benefit from such a group include those who cannot ask for what they need, those who cannot say "no," those who feel that they are pushed around or taken advantage of by others, those who are overly apologetic in their dealing with others, and those who feel guilty when they are angry.

An assertiveness training group is structured as follows:

1. All patients begin the group at the same time. The group is planned to last a given number of sessions (e.g., two times per week, one to one and one-half hours per session, for four weeks).
2. At the first meeting, the therapist describes the function and purpose of the group, the expectations of each group member and the therapist role. Each patient is asked to describe briefly in writing five social situations in which he or she feels unable to make his or her needs known. Patients are then asked to order these needs from least to most difficult.
3. The therapist collects all the data provided by each patient, becoming aware of the common features in which patients experience difficulty. Although the situations and the order of difficulty will vary for each pa-

tient, the therapist can establish a working hierarchy of situations that can be simulated and role-played in each meeting. The kind of situations frequently simulated, in a hierarchical order, include dealing with a stranger who pushes ahead of you in a grocery line, asking for a refund at a store, saying "no" when asked to be on a committee, saying "no" to a sexual advance, and asking for a raise. While these situations are quite general, the therapist has the option of individualizing role-plays.

4. In each subsequent group meeting, the therapist constructs one or more situations for practice in role-playing. The therapist may start the session by giving didactic information about what constitutes appropriate assertiveness, the difference between assertiveness and aggressiveness, and so on.

   In some instances, the group may proceed to a brief muscle relaxation exercise. The therapist then describes the first hypothetical situation. For example, "You've been waiting for five minutes at the checkout line at your grocery store. Suddenly, you find a newcomer has squeezed his way ahead of you. Everyone in line with you appears to notice, but no one has chosen to say anything. How might you handle this situation?"
5. Patients take turns playing a variety of roles in the simulations so that they may be both the giver and the recipient of appropriate assertive responses. The therapist may ask for volunteers, but attempts to ensure that all patients have opportunities to try out new behaviors. When appropriate, the therapist might interrupt the process to model an effective assertive response; he or she may coach and encourage as needed. Group members learn not only by their active participation but by the observation of others. In this kind of group, modeling, as conceived by Bandura, plays a significant learning function.
6. After simulations are complete, verbal feedback is exchanged among participants about the effectiveness of others' responses.

---

[5]An assertiveness group is also identified with the cognitive-behavioral framework. Depending on the therapeutic approach of the occupational therapist and the needs of patients in the group, the therapist may give more emphasis to changing patients' thoughts about themselves, as well as increasing assertive behavior[11].

Although feelings may be expressed, they are not the focus of the interaction. The therapist, through enthusiastic praise, reinforces the effective playing out of assertive behaviors. The therapist helps patients to identify other situations that would be quite similar to the one just role-played to facilitate the generalization of learning. The principle of desensitization has an important function, as patients have a chance to try new behaviors in a setting that is typically less anxiety-producing than those outside of treatment. Further, each patient is given the opportunity to build on past learning, as each week he or she encounters increasingly problematic situations in role playing.

7. As the group meeting nears its completion, each patient targets one specific assertive behavior that he or she will endeavor to accomplish before the next meeting. Time is set aside at the end of every subsequent meeting for members to relate in brief whether they attained their weekly goal. The therapist records changes in individual goals and progress made toward their attainment.

Summary

Behavioral therapy is the application of a collection of techniques that have been found empirically to affect behavior. As Franks[20] notes, while individual therapists select from these behavioral techniques to create their own "brand" of behavioral therapy, all behavior therapies are "predicated upon the common, explicit, systematic, and a priori usage of learning principles to achieve well-defined and predetermined goals."[20] Although behavioral therapy acknowledges biological, cultural, cognitive, and emotional influences, it is not primarily concerned with them.

Learning Principles

One can look at the behavioral approach historically and see it in part as a response to the medical, analytical approach to psychosocial problems that preceded it in the 1940s and 1950s. This stance was seen by many as too vague, aloof, and even mystical in its reliance on such metaphorical constructs as id and ego, and tending in practice to promote a concept of mental illness. The behavioral approach offered an alternative explanation for maladaption that pointed to the less menacing and seemingly more manageable problem of faulty learning. Practitioners who continued to struggle with readmitted patients in the field of acute psychiatry and had little to offer the chronically psychiatrically disabled other than medication now had some specific tools that seemed to offer the opportunity for real behavior change. Occupational therapists followed with other health practitioners, leaving the analytical approach and addressing topics such as behavior change, behavioral goal setting, reinforcement and problem-oriented documentation. As tends to occur when any new treatment approach is embraced, however, behaviorism was embraced nonselectively for some time, which led to some inevitable disenchantment. Finally, the behavior approach was viewed more realistically with perspective on its strengths and limitations.

Internal Motivation Versus External Reward

Many practitioners and lay persons have reacted strongly to the implicit suggestions (made explicit by Skinner) that in the application of behavioral principles, the person(s) dispensing reinforcement is ultimately controlling human behavior. Occupational therapists—believing in the importance of internal motivation, striving to allow their patients and clients maximum choice, and seeing the holistic relationship of attitude to the healing process—were left to consider the possibility that freedom of choice was an illusion, and that healing could be reduced to specifiable biochemical units. Those believing in the value of human pleasure in discovery and competence found themselves unable to address these concerns except perhaps tangentially in reference to external reward.

Although not addressed in the literature, it was evident in much of the occupational therapy practice of the 1960s and early 1970s that therapists working in behavioral settings used behavioral rhetoric but continued to function with the same values, purposes and general direction as before. More recently, occupational therapists have spoken out against the dogma of a strongly Skinnerian behaviorism and are including principles of humanism and cognitive, social and developmental theory in their study, dialogue, practice and research. This approach has resulted in an eclectic behaviorism, as once again we confront the probability that no one explanation for the human condition best describes it.

Contributions and Limitations of the Behavioral Frame of Reference

Contributions

Behavior therapists have selected and followed through with behavior change that can be studied and verified objectively. The behavioral approach to psychotherapy and specifically in occupational therapy can be credited for increasing the scrutiny given to treatment goals and the efficacy of treatment alternatives. Many therapists who thought, perhaps intuitively, that their treatment approach was helpful have been forced to look carefully and reevaluate their treatment outcomes systematically. Further, many patients who have sought psychiatric or emotional aid have been given a concrete way to measure their own progress.

Behavioral therapists have been accused of taking too much control of patient behavior. One might counter that, in discarding the use of psychiatric jargon and labels that tended to overpower the average lay person and probably obfuscated much of what was actually occurring in treatment, the behavioral approach gave back to the patient the ability to make understandable choices about his or her own treatment.

Behavioral techniques appear to work with patients with specific problems in daily functioning and can be used successfully for skill building. The improvement of grooming, appropriate speech, work skills, and social skills have all been addressed repeatedly in the literature. These skills have been especially significant in the treatment of patients who have required long-term, habitual or institutional care. Thus, behavioral therapy has been credited for humanizing the conditions of many persons whose lives have been otherwise devoid of success or joy.

The thrust of traditional behaviorism can be credited for spotlighting the importance of attention and approval as reinforcement, and for the significant role of modeling in the learning process. Behaviorism has acted as a springboard for those investigators who have since sought to understand better the probable intervening process of cognitive structuring and the heretofore undeveloped understanding of social learning.

Limitations

The behavioral approach does not appear to work as well when there is a lack of specific deviant behavior. For example, if a young man is doing well in school and fulfilling his societal obligations, yet expresses the sentiment, "What is life all about?" the behavioral approach has to strain to address the issue, and may, many feel, address it only tangentially. Actually, the therapist can address even these so-called high functioning issues behaviorially, but it is worth noting that the occupational therapy literature does not document treatment with higher functioning individuals or groups.

The behavioral approach appears to work best in a closed or self-contained environment, and gains made in the closed system do not necessarily translate to long-term gains at home. In a closed therapy system, as in an institution, patients are more likely to be influenced by treatment staff injunctions and reinforcements. Further, there is more likelihood that reinforcement will be judiciously given, modeling carefully provided, and progress nurtured. Although any behavioral therapist acknowledges that internal motivation and self-reward must at some point take over if a patient is to make a successful transition to an unsystemized community, this intervening step frequently does not occur. In the everyday world, our fellow human beings may again reward our aberrant behavior or fail to notice our accomplishments, and many behaviors will revert to pretreatment levels. The occupational therapy literature provides evidence of success within a highly structured setting, but has less to point to in terms of carryover to nontreatment environments or to cases of behavioral therapy in which the patient was receiving intermittent outpatient therapy.

Designing and implementing an effective behavioral program for one or many patients are not necessarily as simple as they might appear. Whereas targeting inappropriate behaviors may not be difficult, isolating these behaviors and rewarding only the appropriate responses can be difficult, especially when many patients are working together at one time. Identifying suitable rewards can also be difficult. If all patients desired candy and cigarettes along with hugs and smiles, there would be no dilemma. For many depressed and regressed individuals, however, the secondary, and at times unclear, gains that they receive from maintaining their regressed behavior seem to be more rewarding than anything staff have to offer. The therapist finds himself or herself offering time alone as a reinforcement to a patient whose goal is to spend less time alone, or food to an adolescent with eating problems whose goal is to spend less time involved with food. Further, it is difficult to achieve the kind of generalization desired, while not promoting undesirable response generalization. For example, a specific therapist might elicit increased verbalization from a patient, but this social gain may not be generalized to other staff or to significant others who await the patient's return to home.

Finally, the behavioral position that com-

plex behaviors can be broken down into smaller, discrete units may be true; but in practice the effort to do so can become unwieldy. To define the exact circumstances under which a problem such as depression or diffuse anxiety occurs, one tends to respond to the most superficial issues—the tip of the iceberg. To do otherwise requires the kind of lengthy, extensive therapy that behaviorism has sought to replace.

Traditional behaviorism has not addressed many variables. It has spoken little, for example, to the role of internal motivation in human behavior—the motivation to excel where simple competence might have otherwise sufficed, the motivation to practice until perfect, the pleasure of activity for activity sake. In failing to do so, traditional behavioral concepts seem self-limiting. The role of curiosity (e.g., the pleasure of a child in discovery, and the joy of learning to speak a first word) is not the concern of behaviorists, yet it seems so integral to our understanding of purpose when as occupational therapists we use the term "purposeful activity."

The traditional behaviorist also does not address the issue of cognitive structuring as an intervening variable in learning and in problem-solving. With much of the early impetus coming from those who studied the function of language,[12,13] scientists and practitioners have increasingly felt that such cognitive processing is necessarily conceived and is a separate and meaningful activity in itself.

One might see many of the oppositions to behavioral thinking as philosophical. Behaviorism is a reductionist approach to understanding the human being. If we describe all the pieces–all the exhibited behaviors exhibited–have we really described the person? Or, are behaviors the external display of a far more complex internal process that cannot be as easily discerned? Does behaviorism trivialize the human condition, or is it an honest, practical approach to complex problems? With these questions in mind, we turn to the cognitive behaviorists and others who are concerned with the role of cognitive structuring in learning and in treatment.

Recommended Reading List

Ayllon T, Azrin N: *The Token Economy: A Motivational System for Therapy and Rehabilitation*. New York, Appleton-Century-Crofts, 1968.

Ellsworth P, Coleman A: The application of operant conditioning principles to work group experience. *Am J Occup Ther* 24(6):495–501, 1969.

Duncombe LW, Howe MC, Schwartzberg SL: *Case Simulations in Psychosocial Occupational Therapy*. Ed 2. Philadelphia, F.A. Davis Company, 1988.

Wolpe J: *Psychotherapy by Reciprocal Inhibition*. Stanford, CA, Stanford University Press, 1958.

References

1. Abildness A: *Biofeedback Strategies*. Rockville, MD, The American Occupational Therapy Association, Inc., 1982, p. 8.
2. Anthony WA: *The Principles of Psychiatric Rehabilitation*. Amherst, MA, Human Resource Development Press, 1979.
3. Bandura A: *Social Learning and Personality Development*. New York, Holt, Rinehart and Winston, 1963.
4. Bandura A: *Psychological Modeling: Conflicting Theories*. New York, Adine-Atherton, 1971.
5. Bandura A: *Social Learning Theory*. New York, General Learning Press, 1971.
6. Banus B (Ed): *The Developmental Therapist*. Ed 2. Thorofare, NJ, Slack, Inc., 1979, p. 260.
7. Becker M, Banus B: Sensory-perceptual dysfunction and its management. In Banus B: *The Developmental Therapist*. Thorofare, NJ: SLACK Inc., 1979, pp. 239–273.
8. Bloomer J, Williams S: *Bay Area Functional Performance Evaluation (BaFPE): Task Oriented Assessment and Social Interaction Scale Manual*. San Francisco, CA, USCF, 1986.
9. Boronow J: Rehabilitation of a chronic schizophrenic patient in a long term private inpatient setting. *Occup Ther Mental Health* 6(2):1–20, 1986.
10. Brayman S, Kirby T: The Comprehensive occupational therapy evaluation. In Hemphill B (Ed): *The Evaluative Process in Psychiatric Occupational Therapy*. Thorofare: NJ: SLACK Inc., 1982.
11. Burgess P, Mitchelmore S, Giles G: Behavioral treatment of attention deficits in mentally impaired subjects. *Am J Occup Ther* 41(8):505–509, 1987.
12. Chomsky N: Review of Skinner's "Verbal Behavior." In Jakobovits L, Miron M (Eds): *Readings in the Philosophy of Language*. Englewood Cliffs, NJ, Prentice-Hall, 1967.
13. Chomsky N: *Language and Mind* (Enlarged Edition). New York, Harcourt Brace Jovanovich, 1972.
14. Clark E, Peters M: *Scorable Self Care Evaluation*. Thorofare, NJ, SLACK Inc., 1984.
15. Cormier W, Cormier S: *Interviewing Strategies for Helpers*. Belmont, CA, Wadsworth, Inc., 1979, p. 430.
16. Corey G: *Theory and Practice of Counseling and Psychotherapy*. Monterey, CA, Brooks/Cole Publishing Co., 1982, pp. 135, 119.
17. Diasio K: Psychiatric occupational therapy: Search for a conceptual framework in the light of psychoanalytic ego psychology and learning theory. *Am J Occup Ther* 22(5):400–414, 1968.
18. Dollard J, Miller N: Reinforcement theory and psychoanalytic therapy. In Patterson CH: *Theories of Counseling and Psychotherapy*. New York, Harper and Row, 1973, pp. 89–124.
19. Fine S: Working the system: A perspective for managing change. *Am J Occup Ther* 42(7):417–419, 1988.
20. Franks CM: Introduction: Behavior therapy and its Pavlovian origins: Review and perspectives. In Franks CM (Ed): *Behavior Therapy: An Appraisal and Status*. New York, McGraw-Hill Book Company, 1969, p. 22.
21. Geiser R: *Behavior Modification and the Managed Society*. Boston, Beacon Press, 1976, p. 42.
22. Giles GM: A behavioral approach to the treatment of the severely brain injured adult. *Occup Ther Forum* 2(5): February 4, 1987, p. 3.
23. Gorman P: Mental retardation and mental illness- Behavioral approaches. *Occup Ther Forum* 6(5): February 4, 1991.
24. Hemphill B: *The Evaluation Process in Psychiatric Occupational Therapy*. Thorofare, NJ, SLACK Inc., 1982.
25. Hilgard E, Bower G: *Theories of Learning*. Ed 3. Englewood Cliffs, NJ, Prentice-Hall, Inc., 1974.
26. Hilgard E, Bower G: *Theories of Learning*. Ed 4. Englewood Cliffs, NJ, Prentice-Hall, Inc., 1975, pp. 601–605, 136.
27. Jodrell R, Sanson-Fisher R: Basic concepts of behavior therapy: An experiment involving disturbed adolescent girls. *Am J Occup Ther* 29(18):620–624, 1975.
28. Kanfer FH, Phillips J: *Learning Foundations of Behavior Therapy*. New York, Wiley, 1970.
29. Kaye J, Mackie V, Hitzing E: Contingency management in a workshop setting: Innovation in occupational therapy. *Am J Occup Ther* 24(6):413–417, 1970.
30. King LJ: A sensory integrative approach to schizophrenia. *Am J Occup Ther* 28(9):329–336, 1974.
31. Mager R: *Preparing Instructional Objectives*. Palo Alto, CA, Fearon Publishers Inc., 1962.
32. Mann W, Sobsey R: Feeding program for the insti-

tutionalized mentally retarded. *Am J Occup Ther* 229(8):471–474, 1975.

33. Martin GL: *Behavior Modification*. Englewood Cliffs, NJ, Prentice-Hall, 1978, pp. 22, 58–59, 173.

34. Martin M: Behavior modification in the mental hospital: Assumptions and criticisms. *Hosp Community Psychiatry* 28:292, 1972.

35. Mischel W: Toward a cognitive social learning reconceptualization of personality. *Psychol Rev* 80:252–283, 1973.

36. Mischel W: *Personality and Assessment*. New York, Wiley, 1968.

37. Mosey AC: *Three Frames of Reference in Mental Health*. Thorofare, NJ: SLACK Inc., 1970.

38. Mosey AC: *Activities Therapy*. New York, Raven Press, 1973.

39. Mosey AC: *Components of Psychosocial Occupational Therapy*. New York, Raven Press, 1986.

40. Norman C: Behavior modification: A perspective. *Am J Occup Ther* 30(8):491–497, 1976.

41. Nuse-Clark P, Allen A (Eds): *Occupational Therapy for Children*. St. Louis, Mosby-Year Book, 1985, p. 271.

42. Ogburn K, Fast D, Tiffany D: The effects of reinforcing working behavior. *Am J Occup Ther* 26(1):32–35, 1972.

43. Overbaugh T, Bradley B, Bucher M: Use of operant conditioning to improve behavior of a severely deteriorated psychotic. *Am J Occup Ther* 24(6):423–427, 1970.

44. Palmer F: Present context of service delivery. In Robertson S (Ed): *Mental Health Focus: Skills for Assessment and Treatment* Rockville, MD, American Occupational Therapy Association, 1988, pp. 1.28–1.36.

45. Rotter JB: *Social Learning and Clinical Psychology*. Englewood Cliffs, NJ, Prentice-Hall, 1954.

46. Sieg K: Applying the behavioral model to the occupational therapy model. *Am J Occup Ther* 35(4):243–248, 1981.

47. Skinner BF: *The Behavior of Organisms: An Experimental Analysis*. Englewood Cliffs, NJ, Prentice-Hall, 1938.

48. Skinner BF: *Science and Human Behavior*. New York, MacMillan, 1953.

49. Skinner BF: *The Technology of Teaching*. Englewood Cliffs, NJ, Prentice-Hall, 1968.

50. Skinner BF: *Beyond Freedom and Dignity*. New York, Knopf, 1971.

51. Spiegler M, Agigian H: *The Community Training Center: An Educational Behavioral Social Systems Model for Rehabilitating Psychiatric Patients*. New York, Brunner/Mazel, 1977.

52. Stein F: A current review of the behavioral frame of reference and its application to occupational therapy. *Occup Ther Mental Health* 2(4): 35–62, 1982.

53. Stein F, Nikolic S: Teaching stress management techniques to a schizophrenic patient. *Am J Occup Ther* 43(3): 162–169, 1989.

54. Stein F, Tallant B: Applying the group process to psychiatric occupational therapy. *Occup Ther Mental Health* 8(3):9–28, 1988.

55. Trombley C, Scott A: *Occupational Therapy for Physical Dysfunction*. Baltimore, Williams & Wilkins, 1984.

56. Wanderer Z: Therapy as learning: Behavior therapy. *Am J Occup Ther* 28(4):207–208, 1974.

57. Watts F: Modification of the employment handicaps of psychiatric patients by behavioral methods. *Am J Occup Ther* 30(8): 487–490, 1976.

58. Watts F, Bennett D: Introduction: The concepts of rehabilitation. In Watts F, Bennett D (Eds): *Theory and Practice of Psychiatric Rehabilitation*. New York, John Wiley and Sons, 1983, pp. 3–14.

59. Weed L: *Medical Records, Medical Education and Patient Care*. Cleveland, OH, Case Western Reserve University Press, 1969.

Chapter 5

LIFE SPAN DEVELOPMENT FRAME OF REFERENCE

Focus Questions

1. What differentiates the life span frame of reference from previous developmental frameworks applied in occupational therapy?
2. In what life stage are you? Cite two developmental tasks of this stage.
3. What transitional stage are you approaching?
4. In what ways might goal setting in this framework combine behavioral and developmental tenets? How might this create a theoretical and practical dilemma for the therapist?
5. In what way does life development intervention empower the individual?
6. What are the limitations within the research and theory base cited in support of life span development?

Introduction

Originally, a developmental approach in occupational therapy connoted treatment with adults who had either regressed or had never mastered skills that are normally attained in childhood. This focus continues in many instances of cognitive disabilities and movement-centered treatment. As information grows in the area of life span development, it is recognized that stage-specific periods in adulthood can be expected to create rough spots that the adult must negotiate. Neither regression nor illness is implied, although adults who have been marginally adaptive throughout their lives might be expected to have particular difficulty with life stage changes.

This revised edition reflects a more exclusive life span development emphasis. Developmental treatment specific to cognitive dys-function and movement-centered approaches are addressed in chapters 9 and 10.

In looking at the entire life span developmentally, one is given an excellent basis for conceptualizing not only the changing role that activities serve as the individual matures, but also for appreciating the ever-changing strengths and limitations that need to be considered in relation to skill building.

Such a life span developmental approach suggests beyond the everyday events that may seem fragmented, an underlying order, or evolution in the development of personhood. Working within a life span developmental understanding allows the patient and therapist to cope not only with the patient's presenting or immediate demands for change, but also to anticipate and prepare for expected changes.

Consistent with this text's focus on the adult, this chapter summarizes pertinent work in the area of adult development, relates this work to treatment and proposes avenues for further study.

Definition

The life span development frame of reference is a biopsychosocial framework for occupational therapy assessment and intervention. Adult development is conceived as following a predictable, sequential pattern of age-related stages or phases. These phases are shaped by and respond to physical maturation, cognitive maturation, psychosocial and intrapersonal needs as well as environmental expectations, resources and barriers. Within the context of biological, psychosocial and cognitive development theories, age appropriate life tasks and enabling adaptive skills and behaviors are identified. These behaviors, skills and tasks are stage-specific and interdependent and occur sequentially during the life cycle.

During assessment, the occupational therapist identifies behaviors, skills, and specific accomplishments that permit normal development and promote well-being as well as identifies skills that are lacking and circumstances in the environment that create barriers antagonistic to development. Through the use of purposeful activities, occupational therapy promotes integrated learning and personal competence in sensorimotor-integrated functioning, academic skills, self-care and daily living activities, social interaction, leisure activities, and work performance. Through skill development the patient gains personal competence and confidence to meet life's challenges and master life's tasks.

Theoretical Development

The occupational therapy literature in development weighs heavily at each end of the life span continuum, both in pediatric and gerontology speciality areas. There are theoretical and applied discussions of occupational therapy evaluation and treatment and research with some infant, childhood, adolescent, and elderly populations and fewer that emphasize adult psychosocial development and life span development concepts. Some of the contributors to occupational therapy developmental theory include Gilfoyle and Grady,[24] Llorens,[41,42] Cutler Lewis,[15] Ayres, Mosey,[44,45] Moore, Fiorentino,[23] Hasselkus, and Rogers. In general, the literature proposes physical or holistic approaches in which multimodalities are used as purposeful activities to facilitate normal development, treat or prevent disease and disability, respond to developmental delay, minimize chronic disability, improve physical psychosocial function, promote adaptation, and maintain quality of life.

Developmental treatment models may focus on the acquisition of skills in one particular area, for example, in the acquisition of sensorimotor skills, or may be concerned with skill development across all life skill areas. This chapter addresses the multidimensional development of skills throughout the adult life span.

In mental health, Mosey's adult developmental framework, Lloren's developmental approach, and Fidler's life-style performance framework are frequently referenced in the occupational therapy literature.[21,42,44,45]

Defining Terms

To place theory into a meaningful framework, this chapter organizes theory according to the following format. First, development will be discussed in terms of the adult's life stages. **Life stages** are consecutive time spans in the individual's life that provide an overarching structure for understanding development. Each life stage has a unique flavor or character, as fashioned by both the internal priorities of the individual as well as societal expectations. Integral to life stages are developmental tasks and marker events.

Developmental tasks are the "physiological, psychological and social demands a person must satisfy in order to be judged by others and judge himself or herself to be a reasonably happy and successful person."[14,53] These tasks include such major accomplishments as establishing a marriage relationship, beginning a career, and formulating guiding religious or political philosophies. Developmental tasks have an open-ended quality in that they often evolve to other tasks or need to be reworked in subsequent life stages.

Marker events are more circumscribed in time and are pivotal events within life stages. Such events include marriage; the death of a parent, spouse, child, or close friend; or graduation from college.

Finally, we address what we refer to as **enabling skills**. These are the specific physical, cognitive, psychosocial and spiritual learned behaviors that enable everyday activity and serve as a basis for the accomplishment of the more encompassing developmental tasks. We have selected the term *enabling* to indicate that these skills make it possible for the individual to meet his or her developmental needs. These skills are also seen as adaptive in that they allow the individual to respond to change.

Enabling skills include, for example, the ability to read and write, the ability to speak comfortably in front of peers, the ability to drive a car or find one's way about town. Enabling skills also include broader, less well-differentiated skills, such as some of those identified by Fidler[21] (e.g., coping with ambiguity, differentiating self from others and sublimating drives). Obviously, some enabling skills and their components may be relatively easy to identify, for example, the ability to read and write, whereas other skills, such as those related to the integration of self-esteem, may be much more open to interpretation and consist of virtually an endless number of component skills. Skill building and the assessment of skill level have been the primary goal of occupational therapy in developmentally oriented practice models. The fields of psychology and social psychology provide a conceptual picture of the life span and the developmental tasks to which enabling skills contribute.

Theories of Life Span Development

Life Stages

Data Collection

The psychology literature has contributed significantly to life span developmental theory. Of these, the more frequently referenced in occupational therapy literature are Erikson, Freud, Jung, Gesell, Havinghurst, Neugarten, Bruner and Buhler.

Farrell and Rosenburg[20] summarized the process by which adult developmental theories have most often been formulated. Typically, the theory starts with a descriptive study of adults. In this study, which may be cross-sectional or longitudinal, adults are observed and interviewed extensively. They are asked to give a phenomenological account of themselves, their life history, and their goals. Spouses and significant others may also be interviewed; and pertinent data regarding occupation, health, social affiliation, and so on are obtained. The researcher then compiles the data and looks for discernible patterns or clusters that can be verified through other similar studies.

Many of the theories discussed here are based on the conclusions of a researcher or clinician who has studied rather limited populations. Levinson,[38] for example, studied 40 men. Jung[33–35] based his conclusions on the observation of his clients plus his interviews with some individuals from other cultures. Buhler's work is based on the biographical case study of 200 elderly Viennese in 1930.[8] Erikson's conclusions are based on the observation of his own patients plus the retrospective study of several well-known, accomplished individuals.[17–19] Other recent studies, including those of Gould[26,27] and Vaillant[56,57], involved less than 300 people. Despite this limitation, the reader will discern enough similarity across theories as to be convinced, we believe, of their essential viability. We begin by looking at the seminal work of Jung on life stages and then discuss the more recent study of Levinson.

Jung

Jung made a significant departure from Freud in his conceptualization of adult life span development. Freud believed that primary development ended with adolescence, and he viewed adult behavior as a repetition of patterns established during childhood and as living-out of beliefs gained through early experiencing. Jung envisioned a life span structure in which adults continued to develop, reassess goals, give up old values and embrace new, make new commitments and develop parts of the self that had been undeveloped.[12]

Jung identified four primary stages of life: 1) childhood, 2) young adulthood, 3) middle age and 4) old-age. He was cognizant of the extrinsic or social parameters of each stage and was interested in social institutions such as religion as well as the internal or intrapsychic activity throughout development. Jung's stages are reviewed here because his work made a clear and significant impact on more recent research in adult development.

Childhood.   (birth to puberty). During this stage, the individual is typically protected by and lives within his or her parents' world. The child's sense of "I-ness" is shaped by the beliefs, values and psychic atmosphere created by parents.

A transition to the next stage begins in adolescence. The adolescent has an increased sense of self as separate and independent from parents. He or she must give up childish behaviors and fantasies, must test out new decisions, and must be able to envision the self as separate from parents. The individual achieves this transition partly by questioning the givens of their world and by reassessing these precepts from a personal perspective.

Young Adulthood. (puberty to 35 to 40 years). As adolescence concludes and the individual embarks into the world, he or she must adapt to social demands. The person will

select and pursue a suitable career, marry, and often establish a stable family. The young adult continues to redefine the relationship to one's parents, although he or she will never be entirely separate from them. Adaptation is primarily to outer or environmental demands, as the individual tries to gain status and be recognized as accomplished by his or her peers.

Young adulthood ends at midlife. The individual has adapted, more or less, to societal expectations, but finds himself or herself beginning to question personal accomplishments and values. The individual asks, "What have I done with my life? Has it really been worthwhile?" Even where accomplishments and youthful strivings have been attained, mere revelling in success is not enough. The individual feels the need to take stock and consider where his or her life is going.

Middle Age.   This stage begins somewhere around the age of 40 and with it begins what Jung called the second half or afternoon of life. During this phase the individual begins to know the self more deeply and to respond to inner callings rather than societal expectations. Jung had special interest in this stage.

As discussed earlier with object relations theory, Jung conceived of the self as comprised of polarities. These polarities included a tendency to relate to the world in a fashion either viewed as **extraverted** (interested in others and the environment) or **introverted** (tending toward contemplation and introspection); the existence of both a masculine and a feminine side in all individuals; and a tendency to evaluate information either through rational (logical; discernible means) or nonrational (intuitive) means. Whatever polarity is favored in the individual's outward behavior and conscious thinking, the opposite polar function is latent in the self.

During the second half of life, these unexpressed parts of the self are believed to emerge and develop. For example, a man who tended to act quickly and relate superficially to others during the first half of his life, might in the second half become more thoughtful and introspective. Likewise, a man who was very masculine during the first half of life (**masculine** as used by Jung was in the traditional sense of strong or aggressive) might in the second half of life allow his more **feminine** (sensitive, intuitive, creative, vulnerable, nurturing) side to emerge. This man might develop a wish to be emotionally closer to his wife and children or may develop a desire to garden or to create through the arts. For women, the opposite process will occur. The nurturing, vulnerable woman will allow herself to exert more direct control and authority and will feel more comfortable with taking more responsibility outside of the home.

Although it was not believed that one preference or polarity would be totally replaced by its opposite in the second half of life, the task of midlife and beyond was to allow these latent potentialities to be given some expression. Two processes needed to occur. Each part of the self needed to be given expression through the process Jung called **individuation**; then all parts, all polarities, needed to be united into a unified whole through the process Jung called **integration**.

Another important need in the second half of life was to respond to what Jung called spiritual values. The individual becomes more concerned with philosophy and belief systems and less concerned with materialistic comforts or accomplishments related to physical prowess. Along with individuation and integration, the response to spiritual values helps move the individual toward the ultimate development of selfhood Jung called **transcendence.†** Whereas the individual in the first half of life might be especially concerned with his or her own accomplishments and, for those in the

work place, climbing the ladder of success, he or she might in the second half of life use his or her knowledge to teach or enhance the accomplishments of those younger. This person has more leeway because he or she is established in a career or because children are older; however, the need to respond in a new way comes from an inner urge. A failure to respond to these issues and engage in reappraisal renders the individual increasingly narrow and ultimately unfulfilled as increasing age brings more demands for change.

Toward the end of this stage, as the person moves toward very old age, he or she must face bodily decline. The person leaves the formal work setting, if he or she has not already done so, and generally moves from positions of authority, both in the larger society and within the family. The individual must seriously confront the inevitability of his or her own death, which is reflected in the death of many associates.

Old Age. Old age for Jung was extreme old age. No exact years are given. The individual is typically infirm and is often taken care of by others. He or she actively contemplates his or her own death as well as the prospect of life after death. Jung saw the belief in a hereafter as **archetypical**, or innately present in all persons; and considered the continuation of life through the soul as a reasonable possibility.

A Jungian influence is seen in the work of Levinson[38] and Sheehy,[55] and is compatible with the findings of Erikson,[17–19] Neugarten,[46–50] Buhler,[8–11] Havighurst,[29] Gould,[26–28] and other well-respected developmentalists.

Levinson

Daniel Levinson and his associates at Yale expanded on Jung's thinking and furthered his stages. Levinson's work was based on an in-depth study of 40 adult men and gives special emphasis to the early and middle adult years or late teens to late 40s, a period that Levinson believes has historically been handled vaguely by those in the human sciences.[38]

---

†An example of this movement toward transcendence is found in the story of *Siddhartha*, by Herman Hesse,[31] which abounds with Jungian metaphors and allegory, as do all of Hesse's novels. The reader interested in gaining a feel for Jungian philosophy and symbolism in an enjoyable way is encouraged to read Hesse's works. It should be noted that Hesse and Jung were contemporaries in Europe, and Hesse was at one time in psychoanalysis with Jung.

Levinson states that in shaping his life the male must constantly make choices in the area of occupation, family, friendships, leisure and belief systems. The individual must commit to his choices and ultimately exclude from his attention that which he has not chosen. These choices will mutually determine and be determined by the roles each individual assumes, his unique manner of relating within these roles, and activities specific to role fulfillment.

Stage Cycles. Levinson found that the life structure is an alternating sequence of stable and transitional stages. During a **stable stage**, believed to last from five to seven years, the individual commits himself to the developmental tasks of that stage (Table 5.1). These developmental tasks include accomplishing externally oriented goals (e.g., building a career and establishing one's niche in society, as well as grappling with internal reappraisals and developing intrapsychic polarities, such as those conceived by Jung). As a part of task accomplishment, the individual assumes social and occupational roles specific to each stable stage. He may, for example take the role of novice or apprentice in early adulthood, and be the authority or elder statesman in middle adulthood. Having accomplished the developmental tasks of a given stable stage, or having reached an age where task expectations change regardless of what has been previously accomplished, the individual moves into a transitional stage (usually lasting three to five years) during which life is reviewed.

During a **transitional stage**, decisions are made to discard elements of the former stage no longer experienced as meaningful, to retain those elements still viable, and to move on to the tasks and roles of the next, stable stage. During a transitional stage one is, according to Levinson, "suspended between past and future."[38]

Seasons of the Life Cycle. Levinson found little variability in terms of the ages in which periods begin and end, and he found that the stages occurred in a fixed sequence. It is not, however, that one stage is better or higher than those preceding. Levinson suggests the metaphor of the four seasons: spring, summer, fall, winter. None is intrinsically better than another, but each is essential to the unfolding life cycle.[38]

Midlife. Levinson discusses at length the midlife transition, occurring around ages 40 to 45. Like Jung, he see it as an especially significant time during which internal polarities must be reworked. Levinson identifies opposing inner forces within the individual pertaining to 1) **destruction-creation**, 2) **feminine-masculine**, 3) **attachment-separation** and 4) **young-old**. Levinson describes the midlife as pivotal in terms of the individual's need to confront his own loss of youth and to deal with the recognition that he is not going to live forever. In confronting his own mortality, the individual experiences more urgently the need to give expression to all aspects or potentialities of his being.

Common to all transitional periods are feelings of inner conflict. Often, grief ensues as sadness is felt at what must be given up, and anxiety is experienced regarding the uncertainty of the future. Some preoccupation with death is common in all transitional stages because the process of termination and reengagement is evocative of death and rebirth.[38] For the transition to end successfully, the individual must make new, critical choices. Once choices are made and commitment given them, the next stable stage ensues. However, Levinson emphasizes that certain issues (e.g., separation-attachment or finding a place among peers) will continue to emerge and need to be readdressed throughout the life span.

Mentor Relationship. A concept introduced by Levinson in relation to the male experience and now in popular use for men and women is that of the **mentor**. The mentor relationship is seen as an important, complex relationship during young adulthood. Most often viewed in relationship to the work setting, the mentor is usually several years older than the younger individual, although not old

TABLE 5.1   LEVINSON'S LIFE STAGE AND DEVELOPMENT TASKS

	Ages	Stage	Key Tasks
E A R L Y A D U L T H O O D	17	Early Adult Transition	Question pre-adult world, imagine self as member of adult world; Give up adolescent behaviors; make some preliminary choices for adult life; change nature of relationship to parents; gain more training; learn more about oneself.
	22	Entering The Adult World	Establish own home base; make and try out choices related to occupation, love-relationship, and peer friendships; find a balance between creating a stable life structure and keeping a sense of adventure. Begin to form a "dream"; begin to establish mentor relationship.
	28	Age Thirty Transition	Take steps to modify areas not satisfactory. Find out what is "missing" and either take new steps or strengthen commitments. Continue to develop one's dream; establish mentor relationship.
	33	Settling Down	Invest self in major components; work, family, community activities; settle for a few key choices; work at "making a niche" and climbing the ladder of success; develop a firm sense of authority; change mentor-relationship; feel more self-assured and independent while being tuned into the needs of others.
	40	Mid-Life Transition	Reappraise life structure; redefine goals, values; deal with polarities within self (midlife individuation); polarities related to (1) young/old, (2) destruction/creation, (3) masculine/feminine, and (4) attachment/separation; Accept own mortality. Become mentor to another.
M I D D L E A D U L T H O O D	45	Entering Middle Adulthood	Commit self to new choices.
	50	Age 50 Transition	Modify life structure; can continue to work further on tasks of midlife transition.
	55	Culmination of Middle Adulthood	Build a second middle adult structure. Prepare to face a new era where physical decline and loss of status must be squarely met.
L A T E A D U L T H O O D	60	Late Adult Transition	Deal with physical decline; give up (or prepare to give up) formal authority; firm up values that maintain integrity.
	65	Late Adulthood	Give up formal authority and status; form a broader life perspective; be less concerned with external rewards; contribute wisdom as elder in a supporting role; rely on inner resources. Face prospect of death.

This information is summarized from Levinson, D. *Seasons of a Man's Life*, New York, Alfred A. Knopf, 1978.

enough to be a parent. He or she acts informally as a teacher or sponsor, helping the individual to enhance skills and abilities and acquainting him or her with the customs and values of the occupational and social world. Frequently, through his or her own accomplishments, the mentor may inspire and serve as an example for the younger individual to emulate.[38] Although one tends to hear of the mentor in relation to higher status occupations, Levinson found this relationship evident across social and economic boundaries. Recent research with minority groups suggests that the mentor relationship may occur in the family as evidenced by the relationship between the young adult and respected family elders.[54]

Transitional Stress. Although Levinson's work is not about therapy, it is evident in the histories of those he interviewed that transitional stages are especially likely to cause the individual to experience stress and to prompt the person to contact others for some assistance with transition. Further, failure to work through or accomplish the tasks of any stage may prevent successful task resolution during subsequent stages and unresolved problems may continue to emerge and plague the person. (Because Levinson's work has been cited in relation to the life span development of both men and women, we will use examples for both men and women in subsequent discussion of Levinson's constructs; however, we recognize that this kind of generalization represents a weakness within the adult life span model.)

As an example of the reemergence of unresolved developmental tasks, we cite the young man or woman who is conflicted about his or her sexuality during the late teens and behaves in a manner that is especially inhibited or conversely, promiscuous. If this individual marries in his or her midtwenties without having integrated a satisfying sexual self-image, he or she may experience difficulties with both the sexual and emotional intimacy necessary for a fulfilling marriage. As the family unit expands to include children, concerns about sexual adequacy or attractiveness may exacerbate, and commitment to the marriage relationship may dwindle. This same person, at the age of 45 to 50 years, if still unresolved regarding the sexual self, may display rigid or exaggerated same-sex behaviors (as in the macho man or sweet, defenseless woman) at a time when his or her peers are comfortable with expanding beyond sexually stereotypical behavior.

The therapist cognizant of a life stage conceptualization such as Jung's or Levinson's perceives an underlying order in the events of the patient's life and can assess the individual's strengths, limitations, and needs from a much broader perspective than the immediate demands of a given stress. Restoring comfort and order are not necessarily regarded as a therapeutic goal, as the need for reevaluation and new commitment brings inevitable turmoil. This perspective on treatment will be discussed later in the chapter.

Developmental Tasks

As defined, **developmental tasks** are the major social, vocational, avocational, philosophical and psychological accomplishments necessary for a person to relate in the world satisfactorily. These tasks are understood within the framework of age-related life stages and include changes within social, occupational, and avocational roles, or adjustments in the style of relating within a role. If developmental tasks are achieved, the individual tends to feel pleased and subsequent developmental tasks are more likely to be accomplished. If they are not accomplished, then he or she tends to feel like a failure, societal disapproval ensues, and there is more likelihood of difficulty with future tasks.

As Levinson suggests, implicit in the idea of any task is the concept that it may be carried out well or poorly. Although some tasks are easily evaluated, developmental tasks usually require the distance of time to be adequately assessed.[38] For example, it is relatively easy to identify if one has gained the necessary formal training prerequisite to enter a profession; it is far more difficult to determine whether one has gained in self-knowledge. (Both of these are generally viewed as developmental tasks of early adulthood.) Speaking very generally, one may assess a task as successful when it is "viable in society and acceptable for the self."[38]

Erik Erikson

Erikson also presented a life span theory of development.[17-19] He conceptualized eight stages, four of them specific to adulthood. He saw each stage as necessitating the resolution of a psychological issue or crisis. Thus, the developmental tasks he outlined might be termed psychological tasks. The individual must resolve the psychological issue at each stage to achieve internal harmony and successfully respond to the emotional issues of subsequent stages. Each major task is viewed in terms of a polarity. At each stage the task is mastered within a particular context, which Newman and Newman[51] have referred to as the central process and which frequently identifies the social network in which the person operates to resolve the crisis e.g., within a peer group, in school, or within the family (Table 5.2).[51]

Adulthood begins with the need to resolve "identity versus role confusion." The adolescent must struggle to see himself or herself as separate and meaningful, with some sense of direction, aims and goals for the future. From ages 20 to 40, the issue is between "intimacy versus isolation." The individual must see the self as worthy of love and capable of loving, and develop the ability for close friendships as well as a love relationship. Failure to do so leaves the person feeling alone and isolated. From ages 40 to 65, in middle adulthood, the individual needs to develop concerns beyond his or her own family. The person struggles with "generativity versus stagnation." He or she desires to be more creative—to create products of value, to contribute ideas, and to contribute to the general well-being of others. This psychological adjustment requires a reappraisal of work and relationship goals, so that new directions responsive to inner values

can be pursued. Failure to do so or attempting to stick with old goals results in a feeling of stagnation, and accomplishments lose their meaning.

The psychological task of late adulthood (65 years and later) relates to the need to achieve a sense of "integrity versus despair." Integrity comes about when one can reflect on his or her life and see one's own progression. It means looking realistically at success as well as failures and accepting that failures can no longer be corrected. Although there may be some realistic disappointment at what cannot be accomplished and cannot be remediated, the person feels that he or she has done reasonably well and sees his or her good qualities as outweighing the bad. Failure to achieve integrity finds the individual desperately trying to make amends, making unreasonable demands on others to ease one's discomfort, or withdrawing from all involvment with others in a gesture of defeat.

In summary, Erikson's psychological tasks, if successfully accomplished, result in an autonomous person who is able to value the self while achieving closeness and relatedness to others, is able to look realistically at one's own successes and failures, and to ultimately feel that life has been worthwhile.

Although Erikson's tasks are compatible with those of Levinson and Havighurst (to be discussed), Erikson's tasks are essentially intraspychic or internal. Havighurst's are external (oriented to society), and Levinson's are both intrapsychic and externally oriented.

Erikson's theory is implied or evident in occupational therapy literature. For example, Zemke and Gratz[59] use Erikson's eight stages and developmental tasks as a guide to assess the patient's adjustment to a psychosocial or physical disability. They remind the reader to be sensitive to the impact of disability on the time line that is identified for the resolution of psychosocial crises.

Robert Havighurst

Robert Havighurst[29] identifies six stages of periods in the life span: infancy and early childhood, middle childhood, adolescence, early adulthood, middle age and later maturity. In each period, specific tasks are mastered in response to a combination of forces: physical maturation; the pressures of society; and the desires, aspirations and values of the person and his or her personality, which forms from daily interactions throughout the life span.

The tasks may be universal (e.g., walking or talking) or culturally defined such as those tasks required for role expectations and social skills. Some tasks are recurrent and others are not. **Recurrent tasks** are the ongoing challenges thoughout life such as making friends and defining masculine and feminine roles. Developmental tasks that are not recurrent are associated with time-limited learning periods. These are periods in which the person is physically prepared and psychologically motivated to meet the demands of society.

TABLE 5.2 LIFE DEVELOPMENTAL TASKS

Life Stage Process	Developmental Tasks	Psychosocial Crisis	Central Process
Infancy (birth to 2 years)	1. Social attachment 2. Sensorimotor primitive intelligence causality 3. Object permanence 4. Maturation of motor functions.	Trust versus mistrust	Mutuality with the caregiver.
Toddlerhood (2-4 yrs.)	1. Self-control 2. Language development 3. Fantasy and play 4. Elaboration of locomotion	Autonomy versus shame and doubt	Imitation
Early school Identification age (5-7 yrs.)	1. Sex role identification 2. Early moral development 3. Concrete operations 4. Group play	Initiative versus guilt	
Middle school age (8-12 yrs.)	1. Social cooperation 2. Self-evaluation 3. Skill learning 4. Team play	Industry versus inferiority	Education
Early adolescence (13-17 yrs.)	1. Physical maturation 2. Formal operations 3. Membership in the peer group 4. Heterosexual relationships	Group identity versus alienation	Peer pressure
Later adolescence (18-22 yrs.) Experimentation	1. Autonomy from parents 2. Sex role identity 3. Internalized morality 4. Career choice	Individual identity versus role diffusion	Role
Early adulthood (23-30 yrs.)	1. Marriage 2. Childbearing 3. Work 4. Life style	Intimacy versus isolation	Mutuality among peers
Middle adulthood (31-50 yrs.)	1. Management of the household 2. Child rearing 3. Management of a career	Generativity versus stagnation	Person environment fit and creativity
Later adulthood (51 and older)	1. Redirection of energy to new roles 2. Acceptance of one's life 3. Developing a point of view about death	Integrity versus despair	Introspection

Material in this chart is adapted with permission. Newman and Newman *Development Through Life: A Psychosocial Approach*, Homewood, Illinois. The Dorsey Press, 1979. pp 30-31.

Newman and Newman

Newman and Newman[51] have presented the developmental life span concept in ten stages, which incorporate those periods identified by Erikson and Havighurst. These stages are identified along with the specific developmental tasks of each period and the central process through which development occurs.

The developmental tasks viewed as integral to each stage are more specifically occupational, cognitive, values-related, and relationship oriented (or external) than the internal orientation of either Jung or Erikson. The reader might wish to compare the major tasks described by Levinson with those of Havighurst to see their complementary relationship.

The occupational therapist is concerned about developmental tasks, for they represent the larger or longer-term goals toward which therapy is directed. In selecting activities and building identifiable enabling skills, the therapist strives to enhance the ability of the patient to meet the greater demands of these developmental tasks. Although developmental tasks would not likely be written into a treatment plan, both the patient and therapist use their understanding of these tasks to place treatment in a meaningful life context.

Marker Events

Within the context of life stage structure, and whether the life cycle is perceived as consisting of four to eight or ten periods, the individual is seen as necessarily encountering specific life events, which Levinson calls **marker events**. Certain predictable marker events are experienced within the context of a mental clock that each individual carries internally, which tell him or her when the event should occur.[48] People can state, for example, when they feel is the optimal time to leave home, marry, have a first child, or retire.

These life events necessitate changes in self-identity and reappraisals of values and are regarded as stressful insofar as they require change. However, Neugarten[48] postulates that these events can be reasonably well tolerated when they occur on time; they can be anticipated and rehearsed, and peers may be observed and imitated. For example, having a child may be anticipated and relished by a 28–year-old woman; having a child at age 44 could be very disruptive to a woman who has been enjoying her increased independence. Further, failure to meet a marker event at the time expected may itself be considered a problem. For example, when a young man or woman fails to leave the parent's home by age 30, people, including the parents, often view the behavior as immature or dependent.

On- and Off-Timing of Marker Events. Not all marker events are viewed as positive, nor can they be necessarily controlled by the individual. The death of spouse and forced early retirement, for example, would be marker events that might be both negative and unexpected. Whatever the marker event, the event requires change and adaptation by the individual. The individual's ability to respond effectively is influenced by the extent of successful adaptation in the past, his or her confidence and esteem, and cognitive abilities, as well as by the support and expectations of others, as influenced by role expectations, socioeconomic status, and the nature of his or her peer and broader social network.

To illustrate, if a woman with a high-paying job chooses to have a child off-time at age 40, she may be given a great deal of support by her associates, who find her decision daring but positive. If a woman of low economic status, perhaps receiving government welfare, chooses to have a child at age 40, she may not only be criticized but her very right to childbearing may be questioned.

It is generally agreed that when an event is off-schedule, or non-normative, it is less likely to be anticipated and, therefore, is more likely to have lasting detrimental effects. The early death of a spouse, for example, is generally more difficult for the individual to cope with than when a spouse dies at a much older age. Even positive events, off-time, can be problematic. For example, when a long awaited job promotion occurs at a late age, much of the potential satisfaction may have dissipated, and the individual experiences an almost bitter sense of, "Why couldn't this have happened sooner?"

Marker Events as Landmarks.   Marker events are like the events in a photo album. We can look back and remember the day we got married, or moved to our first home, or sent a child off to college. These events may relate to developmental tasks such as establishing a family or succeeding at an occupation, but are more limited in duration. Even though an event is of limited duration, its effects may be long awaited or long-lasting. As noted by Danish et al,[16] "Events do not occur in a vacuum; they occur in a rich life space of the individual, including competing demands from a variety of areas . . . and people significant to the individual."

Preparedness for Responding to Marker Events. Marker events may or may not contribute to the particular stress that leads a patient to seek occupational therapy. When a patient appears to be having difficulty coping with a marker event, the therapist will pay special attention to the patient's internal and external resources for coping with the event. Whether or not the event is on or off time influences the individual's preparedness to respond to the event and the availability of support from friends, family and community to meet the challenge of the marker event confronting the patient. As with developmental tasks, marker events provide a background for the selection of activities that are chosen according to their ability to enhance or build needed enabling skills.

Mediating Factors in Understanding Development

Before we proceed there are several thoughts we would like the reader to bear in mind as he or she considers the life span development approach in understanding adult behavior.

Tasks Readdressed

Developmental tasks are not like chapters in a book to be read and completed. They better approximate themes in a novel, weaving themselves throughout the story to be constantly reconsidered. Therefore, while one may speak of the ability to engage in give-and-take peer relationships as emerging in middle childhood, the adult needs to consistently readdress the task of establishing meaningful peer relationships, redefining his or her roles with peers in each developmental stage.

To cite other examples, marriage is not simply an event to be accomplished; the marital relationship is reworked in each developmental stage as each partner brings unique, evolving needs and perceptions. Separation from parents is never fully emotionally achieved, but the nature of the parent-child relationship is renegotiated in each developmental stage, from birth of the child to death. Sexual identity is not simply established by a given age, but it is periodically redefined in accordance with biological, emotional and social changes.

Development may be viewed as an ongoing, unfolding process that ultimately moves the individual toward greater wholeness. As a part of that ongoing process, the individual renegotiates the self's relationship to the world. A life span developmental approach assists one in keying in on the nature of this renegotiation, and it provides some guidelines for affirming that this renegotiation is occurring. But the life span approach should not be used to create artificial boundaries or suggest unyielding closures.

Adult Developmental Hierarchy

The degree of flexibility within developmental hierarchies is not clear with many dimensions of adult development. It may be apparent, for example, that a child who has not learned to walk is not going to be able to run; but can one state uncategorically that a person who has not been able to settle on and satisfactorily pursue an occupation or career by the age of

45 or 50, will therefore be unable to deal with the subsequent development tasks of being creative and passing on his or her ideas? Or, one might ask, what if a woman becomes divorced at age 38? Will she be able to address the issues usually predicated on stability? If one needs to start over and find a new job or new career, or become part of a new family, how might this be experienced at age 38 or 44 or 64?

Atypical Life Course

Whether a life stage development framework based on experiences common to adults is as useful for understanding the needs of individuals whose life course has been atypical is uncertain. From the standpoint of the mental health treatment community, one might ask how the life span conceptualization is applied with individuals who have been marginally functional throughout their lives, perhaps even requiring residential or parental care. Does any of the hierarchy apply? Life span theory addresses normative constructs and events, and these questions are not easily answered. The therapist using a life span framework must determine how disruptive events or an unusual life-style mesh with the expectations of society to affect the individual, influence his or her perceptions of self, and determine the options available for meaningful activity.

Changing Norms

Finally, one needs to consider that societal expectations for adults are not static and change as a society itself develops. The adult life span approach to understanding psychosocial development is in a somewhat ironic position. Only recently, especially in the 1970s and 1980s, an adult life cycle was vigorously postulated. But, just as clinicians and researchers are consolidating their information and offering viable, conceptual frameworks, our society is at a stage of reevaluating many of its own age and gender related expectations.[36]

Women, for example, are becoming more career-oriented at an earlier age; many relatively older women are bearing first children; men are becoming more active in the parenting of young children. Older grandparents are more often starting second careers; young men and women are moving into professions and positions of authority (e.g., as judges, lawyers and mayors). It is not just that these age disparate events are occurring; equally important, society and the individual are becoming more tolerant and indeed supportive of such change. Thus, when one speaks of the on or off timing of a marker event (e.g., marriage, job change or birth of child), the criteria for using such a label are becoming questionable. Although it is not clear at this point to what extent age and stage expectations or timetables have actually been altered, it is imperative that the therapist working with an individual understand the patient's internalization of a timetable and that the therapist not see developmental guidelines as inflexible standards.

Enabling Developmental Skills

If the developmental tasks of the life span are to be accomplished, the individual must successfully learn the broadest spectrum of enabling skills. That is, the person must be able to use his or her senses, muscles and skeletal system efficiently and effectively; must be able to manipulate ideas; needs to develop guiding philosophies; needs to perceive the self as a meaningful, separate and influential being; and must establish a way to communicate and cooperate with others. Just as the developmental tasks of Jung, Erikson, Levinson, and others are conceived as sequential and hierarchical so are the enabling skills viewed as logical and sequential in their development.

Mosey's Seven Adaptive Skills

In 1970, Mosey[44] articulated a developmental frame of reference for adults. She identified seven clusters of enabling skills and subskill components that must be sequentially mastered in order for the person to satisfy personal needs and meet society's expectations. The skills were grouped as perceptual-motor,† cognitive, drive-object, dyadic interaction, group interaction, self-identity and sexual identity skills. The skills and their subskill components are listed in Appendix H. For the most part, the adaptive skills suggested by Mosey are skills that would normally be integrated by adulthood.‡ Developmental difficulties arise, however, when an adult has failed to or is delayed in successfully integrating these skills, or when an adult once capable of using these skills becomes unable to do so. A developmental slip backward is referred to as **regression**.

Fidler's Skill Clusters

Fidler identifies four skill clusters that she believes are critical to achieving social efficacy and personal satisfaction: 1) the ability to care for oneself at a level of greater independence than dependence; 2) the ability to engage in a variety of experiences that satisfy the self and provide intrinsic gratification; 3) the ability to contribute to the welfare of others and 4) the ability to enter into and sustain reciprocal interpersonal relationships.[21,22]

Fidler also emphasizes the influence on performance by factors in the external environment, including, for example, the culture, economics, family constellation, housing and geography. Less emphasis is placed on regressed or infantile adult behavior, and more is placed on looking at the nature of the adult's current life-style and its relative utility for enhancing life experiences.

---

[2]Since Mosey's publication, the terms sensorimotor and sensory integration are being used. In this text we refer to sensorimotor-integration.

[3]In a later publication, Mosey acknowledges the limitations of her developmental framework in addressing many problems that arise in adult development. She proposes an alternative treatment framework, role acquisition, which is intended to describe learning by adults of changing adult roles through the life span.[45] Further, she suggests that this model is particularly suited for adults needing to cope with transitional stress. Role acquisition in this case represents a behavioral theoretical and treatment approach.

Current Practice in Occupational Therapy

The Person and Behavior

Innate Motivation

The individual is perceived as a physical-psychosocial being with an organismically determined press to grow and become increasingly complex. The basis for this growth and development is in the physical maturation of the individual as well as in the innate need to experience all aspects of the self and to expand one's intellectual prowess. The need to experience and master the challenges in one's world acts as a motivation, nudging the individual to "seek out environmental interactions."[44] In doing so, he or she continually encounters new information, novel experiences, and new demands that disturb the status quo. Tension is created, provoking a process of response to change known as **adaptation**.

Adaptation

When adapting, the person must respond to external expectations as well as one's own feelings as he or she integrates new information, learns new skills, reappraises current beliefs and makes other necessary accommodations. A history of successful adaptation increases the likelihood that future requirements for change will be successfully met because the individual sees the similarity between problems now encountered and those dealt with previously, has increased confidence in his or her own ability to cope with change, can call upon strategies that have been used before, and has established a social support network to which he or she can turn.[16]

Environmental Nourishment

A person needs to develop in the same sense that a plant needs to grow; the environment plays a vital role in the developmental process. From society, the person gains information about what is expected from him or her at various life stages; as these expectations are internalized they help to define the individual's expectations for the self.

The environment, which includes the people, objects, ideas and activities one encounters, provides the fertile ground in which learning and ultimately development can occur. The individual must have the opportunity not only to observe the actions of others but also to actively participate with objects (tools or materials), to exchange ideas and personally interact with others.

This way of developing is ultimately satisfying to the person and increases his or her sense of competence, even if the process brings periods of disruption or dissonance. From persons in his or her social network, the individual may gain support and encouragement for attempts at change, and finally, approval when he or she has succeeded in meeting their expectations.

Stage Specificity of Successful Function

The individual progresses through identifiable life stages, which have accompanying developmental tasks. These stages have been discerned across a variety of cultures and in the life histories of those who lived long ago, as well as in people today. The broad stages are characterized as orderly, sequential and invariant.

Skills specific to the biological, cognitive, social, and psychological development of the individual develop in a manner also conceptualized as orderly, sequential and hierarchical and similarly across cultures. These skills are not only quantitative (measurable) but qualitative, or given life by the individual's subjective experiencing of them. These skills enable the individual to meet the greater demands of developmental tasks and to ultimately function in a stage-appropriate manner.

Readiness

Implicit in the stage concept of life and skill development is the supposition of readiness. That is, there appear to be specific normative ages or age ranges at which the individual's physical endowment, psychological need, and societal demands combine to create a climate in which certain issues are best addressed, skills developed, or commitments to change made.

Trying to encourage the person to build skills before he or she is ready, as with pushing a child, is believed either to be futile or to build skills that will prove unstable. Failure to build developmental skills during the time of optimum readiness may impede this and future skill development or lead to a sense of failure or lessened satisfaction with self.

Task Renegotiation

It should be emphasized, however, that many tasks and issues will need to be addressed and then reworked during another stage. As our society becomes more complex and tumultuous, for example, a man or woman may find himself or herself making career decisions, not just in early adulthood, but several times during the life span. On a feeling level, developmental tasks may be experienced quite differently when they are addressed in one stage as compared to another. A new career, a new spouse, or an altered style of living all may be responded to somewhat differently depending on age and place among peers.

Dysfunction

Dysfunction results when stage-specific enabling skills have either not been learned or can no longer be used effectively. Sometimes dysfunction suggests a time of temporary difficulty as the person copes with life's transitions; other times, it may reflect inflexibility, or holding on to old ways of doing things when new ways are needed.

Because life stages and developmental skills are viewed as hierarchical, typically it is felt that no one stage or step in skill building can be skipped. At times, however, both the therapist and patient recognize that past opportunities have, indeed, passed. A 40-year-old man who didn't experience the carefree life of a young man can't realistically go back and recapture that period. Skills lacking during one life stage, if learned or developed during another, need to help prepare the person to respond to and cope with what lies ahead.

Barriers to Development

Barriers to adult learning and development can be broadly categorized as follows:

1. Situational barriers (e.g., lack of time, funds or information);
2. Dispositional barriers (e.g., biological or physical limitations, attitudes and perceptions one holds, or past experiences with previous developmental issues);
3. Institutional barriers (e.g., those that arise from policies that limit certain people from taking advantage of opportunities for advancement).[2,53]

The developmental therapist perceives the need to evaluate and address these barriers and to establish goals that will lead to successful skill accomplishment in accordance with the developmental priorities of the individual.

Function of Activities

Education

A life span development framework has a strong educative thrust in terms of laying a foundation for skill building, teaching performance or remedial skills, or planning for anticipated skill requirements. Activities are analyzed according to their component skill requirements. Activity selection is a matchmaking process in which the individual's life stage, level of function, and developmental needs are matched to activities that use skills already in the person's repertoire while providing a chance to learn new skills or means of compensation. No illness is implied in the life span development framework, and activities are not predicated on diagnosis.

When possible, activities may be selected

for their ability to increase insight and help the individual to generalize learning across past, present and anticipated life experiences. The developmentally oriented therapist, however, recognizes the individual differences in cognitive skill; no particular emphasis on insight as in the object relations framework, or on thoughts, as occurs in cognitive-behavioral treatment, is evident. The specific activities chosen and skills targeted for learning vary according to the emphasis of the treatment program and the individual's particular learning goals.

Practical Limits

Skill building overall usually requires ample opportunity within an activity format for experimentation, repetition, practice and finally refinement of given schemes. Some skills, such as learning to plan a budget, learning basic meal preparation or learning the skills in hand sewing, although not perfectable, can be reasonably acquired in a relatively short period.

Other skills, such as being able to interact comfortably in a diverse social group or skills specific to anticipated employment (e.g., secretarial skills or computer skills), are not likely to be mastered in a short time. An individual who wishes to learn skills that are more extensive or require much practice often begins the process of learning component skills or practicing them in occupational therapy and eventually is directed to other educational facilities for further skill development.

In some instances within the therapy setting, information may be given in a classlike format by a therapist or other professional. In this structure, the individual is taught along with others with similar learning needs.

Purposefulness

The therapist is always aware of the individual's need to feel a sense of purposefulness in whatever activity is selected. In the life span development framework, this purpose is couched in terms of intrapsychic, interpersonal and environmental changes that accompany life stages. Most people have a need to be contributing members of their family or society; however, the way in which they can contribute changes. For example, little children love to help Mom sweep, polish furniture or wash the car; the school-aged child delights in cleaning blackboards or running errands for the teacher; the adolescent likes to help peers; the adult may be concerned with how to help in church or in the community; the older adult is pleased in teaching those that choose him or her as a mentor or giving a helping hand to family members in need.

Everyone has a need to contribute. In physical medicine and rehabilitation settings, patients often give suggestions to one another regarding wheelchairs or equipment, as well as support for enduring the pain and frustration that each experiences during the rehabilitation process. The need to contribute is evident also in those who experience emotional or psychiatric problems, and at times these individuals are baffled as to how they can contribute to anyone else when, as one patient put it, "I can't even take care of myself."

When individuals cannot identify activities that seem purposeful or directions their lives will take, the therapist uses his or her knowledge of adult development to make some educated guesses about what activities would help the individual to make necessary adaptations and accomplish meaningful tasks. The following example comes from the author's practice.

**Case Illustration
A Struggle for Integrity**

A 76–year-old woman, never married, was being seen as a homecare patient. She was incapacitated by a series of strokes that left her unable to walk, with impaired speech, and in a generally weakened condition. She was markedly depressed, stating that she felt useless because she was unable to participate with her family in a way she perceived as helpful and normal. The therapist was called in because family caretakers were unable to meet the incessant demands they felt this woman made on them. The therapist talked with the patient about the ways in which she, as an elder in the family, might pass on to others, in this case to

---

grandnieces and nephews, the wisdom she had gained over a lifetime. Although she was no longer interested in pursuing a hobby she had once enjoyed, painting greenware, she did follow up the suggestion that she could pass this skill on to a grandniece. When the therapist queried whether this woman might want to save her philosophies and knowledge of family history in a written or taped diary, to be read later by younger kin, the woman could not see the usefulness of such an endeavor, calling it presumptuous.

In the therapist-directed process of looking at family momentos and recalling life experiences, however, the woman made an informal life review; evaluating where her life had gone, considering which decisions had been positive and where she had erred. This woman is not cited to illustrate any magic cure, as she continued to have bouts of depression. But, the severity of her depression appeared lessened. According to family members, she was less demanding, slept more restfully, and seemed more accepting of her own limitations.

Significantly, this woman could not articulate any need to engage in life review. She continued to perceive her usefulness in much the same way as she had 20 years earlier. When those earlier avenues became closed to her, she could generate no other possibilities. It should also be mentioned that this woman displayed some cognitive impairment, and her ability for insight and abstraction appeared limited. Still, the need for Erikson's integrity was quite evident.

Individualizing Activities

In summary, as suggested by the examples given, activities are purposeful within a patient's life experiences when they use the individual's skills, are consonant with the perceptions he or she has of the self within given roles, and allow the person to meet changing internal and external expectations. The patient may or may not be able to articulate personal needs in relation to activity, but will often experience a feeling of discomfort when he or she tries to fulfill new challenges with old ways of doing things. With a knowledge of life span development, the therapist can assist the patient to select activities that will more effectively meet his or her changing priorities or circumstances.

Theoretical Assumptions

When applying the developmental frame of reference in occupational therapy, the therapist bases evaluation and treatment on the following assumptions, which have been derived from life span development theory and are summarized here.

1. Human development occurs in an orderly fashion throughout the life cycle.
2. Steps within the developmental process are sequential and none can be skipped.
3. The person has an innate drive to encounter the world and master its challenges.
4. The environment also bears upon motivation by acting to sanction and reward certain behavior and discourage other.
5. As a person proceeds through the life cycle, he or she encounters life events and changing internal and external conditions that necessitate reappraisal and change.
6. Confrontation with change creates tension, disequilibrium and stress; this process is not, of itself, pathological, and in fact is often a necessary part of the change process.
7. The person's response to demands for change can result in adaptation and mastery, attempts to maintain the status quo, or regression and dysfunction.
8. The person's ability to master developmental tasks is influenced by physical capability, learned skills, his or her life experiences, the availability of resources and opportunity.
9. Successful adaptation tends to lead the individual to feel self-satisfaction and to gain societal approval.
10. A history of successful adaptation promotes future success in meeting challenges.
11. Through the use of purposeful activity in occupational therapy, the individual can learn, relearn, or adapt skills requisite to coping with developmental demands.
12. Activities are purposeful when they accommodate the patient's needs, interests, abilities, and place within the life span and when they provide sufficient opportunity for development.
13. As in life, during treatment the patient has responsibility for his or her own development.

Role of the Occupational Therapist

Providing a Growth-Facilitating Environment

As he or she adjusts to the developmental needs of the patient, the occupational therapist must be flexible, acting sometimes as a teacher, facilitator, participant, or supporting agent. As a teacher or facilitator, the occupational therapist selects or creates a growth-facilitating environment and provides purposeful activities that will enhance the acquisition of knowledge and skills necessary to maintain optimum function, prevent regression, and promote developmental change in the treatment and later community environment.[44] In some instances, the therapist may use a class-like structure or groups to disseminate knowledge and promote skill building while remaining sensitive to the uniqueness of each patient. When possible, the therapist identifies and helps to mimimize environmental barriers.

Being Well-Informed About Life Span Development

When the therapist identifies specific areas in which enabling skills are lacking, a key function of the therapist is to design or select experiences, or help the patient select experiences, that will provide a vehicle for him or her to learn and practice essential skills. The therapist must be familiar with the developmental requirements in a range of human endeavor, as well as hold a conceptual picture of the ebb-and-flow of life span development.

Although change necessitates a period of moderate disequilibrium, the therapist can assist the patient, if he or she is cognitively able, to understand these changing needs and to place immediate stress in a larger perspective by providing the patient with information about life stages, transitional periods and developmental tasks. Often when individuals learn that transitional periods can be expected to create some stress, they are less likely to be alarmed by the disequilibrium that they feel. In providing the patient with a life span conceptual framework, the therapist also gives the individual landmarks against which he or she can assess occupational, avocational and social options.

Acting as a Liaison

In a supporting role, the therapist conveys to the patient his or her confidence in the individual's ability to meet the demands of normal developmental stress, to accommodate to the changes that ensue and to meet the challenge of life's tasks. The therapist is a resource that helps patients make the transition from the treatment setting to the community setting. Throughout the treatment process, the occupational therapist is conscious of environmental/cultural expectations and assists the patient to adopt strategies and behaviors that will promote physical-psychosocial maturity and motivate performance that meets cultural, environmental and developmental expectations.

Evaluation

Impact of Life Span Imperatives Across Theoretical Frameworks

Whether consciously or unconsciously, each of us uses a developmental stance in assessment, no matter what our frame of reference. When an individual indicates that he or she is in distress, we ask ourselves, "How does this person function as compared to the expectations of society and himself or herself?" For example, if a patient is 23 years old, we want to know if he or she is going to school, or pursuing a career, or living at home; and although we may be flexible and avoid judgments, we are nevertheless interested in this information because we know what is expected of a 23-year-old. Much of what each of us consider healthy or constructive is related to the life span expectations that all of us within a given culture hold in common. In that sense, each of us makes developmentally based assessments.

Movement from Global Constructs to Specific Skills

Some emphases are particular to the life span developmentally oriented assessment. A review of the earlier discussion of developmental theory will reveal movement from global or broad constructs to specific and a holistic concern for all areas of function. The process of assessment can move quite naturally in much the same way.

For example, the therapist might meet a new male patient, age 37, and ask him to describe what he perceives as his present difficulties. The therapist would note the stage within the life span, as suggested by Jung, Levinson, Erikson, or other life span theorist and would wonder if the individual was in or approaching a period of life reassessment. He or she would realize that societal expectations for this individual included that he have a job, live independently from parents, be dating if not in a marital relationship, and have peer affiliation. The therapist could ask for a brief history from the patient or his family, with special emphasis on his current status regarding occupation, self-care, social affiliation, roles and pastimes. The therapist could then determine whether the individual was in or out of synchronization with the developmental tasks of his stage.

Characterizing the Life-style

During the assessment, the occupational therapist is sensitive to the specific life course that the patient has experienced and to the individuality that it represents. Fidler[21] refers to this as the need to identify the person's "characteristic life-style" and stresses the importance of appreciating the individual's values, and the way in which the family culture and environment enhance or hinder the development of skills.

When organizing and evaluating the data from the patient's life history as well as assessing the patient's present level of function, the therapist may keep the following questions in mind:

1. Based on chronological age, in which life stage of development is the patient?
2. Does the patient's life history and skill performance suggest adequate functioning in this stage?
3. How do biological endowment and limitations bear on performance?
4. Does the patient demonstrate the skills that suggest mastery of the developmental tasks identified with each of the stages before the present developmental level at which the patient is presently functioning?
5. What present stresses and expectations confront the patient to which he or she must respond and cope to continue to grow, change and adapt in life?
6. Is the patient's interpersonal network adequate to help the patient confront stress, resolve the psychosocial crisis, and meet the challenges of his or her life course?
7. Does the patient demonstrate coping strategies rather than defensive patterns?
8. How does the patient respond to both stress and change? Is the patient challenged or overwhelmed by stress?
9. Can the patient identify and use personal, interpersonal and environmental resources to respond to change and/or stress?
10. What barriers exist in the environment?

When it appears that the patient has not been able to succeed at tasks specific to life stage expectations, the therapist will use assessment to determine 1) which enabling skills are deficient or weak and which are strong, 2) which barriers (environmental or intrapersonal) are keeping the individual from developing or utilizing his or her skills, and 3) in what situations and under what conditions is the individual most likely to function best.

Variability in Performance

Throughout assessment, the therapist identifies areas of strength and potential means of building on available resources. Therapists recognize that adults, like children, do not function optimally or necessarily in a stage-consonant manner in all areas of endeavor or equally well in all situations. We have all seen persons who are able to think clearly and effectively until they encounter a stress (e.g., an illness or accident), at which point they become confused and childlike. The same fluctuation can be true of more dysfunctional patients.

Most therapists working with psychiatric patients can recount experiences in which individuals were able to function well within the treatment setting but not outside the setting. For instance, a patient could sit for long periods in occupational therapy cooperating with other patients to accomplish a group mural, laughing spontaneously and appearing at ease. Once back into the community, the individual became anxious, unable to concentrate, and fearful of making mistakes. Although one can use such an example to document that higher social skills did not truly exist, one could also question whether the difference in function depended largely on the degree of acceptance and support the patient felt. When the person felt accepted, anxiety was lessened and the ability to use his or her own skills increased. In an environment in which others are generally oblivious to this same person's need for encouragement, doubts set in, anxiety ensues and function declines.

Developmental Profile

To identify the boundaries of performance for specific enabling skills, the therapist uses interview or observation during task performance and interprets the observation findings.[44] Fidler[21] has designed a lifestyle performance profile to help the therapist organize his or her findings from the interview and social history (Table 5.3). In Fidler's opinion, assessment instruments that evaluate functional skills in leisure and work may be helpful, but most data is best obtained from the patient interview. By getting a picture of the history of performance, it becomes possible to characterize the indivi-

TABLE 5.3

THE LIFE-STYLE PERFORMANCE PROFILE

**Skill and skill level, "appropriate" balance
determined by age, culture, and biology**

Self-care and Maintenance	Self-needs/Intrinsic Gratification

Self-care:
  Washing
  Dressing
  Eating
  Toileting

Self maintenance:
  Food preparation
  Shopping
  Money management
  Transportation
  Daily schedule—time
  Care of:
    Living area
    Personal belongings

Self support

Existing skills

Skill deficits

Self care values and attitudes

External resources/barriers:
  Family/social
  Culture
  Economics
  Environment

Acknowledgment of own personal needs and interests

Interests manifested

Interests actually pursued

Abilities and skills being used

Skill deficits

Intrinsic gratification values and attitudes

External resources/barriers:
  Family/social
  Culture
  Economics
  Environment

Service to Others	Reciprocal Relationships

Role identity and responsibilities:
  Household and financial management
  Job market role
  Support/care of dependents
  Student role
  Family member role

Role/job demands and pressures

Skills required

Existing skills

Skill deficits

Appropriateness of role identity/responsibilities

Service values and attitudes

External resources/barriers:
  Family/social
  Culture
  Economics
  Environment

Patterns of relating
  Friends
  Peers
  Family
  Groups
  Intimacy

Interpersonal
  Values
  Expectation of self/others
  Roles and responsibilities

Skills required
  Existing skills/assets
  Skill deficits

External resources
  Family
  Culture
  Economics
  Environment

Adapted from FOCUS: Skills for Assessment and Treatment. ed. by Susan C. Robertson, Rockville, MD: American Occupational Therapy Association, Inc., 1988.

dual's whole pattern of activity, values and attitudes.

Therapist-Patient Collaboration

As the interview progresses and the occupational therapist observes the patient's behavior during the assessment tasks, the therapist also makes assumptions and draws inferences from that behavior. These interpretations are then discussed with the patient in a manner that considers the patient's ability to understand and the therapeutic benefits of sharing. The outcome of this patient-therapist discussion can clarify the developmental profile and affirm or negate the therapist's interpretation as well as pose questions that will identify additional assessment needs. The therapist's interpretations are based on physical and psychosocial developmental theories and the normal pattern of development and change that occurs throughout the life span.

Assessment Batteries

To date, no standardized occupational therapy tests accurately reflect adult skill performance based on a continuum of normal life span development. Standardized tests are available to assess enabling skills primarily in the area of sensorimotor-integration function, but most have been standardized only for the child population and in the area of cognitive dysfunction. These tests have been used by therapists as screening tools to identify adult performance problems and possible directions for treatment of the adult patient.

Screening Tool. A **screening tool** is a test, or specific activity, that is used to distinguish an individual patient who has a particular skill, or more often, deficit, from those individuals who do not. It is used to identify the patient's skills, abilities and problems in a particular area.

Other assesssment instruments are also available both within occupational therapy and from related fields specific to given skills outlined in Fidler's performance profile. If the occupational therapist chooses to use any of these as screening tools with adults, we recommend that the therapist research the literature that summarizes assessment protocol, reliability and validity studies and the neurological, psychological and occupational therapy views and critiques of these instruments.

The following assessment batteries with the life span development framework are presented here because each elicits or helps to organize developmental data that has been identified with this frame of reference. However, none of these assessments address directly the life stages and transitional stages described in the earlier theoretical review.

Life-style Performance Profile: An Organizing Frame. Authored by Gail Fidler, the profile suggests guidelines for gathering and organizing data to describe physical and psychosocial skills that reflect adaptive performance and mastery of life tasks. This profile is outlined in Table 5.3 and also discussed in Hemphill and Fidler.[21,30]

Adolescent Role Assessment. The author Maureen Black states that this assessment is not a diagnostic tool and proposes this assessment as a guide for evaluation and treatment planning. An interview format is described to elicit data to indicate past, present and future role adjustment based on occupational choice.[5,30]

Role Change Assessment. This interview tool is used to assess older adults. It elicits information regarding the roles of the older adult. The adult chooses from major categories (e.g., family and social, organizational, vocational and leisure) and identifies the value of the role, the environment in which the role is practiced, and the type of activities the role encompasses.[32]

The Occupational Performance History Interview. Described in more detail with the assessments for the model of human occupation, this semistructured interview guide, available from the American Occupational Therapy Association, is designed to act as a generic history taking format. It poses questions in five content areas: environmental influences, life roles, organization of daily routines, perceptions of ability and responsibility, and interests, values and goals.[37]

Role Checklist. The Role Checklist was developed by Oakley for use within the model of human occupation. The patient is asked to respond to a list of ten possible roles, indicating whether or not he or she has assumed these roles (past or present, or anticipates doing so in the future) and indicating if each role is perceived as very valuable, somewhat valuable or not valuable.[4]

Treatment

Treatment Goals

As with all the treatment frameworks presented in this text, the developmental frame has been strongly influenced by the general acceptance in health care of behavioral goal setting.

Behavioral Goal Statements. Mosey speaks to this behavioral influence when she suggests that goals should be carefully identified and promoted through judicious and selective reinforcement by the therapist.[44,45]

Danish et al,[16] in their discussion of life development intervention, stress that problems must be viewed in terms of "behaviorally oriented positive goal statements," and they cite the necessity for a delineation of "behavioral components of a skill" in skill development.

Goals for Prevention. As mentioned earlier, previous occupational therapy intervention in the area of development has tended to emphasize goal setting to counter regressed or childlike behavior by adults and has not been aimed at helping adults to pass through transitional and life stages. This focus appears to be changing, however, as evidenced in Mosey's more recent theoretical discussions and in the increasing emphasis in the model of human occupation on life span development. As

information pertaining to life span development (especially the adult's middle years) becomes more influential in occupational therapy, one might expect to see more goal setting aimed at preventive intervention.

Attainable Steps Toward Long-term Goals. Whatever goals are established, they must be stated in terms of desired behavior or preformance skills and subskills, be attainable and understood as such by the individual, and be achievable within a reasonable period. Short-term goals allow the individual to recognize his or her own progress and increase confidence and may be viewed as steps to long term goals, some of which may or may not be realized during the course of treatment.

Treatment Process

Remediation-to-Prevention Continuum. Throughout the text, we have used a patient-treatment model, but the reader will recognize that much of the discussion regarding life span development has focused on the normative process. Although many individuals do not function within the norms and become identified as needing professional assistance, not all therapists conceive of developmental skill building as a matter of treatment; some approach it as a process of education or reeducation. This approach has been less apparent in occupational therapy than in counseling.

In the discussion of life span intervention, we first discuss treatment as it has been typically conceived in occupational therapy. An emphasis has been placed on remediation or stabilization with individuals identified as patients. The focus has been in what might be called "catch up" skill building.

In contrast are some preventive treatment principles emerging in the area of counseling and the community mental health system. In many instances, activities such as those familiar to occupational therapy are used. Rather than suggesting that remediation, stabilization or prevention is necessarily a better treatment goal (all have their place and one process is often difficult to separate from the others), it may be that as treatment progresses the therapist and patient will profit by changing their treatment emphasis.

Although prevention or preventive medicine has not been the predominant arena for occupational therapy practice, prevention is being given increasing attention in health care. No one is certain just how committed in dollars the government or the public is to preventive care. It seems important, however, for occupational therapists to assess what role they can play in this area.

Building Adaptive Skills in Occupational Therapy. Developmental skill building follows logically given the postulates presented thus far. The therapist provides an environment that enhances the opportunity for the individual to follow a normal developmental pattern and selects activities that bridge the gap between the individual's present skill level and the skills he or she needs to learn and master. Once new skills have been attained, the next, successively higher step in skill development is approached. While enabling skills across all areas are interdependent, the person often presents an uneven developmental picture; that is, he or she has achieved some age-appropriate developmental tasks, but not others; or has strong skills in some areas, but not in others. The process of developmental skill building is one of maximizing strengths and building on previous accomplishments while developing new skills.

Depending on the specific nature of the deficits or delays, projected learning needs, or the treatment philosophy of the therapist, skill building may be approached quite differently in one treatment center than in another, even when the clinicians all espouse a developmental approach.

Mosey gives general treatment guidelines for developing adaptive skills. In agreement with other developmental theorists, she states that the therapist needs to begin with the most primitive subskill a patient has not yet learned or needs to learn and create a learning ex-perience in which this learning can oc-

cur. The therapist's task is to identify what skills are lacking and to envision experiences in which these skills might be learned and well practiced.[44]

Other theorists, however, would not recommend building more primitive skills if this proved approach impractical. We can cite, for example, the new mother who seeks treatment because of extreme depression or anxiety after the birth of her first child, and describe a typical, though abbreviated, developmental approach. Upon assessment, the therapist finds that the young woman has limited experience with infants and lacks both basic skills and information related to meeting the physical and emotional needs of an infant.† The developmental therapist would note the particular skills and areas of knowledge that were lacking and would provide learning experiences in which these could be acquired. She might have the woman practice feeding, dressing and bathing a doll or the woman's own infant if possible until the patient felt comfortable with her own skills. Further, the therapist might identify resources (e.g., literature, experts in the area of child care, or adult classes) that could be used to help the patient learn more about children's growth and developmental needs. The therapist would also think it important for the patient to identify resources and learning means to meet her own need for recreation or time away from the child; but depending on the amount of time available for treatment, treatment goals might be aimed at increasing the mother's ability to care for the needs of the infant.

Relative Emphasis on Behavioral Reward. Mosey[44,45] offers a model in which given subskills (enabling skills) are conceived as behavioral goals and suggests using the behavioral method of giving positive or negative reinforcement to promote skill building. Although the use of a behavioral model of rewarding is not particular to Mosey, her conceptualization

---

†This same situation may also be viewed in behavioral terms as an overreliance on external, behavioral reward, or a failure to generalize learning.

of external, therapist-given reward is not consistent with the developmental postulates of some theorists, for example Piaget and Kohlberg, who state that the need for development is innate, satisfying, and self-regulating and does not need behavioral reward to be sustained.†

Limited Opportunity for Follow-Through. As stated by Briggs et al,[7] "Few therapist have the opportunity to follow a client through developmental stages or adaptive skill learning, over an extended period of time." Therefore, when one speaks of developmental skill building, there is often only a speculative movement through developmental stages. Actual treatment may focus on demonstrable, shorter-term goals and is more often conceived as maintaining function, setting the wheels of skill building into motion, increasing patient's self-confidence, and off-setting remission.

Life Development Intervention

The model of life development intervention offers a slightly different perspective. Coming from the counseling literature, it has a strong educative and preventive component.

Life development intervention (LDI) works to "help people encounter routine and unexpected life circumstances by developing their personal competence in life planning and their interpersonal competence in developing a caring social network. The intent is to encourage individuals to be producers of their own development, to be active problem solvers and planners and to develop a sense of self-efficacy."[16]

Danish et al[16] suggests a generic model of LDI for responding to a variety of life events. They delineate six stages in the helping process:

1. Goal assessment—Translating problems or inadequacies into positive, attainable goal statements as well as analyzing barriers to goal attainment.
2. Knowledge acquisition—This may include formalized information given by the helper or designated others.
3. Development of decision-making skills—A hierarchy of steps for successful decision making is taught, and emphasis is given to the fact that indecision is a decision in favor of inactivity.
4. Risk assessment—This is a planned review of alternative and roadblocks and a weighing of benefits as well as potential costs of a selected plan of action.
5. Creating social support—Especially important for future problem-solving is the ability to recognize, gain access to and make use of social and community resources.
6. Planning skill development—This includes developing a rationale for learning a given skill, determining the behavioral components of a skill, developing criteria to establish when a given skill is accomplished, determining how the skill will be learned, evaluating skill attainment, and considering how the skill development model might be applied to other, perhaps future goals.

The individual who needs assistance may be initially helped to identify the particulars of a given, stressful situation. Special attention will be paid to his or her manner of problem-solving, and the person may be taught a more successful problem-solving strategy. Specific goals are determined and skills targeted or taught to attain these goals. Once a current stress is handled, the therapist works to draw analogies between this stress and its demands for change or adaptation and past as well as future events.

Empowering the Individual. The therapist believes that when a future crisis requiring change is encountered, the individual will more likely handle it effectively if he or she can 1) see similarities between this crisis and

---

§The authors are aware that in her discussion of developmental treatment Mosey describes the judicious application of positive and negative reinforcement by the therapist.[44] However, the authors do not find this aspect of behavioral therapy to be consistent with the basic tenets of developmental theory.

past, successfully accomplished problem-solving situations and 2) generalize problem-solving skills. As more and more changes are accommodated successfully, new events are approached with increasing confidence.[16]

As proposed by Danish et al,[16] LDI becomes the ability to identify and set life goals. The issue for the individual is not "Where have I failed," but "What do I want to learn?" and "What course do I wish to set?" This approach is described as proactive not reactive and is believed to give a sense of empowerment.

We can refer to the example given earlier of a classically developmental approach designed to teach necessary skills to a young mother with a newborn. In LDI, the mother would be taught skills related to child rearing. Then, however, the occupational therapist would help her to look ahead to anticipate future needs. The patient might be asked to think about questions such as, "What will I want to be doing when the child is two or five years old and no longer needs constant care?" Goals of LDI might relate to the woman's wish to increase her level of education or gain occupational skills that can be used three years hence.

LDI Used in a Group Context. Much of the discussion of life development intervention pertains to its use with several individuals, all encountering or expecting to encounter similar life changes. For example, young persons graduating from high school and lacking specific career plans, mothers of toddlers, or older persons anticipating retirement might be contacted through a community outreach program. The ensuing process is one of helping through education, not treatment. If we use prospective retirees and their spouses as an example, they might be brought together in an informal class-like structure and be allowed to participate in the following:

1. Ask about their expectations for change;
2. Receive information about the more common changes they could expect to encoun-

ter (e.g., changes in amount of leisure, changes in spendable income, changes in status, and changes in the amount of time spouses are together);
3. Receive a rationale for learning new skills or learning new ways to balance their time;
4. Select desired skills;
5. Learn specific skills (e.g., how to use community resources; avenues for volunteerism; or skills specific to a new hobby, avocation, or potential source of supplementary income);
6. Practice new skills under supervision;
7. Compare notes and gain encouragement as new skills are put into action. Cantor[13] also gives an example of a proactive program for retirees.

Looking at expected life changes appears to be an effective strategy for an occupational behavior orientation (refer to Chapter 6) and is similar to the educational modules discussed with cognitive-behavioral treatment, the difference being that the emphasis is on prevention and not treatment.

LDI and Dollars. These prevention or proactive programs are made available through community mental health centers because the community health system wants to identify members of the population more likely to experience problems. By not only helping individuals avert a crisis, but also by helping to familiarize them with nontreatment community resources, the teaching agency expects to relieve some of the demand from the health care system, while facilitating community involvement more positively.

It requires foresight to envision the positive outcome of LDI programs and research dollars to substantiate their effectiveness. With the competing demands of individuals already identified as in extreme stress, the occupational therapist might have difficulty finding or creating an opportunity to offer LDI programs. Other professional groups include recreational therapists, nurses, and education specialists who, in given agencies, provide this kind of service. Yet, with LDI, emphasizing as it does choices regarding ones use of time in activities, principles of life development intervention could contribute to the occupational therapist's role in the community and add another dimension to occupational therapy practice.

LDI and the Patient with Chronic Problems. Life development intervention, as described by Danish et al,[16] is used with individuals who have had at least some success in coping with reactive life events, who have some ability for insight, and have demonstrated motivation. It should be added, however, that programs similar in principle to LDI have been instituted by community agencies for the patient who is chronically dependent. The patient with chronic mental illness is assisted to recognize his or her own strengths and limitations, plan for the future, and helped to meet his or her needs through a network of community-based, nontreatment providers. This approach may be useful because many patients with chronic problems find it especially difficult to cope with change and have symptoms that worsen dramatically during times of increased stress.

Life development intervention for persons with physical, cognitive or emotional impairment might involve helping the individual determine reasonable and attainable goals, find resources within the community, and explore avenues for goal achievement. Although many of the typical developmental tasks, as identified by Erikson, Jung, and others might or might not be attainable, goals appropriate to the limited abilities of the individual would be established and could increase the person's sense of dignity, worth and empowerment.

Summary

In many ways, a life span development frame of reference acts as an overarching conceptual structure for organizing diverse constructs, all of which contribute to intervention based on life span theory. There is a developmental core

of knowledge with the individual perceived as moving through identifiable, hierarchical and sequential life stages. When the framework addresses skill building, however, there is a strong influence from behaviorism, as typified by the discussion of life development intervention in Danish et al.[16] Additionally, the enabling skills identified within this framework include psychological skills (often couched in traditional Freudian terms), cognitive skills (which share their theory base with information from cognitive-behaviorism), plus diverse other skills, any of which might be addressed within the other frames of reference presented in this text. What we assess now are the signifcant beliefs and priorties that distinguish the life span development frame of reference.

Contributions and Limitations of Life Span Development Frame of Reference

Contributions

The developmental approach in sociology and psychology and in applied fields, including health and education, have a long history. More recent is the attention paid to the middle of the life span, in contrast to the emphasis on childhood and older adulthood.

What this life span model provides is a larger context in which to place the immediate or presenting problems that bring individuals to treatment. Unfortunately, it is often easy to get so caught up in responding to acute problems that we lose sight of how these immediate problems relate to one's life-style or can be expected to manifest in future problems. Even when the presenting crisis is addressed, gains made during active intervention may not carry over at home after treatment.

By providing patients with a life span context from which to view presenting problems, treatment can often become more meaningful, and patients have a means to anticipate and potentially prepare for future life changes and stresses. When treatment is successful at helping the individual to generalize learning across past, present and future, the person gains confidence that he or she will be able to cope effectively with both expected and unexpected future events.

The life span framework recognizes that there are expected periods of disequilibrium and that certain developmental tasks have to be readdressed as one grows older. Illness is not implied, and the individual is freed from the burden of applying negative labels to himself or herself when in a period of distress. We realize that psychiatric labels may have already been given to the person who seeks professional help, but there is nothing in this frame of reference that necessitates such labeling.

Developmental, sequential skill building contrasts with behavioral skill building and avoids the potential problem establishing unstable splinter skills. One could expect, therefore, that skills built according to a developmentally based hierarchy will be durable and provide a firm foundation for those skills that will be added to meet future demands. As indicated, however, in some instances it is unclear whether sequential skill building is peceived as necessary. The assumption that developmental skill building is necessarily superior to behavioral skill building, including the learning of splinter skills, represents an area of considerable debate between developmentally and behaviorally oriented helpers, and is not adequately addressed by research.

The developmental framework has been described as especially suited for the treatment of those who come into therapy with a low level of function.[1,7,40,44] We see the life span development framework as versatile and applicable across a broad range of individual ability. The nature and emphasis of programs will vary according to the developmental needs of the individual patient.

Limitations

The life span development frame of reference requires extensive application, assessment, research and documentation to clarify its utility. The current frames of reference in occupa-

tional therapy that are developmental in origin have been too exclusionary to serve as adequate tests of a multidimensional life span frame of reference. However, they do provide input into the larger knowledge base and represent compatible practice theories within the greater framework.

There is seldom, if ever, an opportunity to see the individual's progression from one life stage to another or to see the completion of a developmental task during the duration of treatment. Therefore, although one can establish the efficacy of skill building, it is not possible to verify that skill building has led or will lead to satisfying transitions through life stages. These stages must be understood as hypothetical constructs that aid in determining priorities in treatment.

The rules of normal development are used to establish treatment guidelines for individuals whose life courses have often traveled far from the norm. Developmental theory does address the problem of failure to achieve developmental expectations, identifying such failure in general terms as a matter of physical inability, or limited opportunity. However, it becomes difficult in practice to determine why some individuals, physically and cognitively able, have been seemingly incapable of or unwilling to take advantage of opportunity. Although these may be the individuals blocked by the dispositional barriers cited by Aslanian and Bickell, they nevertheless present seemingly intractable treatment dilemmas, and their development needs may be best served by an alternative treatment approach.

It is not yet clear what specific skills are necessary to enable the various developmental tasks, what subskills comprise these skills, or how best to determine if these subskills exist. For exmple, what skills enable an individual to satisfactorily pursue a career? Given a patient who has not been able to settle on a career, how does one determine which enabling skills are deficient? In a closely related problem, the best means for teaching or enhancing skill development is not precise.

The occupational therapist will need to use judgment in deciding which skills and sub-skills are deficient, which would reasonably represent initial and latter goals for treatment, and what constitutes an optimum learning environment. This lack of precision in knowledge about the skill components of given developmental tasks and enabling skills is not particular to a developmental framework. It can be viewed as especially problematic in this frame, however, because of the perceived need to build skills in a stairstep fashion.

There is a danger that an overly rigid interpretation of life stage concepts will lead to unreasonable expectations for conformity. When the individual expresses dissatisfaction with his or her own life, that may be sufficient cause to pursue treatment. When individuals express satisfaction with their life courses, but society or significant others indicate disapproval of their conduct, the problems posed in treatment may be quite different.

This chapter has emphasized the importance of using a life stage concept as a flexible construct, while appreciating the wide diversity in individual experiencing. When life stage constructs are rigidly applied, they lose their utility.

Many in the human sciences believe that adult developmental theory has been built on a lopsided structure in which more has been learned about the experience of men than women and those in the middle and upper socioeconomic class than those of lower incomes. Nor has this structure been adequately studied in varied cultures. Although we can not develop this discussion further here, the interested reader is referred to the chapter references.[3,6,25,39,43,52]

We must reiterate that an understanding of human development can only enhance the therapist's practice, regardless of the frame of reference embraced. The extent to which a life span development frame of reference will be chosen as a guiding structure for occupational therapy practice in mental health is as yet uncertain.

Recommended Reading List

Maeda D: Aging in Eastern society. In Hobman D (Ed): *The Social Challenge of Aging*. New York, St. Martin's Press, 1978.

Thomas M, Kuh G: Understanding development during the early adult years: A composite framework. *Personnel Guidance J* 61:14–17, 1982.

Treiman D, Terrell K: Sex and the process of status attainment: A comparison of working men and women. *Am Sociol Rev* 140:174–200, 1975.

References

1. Allen CK: *Occupational Therapy for Psychiatric Diseases: Measurement and Management of Cognitive Disabilities*. Boston, Little, Brown and Company, 1985.
2. Aslanian C, Bickell H: *Americans in Transition: Life Changes as Reasons for Adult Learning*. New York, College Entrance Examination Board, 1980.
3. Auster CJ, Auster D: Factors influencing women's choice of nontraditional careers: The role of family, peers and counselors. *Voc Guidance Quart* 29:253–265, 1981.
4. Barris R, Oakley F, Kielhofner G: The role checklist. In Hemphill B (Ed): *Mental Health Assessment in Occupational Therapy*. Thorofare, NJ, SLACK Incorporated, 1988, pp. 73–91.
5. Black M: The adolescent role assessment. *Am J Occup Ther* 30(4):73–79, 1976.
6. Bloom DE: Women and work. *Am Demographics* 8:25–30, 1986.
7. Briggs A, Duncombe L, Howe M, Schwartzberg S: *Case Simulations in Psychosocial Occupational Therapy*. Philadelphia, F.A Davis Company, 1979, p. 144.
8. Buhler C: The curves of life as studies in biographies. *J Applied Psychol* 19:405–409, 1953.
9. Buhler C: Meaningful living in the mature years. In Leemeir RW (Ed): *Aging and Leisure*. New York, Oxford University Press, 1961.
10. Buhler C: Genetic aspects of the self. *Annals NY Acad Sciences* 96:730–764, 1962.
11. Buhler C: The developmental structure of goal setting in group and individual studies. In Buhler C, Masserik F (Eds): *The Course of Human Life*. New York, Springer, 1968.
12. Campbell J (Ed): *The Portable Jung*. Hull RCF (trans). New York, Viking Press Incorporated, 1971.
13. Cantor S: Occupational therapists as members of preretirement resource teams. *Am J Occup Ther* 35(10): 638–643, 1981.
14. Chickering AW, Havighurst R: The life cycle. In

Chickering AW (Ed): *The Modern American College.* San Francisco, Jossey-Bass, 1981, p. 25.

15. Cutler Lewis S: *The Mature Years: A Geriatric Occupational Therapy Text.* Thorofare, NJ, SLACK Incorporated, 1979.

16. Danish S, D'Augelli A, Ginsberg M: Life development intervention: Promotion of mental health through the development of competence. In Brown SD, Lent RW: *Handbook of Counseling Psychology.* New York, John Wiley and Sons, 1984, pp. 525, 539–540, 531, 538–540, 533, 532.

17. Erikson E: *Childhood and Society.* New York, W. W. Norton and Company, 1950.

18. Erikson E: Identity and the life cycle. *Psychol Issues* l: 1–171, 1959.

19. Erikson E: *Identity, Youth and Crisis* New York, W. W. Norton and Company, 1968.

20. Farrell M, Rosenburg S: *Men at Midlife.* Boston, Auburn House, 1981.

21. Fidler G: The life-style peformance profile. In Robertson S (Ed): *Mental Health Focus: Skills for Assessment and Treatment.* Rockville, MD, The American Occupational Therapy Association, 1989, pp. 3.35–3.40.

22. Fidler G, Fider J: Doing and becoming: Purposeful action and self-actualization. *Am J Occup Therapy* 32: 305–310, 1978.

23. Fiorentino M: *Reflex Testing Methods for Evaluating C.N.S. Development.* Springfield, Ill, Charles C. Thomas, 1965.

24. Gilfoyle E, Grady A, Moore J: *Children Adapt.* Thorofare, NJ, Slack, Incorporated, 1981.

25. Gilligan C: *In a Different Voice - Psychological Theory and Women's Development.* Cambridge, MA, Harvard University Press, 1982.

26. Gould R: The phases of adult life: A study in developmental psychology. *Am J Psychiatry* 5:521–531, 1972.

27. Gould R: Adult life stages: Growth toward self-tolerance. *Psychology Today* Febuary:26–29, 1975.

28. Gould R: *Transformations.* New York, Simon and Schuster, 1978.

29. Havighurst R: The world of work. In Wolman BB (Ed): *Handbook of Developmental Psychology.* Englewood Cliffs, NJ, Prentice-Hall, 1982.

30. Hemphill B: *The Evaluative Process in Psychiatric Occupational Therapy.* Thorofare, NJ, SLACK Incorporated, 1982, pp. 43–47, 9–53.

31. Hesse H: *Siddartha.* New York, Bantam Books, 1977.

32. Jackoway I, Rogers J, Snow T: The role change assessment: An interview tool for evaluating older adults. *Occup Ther Ment Health* 7(1):17–37, 1987.

33. Jung C: The Stages of Life. In *Modern Man in Search of a Soul*ft. New York, A Harvest/HBJ Book, Harcourt Brace Jovanovich, 1933.

34. Jung C: *Memories, Dreams, Reflections.* Jaffe AR (Recorded and Ed), and Winston C (Trans). New York, Pantheon Books, 1963.

35. Jung C: *Man and His Symbols.* New York, Doubleday and Company, 1964.

36. Kaplan P: *The Human Odyssey—Life Span Development.* St. Paul, MN, West Publishing Company, 1988.

37. Kielhofner G, Henry A: Use of an occupational history interview in occupational therapy. In Hemphill B (Ed): *Mental Health Assessment In Occupational Therapy.* Thorofare, NJ, SLACK Incorporated, 1988, pp. 59–71.

38. Levinson D: *The Seasons of A Man's Life.* New York, Ballantine Books, 1978, pp. 51, 319, 51, 97–101, 53.

39. Levinson D: Toward a conception of the adult life course. In Smelser NJ, Erikson EH (Eds): *Themes of Work and Love in Adulthood.* Cambridge, MA, Harvard University Press, 1980.

40. Levy L: Movement therapy for psychiatric patients. *Am J Occup Ther* 28(6):354–357, 1974.

41. Llorens L: An evaluation procedure for children sixten years of age. *Am J Occup Ther* 21(2):64–69, 1967.

42. Llorens L: *Application of a Developmental Theory for Health and Rehabilitation.* Rockville, MD, American Occupational Therapy Association, 1976.

43. McIlroy JH: Midlife in the 1980s: Philosophy, economy, and psychology. *Personnel Guidance J* l62:623–628, 1984.

44. Mosey AC: *Three Frames of Reference in Mental Health.* Thorofare, NJ, SLACK Incorporated, 1970, pp. 140, 141.

45. Mosey AC: *Psychosocial Components of Occupational Therapy.*New York, Raven Press, 1986.

46. Neugarten B: *Personality in Middle and Late Life.* New York, Atherton Press, 1964.

47. Neugarten B: Continuities and discontinuities of psychological issues into adult life. *Hum Dev* 12:121–130, 1969.

48. Neugarten B: Time, age and the life cycle. *Am J Psychiatry* 136(7):887–894, 1979.

49. Neugarten B, Datan N: The middle years. In Arieti S (Ed): *American Handbook of Psychiatry.* New York, Basic Books, 1973.

50. Neugarten B, Moore J: The change age-status system. In Neurgarten BL (Ed): *Middle Age and Aging.* Chicago, University of Chicago Press, 1968.

51. Newman BM, Newman PR : *Development Through Life: A Psychosocial Approach.* Homewood, Ill, 1979.

52. Peck RC: Psychological developments in the second half of life. In Neugarten GL (Ed): *Middle Age and Aging.* Chicago, University of Chicago Press, 1968.

53. Rodgers R: Theories of adult development: Research status and counseling implication. In Brown SD, Lent RW: *Handbook of Counseling Psychology.* New York, John Wiley and Sons Inc., 1984, pp. 488, 506.

54. Ross DB: Cross-cultural comparison of adult development. *Personnel Guidance J* 62:418–421, 1984.

55. Sheehy G: *Passages*. New York, E.P.Dutton and Company 1976.
56. Vaillant G: Theoretical hierarchy of adaptive ego mechanisms. *Arch Gen Psychiatry* 24:107–118, 1971.
57. Vaillant G: *Adaptation to Life*. Boston, Little Brown and Company, 1977.
58. Wolman B (Ed): *Handbook of Developmental Psychology*. Englewood Cliffs, NJ, Prentice-Hall, 1982.
59. Zemke R, Gratz R: The role of theory: Erikson and occupational therapy. *Occup Ther Ment Health* 2(3): 45–63, 1982.

Chapter 6

MODEL OF HUMAN OCCUPATION

Focus Questions

1. The model of human occupation is recommended for which patient populations?
2. What is human occupation?
3. Describe an open system.
4. What are the subsystems of the human system?
5. Why is the volition subsystem considered the most important subsystem?
6. Compare the role of the therapist in this framework with that in other frameworks.
7. What influences a person's participation (or lack of participation) in a given occupation?
8. What theoretical tenets make the model of human occupation different from other theoretical frameworks described in occupational therapy literature? Which tenets are similar to those associated with other frameworks discussed in this text?

Introduction

As noted previously in this text, theory is not static. It frequently goes through a process of change and refinement as a profession develops, knowledge increases, and clinical practice changes to meet the challenges of health care and rehabilitation. In occupational therapy one example of theory development lies within the model of human occupation. Since our discussion of occupational behavior in the first edition, this framework has evolved and changed to form the model of human occupation. Many constructs have been elaborated and more carefully integrated, and some have been given less importance or eliminated. This frame of reference draws on the work of literally hundreds of theorists, researchers and practitioners in attempting to describe how occupation furthers human well-being.

Definition

The model of human occupation, an outgrowth of the occupational behavior frame of reference, is described as a holistic model for practice, education and research. A highly eclectic model, it incorporates the views expressed by early occupational therapists and proponents of general system theory, with ideas from existential and humanistic psychology, ego pscyhology, cognitive theory, sociology, biology and social psychology. These ideas are combined to describe the nature of human occupation (also referred to as occupational behavior) as it develops and changes throughout the life span. The model emphasizes the occupational nature of the person as a system and the role of the environment in enabling and providing boundaries for human occupation. Human occupation guides the analysis of the system's (person's) function within the environment and influences evaluation and treatment strategies. The role of the occupational therapist is to identify the level of functional performance and to use occupations to develop the adaptive skills and behaviors needed for role performance. Varied evaluation instruments are used to identify occupational performance. The case method of problem-solving guides the analysis of evaluation data and influences treatment planning.[69,73]

Theoretical Development

Occupational Therapy Theory

Occupational Behavior and Mary Reilly

During the late 1960s and throughout the 1970s, occupational therapy theorists, educators and clinicians—many under the leadership of occupational therapist and educator Mary Reilly—emphasized the importance of occupation in one's life and in treatment and developed many of the occupational behavior views that continue to influence occupational therapy today. Through her work, Reilly encouraged the profession to adopt an occupational behavior paradigm. This paradigm emphasizes the biopsychosocial nature of function and the need for human achievement. She suggested that the paradigm become a framework, broader than that of the medical model and applicable for practice, education and research. This model of practice for occupational therapy addresses the healthy nature of a person as well as the problems and incapacities that result from illness.[110,111,112,113]

Reilly urges occupational therapists to focus on occupation as the means of promoting adaption and life satisfaction. She encourages therapists to use the patient's healthy behavior to solve functional problems that result from disease and developmental delay. During treatment, therapists should use healthy behavior and occupations to help patients explore and master their environment and learn to cope with their difficulties in daily living, work and leisure.[110,111,112,113]

These views reaffirm those of Meyer and Slagle, Barton, and Tracy, all founders of the profession. These earliest proponents of occupational therapy expressed their belief in the value of occupation; in the need for a balance of work, play, rest and sleep; and in the importance of sound habits.[10,39,40,41,42,47,95,96,119,120,123,128,129]

During the 1970s, the occupational behavior body of knowledge expanded as Reilly worked with graduate students to develop an understanding of biopsychosocial function and human achievement. During this process, the works of ego psychologist R.W. White, psychoanalyst and developmental psychologist Erik Erikson, and psychologist, personality theorist, educator and researcher David McClelland were used to support the concepts that form the theory of occupational behavior.

Model of Human Occupation

During the 1980s, occupational therapists worked diligently to build on the concepts of the occupational behavior theory. Of these therapists, Gary Keilhofner is most frequently recognized for his leadership in theoretical development and research. Originally, Kielhofner and his colleagues maintained the name, occupational behavior frame of reference, but later extended and refined the concepts to formulate what they called the model of human occupation. Today it may be referred to as *the model* or *MOHO*.

In the previous decade, therapists applied the model of human occupation in many of the specialty areas of practice, used it as the basis for research, and published numerous articles in the occupational therapy literature. A sample of these articles is cited and highlighted here to reflect frequent themes that emerge during the review of this literature.

The majority of MOHO literature describes research in the area of assessment instrument development.[11,16,20,21,54,58,60,61,81,82,106,131,132] The primary focus of these studies has been to identify validity and reliability standards for these assessments.

Other studies have examined program effectiveness, comparative group studies[8,9,43,45,60,61,76,87,122,123] and the model's application in practice. In practice, the model has acted as a framework for programs in community or institutional settings and for child through older adult populations with varied disabilities. It guides practice in physical disability, mental health, work hardening, pediatric, gerontology and developmental disability specialty areas of practice.[74,80,84,85]

Research Designs

Group comparison, correlation and single case studies are the more frequent research designs used to evaluate MOHO in practice arenas. Those with normal children, adolescents and adults are compared with persons of similar age with psychiatric diagnoses, psychophysiological problems, various medical diagnosis or chronic problems. These studies indicate that dysfunctional persons exhibit problems related to level of function, self-esteem, sense of control and activity patterns.

Program Outcome

When MOHO has been used to evaluate program effectiveness, the assessment instruments noted previously as well as multiple standardized assessments associated with physical medicine, education and psychology have been used to identify factors believed to contribute to occupational function and dysfunction. Parameters include the subjects' values, interests, goals, skills, roles, habits, locus of control, temporal orientation and physical and psychosocial abilities and the differences in quality of life before and after occupational therapy treatment. The outcomes of these studies describe the influence of the previously mentioned factors on level of function and dysfunction.

Summary of Occupational Therapy Theory

Of the areas of reseach identified, the majority of research studies focus on instrument development. As West[136] notes, instrument development and the implementation of studies with stronger research designs appear to be the current emphasis in MOHO research. Previous MOHO research has been criticized for its small sample size, lack of reliability and validity measures, nonrandom samples, and unsophisticated statistical procedures.[35] However, because of their focus on occupation, all the studies are believed to have contributed to the theory base of occupational therapy.[27]

System Theory, Behavioral and Social Science Influences

In much of MOHO research, occupational therapy literature as well as system theory, personality theory and behavioral and social science concepts, are frequently referenced. For this reason we briefly summarize the most influential of these studies. Those readers wishing a more in depth understanding are referred to the original works, which are cited in the reference list at the conclusion of this chapter.

System Theory

The term system theory may suggest a model as shown in Figure 6.1. This figure suggests

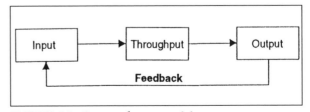

FIGURE 6.1   System theory model.

that human beings are like a machine or computer. Information comes into the system, **input**; is processed by the system, **throughput**; and transformed to become **output**, which produces information that comes back into the system, **feedback**. This model of man-as-machine, used by Heinz Werner[134,135] and Allen Newell and Herbert Simon,[100] fails to convey the complexity, spontaneity, willfulness, and ability for adaptation inherent in the person system.

A more encompassing system theory, general system theory, is described by biologist Ludwig von Bertalanffy.[130] General system theory is used to describe the dynamics of open systems such as the complex human system, which consists of multiple component parts or subsystems. These components have innumerable functional relationships that result from the system's constant interaction with the environment.

Von Bertalanffy distinguishes the open living system from the closed machine system. Open systems have energy for constant interaction with the environment and are able to take what they need from the system to function and change. Machines do not have this capability for control and self-regulation. Von Bertalanffy also recognizes that the open system (person) is a part of greater systems and interacts with them. The person has numerous component subsystems such as the musculoskeletal, digestive and neurological subsystems, while being part of such larger systems as the family, community and culture. All systems within the person and that make up his or her environments are in constant contact and are interdependent. Therefore, anything that affects the part will effect the whole.[130] According to Kielhofner,[70] "Open system thinking seeks to construct a more existential and humanistic view of persons . . ."

In its discussion of systems, the occupational behavior and human occupation literature most often refers to the open system constructs of von Bertalanffy. Ironically, however, MOHO literature usually represents the human system with a constrained or closed system figure similar to that used to depict a machine (Figure 6.2).

Ego Psychology and Developmental Literature

As in other theoretical frameworks in occupational therapy, the model of human occupation has been influenced by the knowledge advanced in the social sciences. In the model of human occupation, the views of R.W. White and David McClelland are[73] influential and are briefly highlighted here.

White. Before pursuing his interest in personality, Robert White taught history and government. Later, when working with Murray at Harvard and while teaching and doing research in psychology, White formed his views about personality and psychopathology. Based on his observations of psychotherapeutic interaction and from research he identified two types of motivation: 1) **effectance motivation**—the person's desire to use one's own actions to cause an effect and 2) **competence motivation**—the person's attempt to become competent through one's experiences.[91]

The need to explore and cause an effect has a biological basis and suggests that a person tries, in a sense, to create or discover challenge. This process can be thought of as the need to create tension and disequilibrium as opposed to desiring balance, equilibrium and tension reduction. Through exploration a person gains experience and knowledge, which helps him or her to perform competently in the environment and achieve a sense of competence. The need to continually explore and become more competent is felt to be innate, or biological, in origin and differs from the other biologic needs that might motivate behavior. These needs evolve and are expressed throughout life, initially through exploration, play and make believe and later, in adolescent and adult behavior, as work and productivity.

McClelland. David C. McClelland has dedicated his career to teaching and research on personality development and more recently the application of his theory of personality in underdeveloped countries. His work focused on the thoughts or cognitions that precede an individual's decision to engage in activity.[91,99]

McClelland offers a rather unusual view of behavior. Although not a simple theory, its core can be simply stated as follows. People desire or crave small amounts of unpredictability in order to offset boredom, but they try to avoid large amounts of unpredictability (which would be perceived as threatening).[91,99]

McClelland describes three factors that influence function and personality development: motive, trait and schemata. A **motive** is "a state of mind aroused by some stimulus situation that signals an imminent change that will be either pleasant or unpleasant."[91,99] McClelland assumes that the person will act either to increase pleasure or to avoid the anticipated unpleasant change. When the person anticipates pleasure, an approach motive exists; when he or she anticipates an unpleasant change, an avoidance motive exists.[91,99] These motives correspond to a person's multiple needs. McClelland has emphasized the needs of achievement, affiliation and power. Each of

these needs may increase the likelihood of an approach or avoidance response.[91,99] For example, in social situations the person who has a need for affiliation may be motivated to approach or participate in situations he or she anticipates will facilitate involvement with others. Those who wish to avoid affiliation may withdraw in social situations or avoid going to events expected to require social interaction. Approach and avoidance responses for achievement are referred to as need for achievement or fear of failure.

McClelland does not address the development cycle per se. Through their history of experiences, however, individuals come to expect particular outcomes. If the outcome expected corresponds to the actual event and is positive, the person will have a pleasant feeling and approach similar experiences in the future. If the outcome expected is very different from the actual experience or is unpleasant, the person may experience anxiety and avoid similar situations. The person's thoughts and experience can produce tension. Too much tension can cause a person to avoid the situation; not enough tension can cause a per-

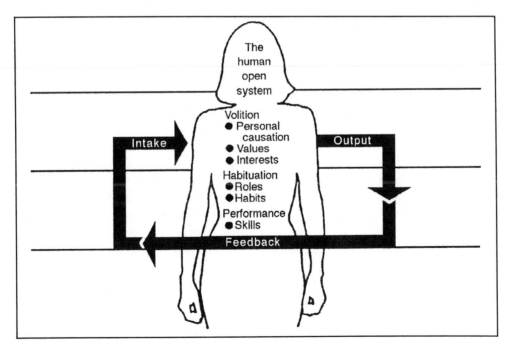

FIGURE 6.2   From Kielhofner G (Ed.): *A Model of Human Occupation.* Baltimore, Williams & Wilkins, 1985. Reprinted with permission.

son to lose interest in the situation; adequate tension motivates the person to act.[91,99] Over time a pattern of thoughts and behaviors develops that may reflect approach and avoidance motives. This motivational pattern gives direction in one's life. **Approach motives** indicate the anticipation of success and lead to planned task behavior, which can produce effective, efficient outcomes and a sense of satisfaction. **Avoidance motives** usually emphasize the barriers to goal achievement and emphasize threats in the environment. They can yield ineffective, inefficient or obsessive thoughts and behaviors; passivity; or a sense of threat or dissatisfaction.[91]

McClelland, unlike other personality theorists, distinguishes between intentional and habitual functioning. **Intentional functioning** is goal-directed behavior and may cause a person to do something they have not tried before. **Habits** are consistent ways of behaving in particular circumstances and are learned through repetition. They are not the result of conscious planning. McClelland calls a collection of habits a **trait**. A trait is a "learned tendency in persons to react as they have reacted more or less successfully in the past in similar situations when similarly motivated."[91,99] Traits differ from motives. Traits are not goal directed; motives are traits and habits influenced by consistent rewards; motives are not. Traits explain habitual functioning; motives explain intentional functioning. A cluster of traits make up a **role**.[91,99]

The third element of personality suggested by McClelland is the schema. The **schema** is a cognitive unit that symbolizes past experience. Schemata house one's values, ideas and social roles, and thereby provide a guide for living and boundaries for the possibilities in one's life. According to McClelland, ideas and values concern primarily economic, aesthetic, social, political, religious and theoretic realms.[91,99] Social roles, previously identified by Linton,[89] are age, sex, family position, occupation and group member roles.[91,99]

In summary, McClelland's writing emphasizes the importance of expectancy in behavior

as the person anticipates what lies ahead. As such it is a highly cognitive, if eclectic, approach to understanding behavior. Although not described here, his work also provides guidelines for measuring the previously noted constructs in order to operationalize them. The reader is referred to the original sources for research approaches and the standard assessments used in these studies.

Erikson. MOHO theorists also frequently reference Erikson's psychosocial developmental theory (see Chapter 5).

Current Practice in Occupational Therapy

As noted, occupational therapy publications reflect a broad application of the model of human occupation,[2,22,30,44,49,50,51,86,88,90,101,103,108,117,121,124,127] suggesting that the model is being used as the theorists intended, as a generic frame of reference for practice. This chapter, however, focuses on the model's application in adult psychiatry.

The Person and Behavior

The person is an open system that interacts with the environment through a cybernetic process or cycle of intake, throughput, output and feedback.

People, objects and situations in the environment or the person's needs and inner tensions produce the stimuli that become **intake**. The term intake is used instead of input, states Kielhofner,[70] to indicate that the organism actively seeks and take in information and is not just a passive recipient. This information is then transformed during *throughput*. During throughput the person uses his or her personal interests, goals and beliefs to evaluate stimuli. After these stimuli are evaluated, the person uses personal skills and habits to respond to input. These interactions (throughput) allow the system to function, thereby maintaining the system and producing new skills. They come together to produce new information and actions, *output*. This output returns to the system as *feedback* and new input. Then the cycle begins again and the system maintains itself through its own actions.[62,64-66,68,70,77-79,83,114]

Occupational Behavior

Output is identified in the literature as occupational behavior and is the primary concern of occupational therapy. **Occupational behavior** has varied definitions, which collectively are described as work, play and self-care activities.[3,25,62,67,73,80,137]

Although definitions of occupational behavior vary, they all identify occupation as follows: 1) a consciously motivated action rather than one that might be conceived as unconsciously motivated; 2) an observable action rather than one with thinking, feeling or reflecting emphasis; 3) an organized rather than a random activity; and 4) an action that is constructive or positive and brings satisfaction to the self. Therefore, activity that brings the self into discredit with others (e.g., intentionally destructive behavior) would presumably not be occupation.

In publications since 1985, the construct of occupation maintains the previous emphases and adds three others: 1) occupation is any activity during waking hours; 2) occupation reflects individual differences based on the person's beliefs, values, and experiences over time; and 3) occupational activities form one's life routines.[73,80]

Hierarchy of Subsystems

The person as an open system has three subsystems, which are arranged in a hierarchy and influenced by the cybernetic cycle. The volition, habituation and performance subsystems interact and determine how the system functions in the environment. Their interrelationship reflects the throughput of the dynamic cycle. This cycle maintains the person system or changes the system.[104,105] According to MOHO theorists, each of the subsystems is responsible for a different aspect of occupational behavior.

Volition Subsystem

At the top of the hierarchy is the **volition subsystem**. It is responsible for motivating behavior and for choosing what behavior will be pursued.

Motivation

The view that motivation for human behavior is the innate need for the person to explore and master the environment is influenced by the views of Berlyn, White, and DeCharms.[13]

Berlyne[13] believes that the person engages in activity for its own sake, experiences pleasurable conflict and arousal when he or she encounters the environment, and seeks activity that meets personal interests.

R.W. White states that the individual has urges for activity of all kinds and that the ego gains satisfaction from exploration and competence, thereby serving as a motivation for the person to encounter the world. White is described by Hall and Lindzey[52,53] as a neo-Freudian ego psychologist. An ego psychologist does not deny the basic Freudian constructs of id-ego-superego, but chooses to focus on the autonomy of the ego in its ability to consciously determine avenues of exploration and to gain (for the individual) conscious satisfaction in personal accomplishments.[52] See articles by White in Recommended Reading List.

DeCharms[37] proposes that the individual's primary motivation is to be effective and produce change in the environment.

We remind the reader that in MOHO the motivation or energizing component for human behavior is the innate need for the person to explore and master the environment.[24,80] This view of motivation is influenced by the views of Berlyne,[13] White, and DeCharms. Also referred to in the literature and slightly different in scope is the idea that the individual needs to have purpose or meaning in life. Basic survival needs are not denied, but the individual's striving to be creative, to move toward greater complexity and self-enhancement, is emphasized.[71]

Using the ability to think symbolically and imaginatively, the person creates a picture of what he or she is capable of accomplishing and is able to consciously choose what actions to take. As the decision maker, the volition subsystem can be called the highest and ruling subsystem in behavior.[80]

Much of conscious thought, as it pertains to decision making relates to values, interests and beliefs, all of which are paid special attention in this framework.

Values are defined as "images of what is good, right and/or important"[80] and further as "commitments to performing in 'culturally sanctioned ways."[80] Values influence the person's use of time, choice of activities, priorities established and standards of performance. Although values have a personal component (e.g., people will value what they believe will help them achieve personal meaning and satisfy personal standards), they are also strongly influenced by society (e.g., the person will value what his or her society values).

One component of values consistently noted is that of **temporal orientation**, or the person's ability to see himself or herself as a potent player in past, present or future time. Being unable to project the self into future endeavors, or course, interferes with occupational goal setting.

Personal causation refers to to the individual's belief in his or her ability to succeed, to meet life challenges, to be in control, and to be responsible for his or her own emotional wellbeing.[80,105] It is important for the person to feel in control of events and others to some degree, but the individual also needs to understand that some things are outside of one's control.

Interests are the individual's propensity to enjoy specific occupations and also helps to establish priorities for activity participation.

Habituation Subsystem

In the middle of the hierarchy is the **habituation subsystem**. This component houses the habits and roles for the person's daily routine. Habits should help to organize behavior so that it is "expected and valued in the environment in which it is to be performed."[80] Habits and roles help to maintain the system, can provide support for adaptation to varied environments, and, when automatic, can release energy for growth and development and intentional pursuits.[80]

For example, an adult's routine of personal hygiene, grooming, and preparing and eating breakfast in the morning when done automatically may require a minimum expenditure of energy. Therefore, energy is available to simultaneously eat and read the newspaper, or to listen to the news and plan the day's schedule. When the person becomes depressed or physically disabled, however, he or she may now need to consciously use much energy in deciding what to wear or may need to mobilize energy to pay attention to safety issues while grooming and preparing breakfast. When the energy required to complete daily routines is increased, the energy within the system is dispersed differently or less energy may be available for intentional pursuits, growth and development, and role responsibilities. This change often leads to a loss of balance in habits, roles and occupational performance.

Roles

Roles are also part of the habituation system. As a person forms habits or patterns of behavior, he or she internalizes expectations that come from society or from within the self. These internal and external behavioral expectations provide the guidelines for one's roles in society. A **role** is a position in society that has a set of expectations, responsibilities and

TABLE 6.1   ATTRIBUTES OF ROLES

1. Roles prescribe the use of time.
2. Roles provide the standards for behavior and competence.
3. Roles change over time throughout the life span.
4. Roles are learned through socialization.
5. A person's history of role performance influences the individual success in roles.
6. Failure to internalize roles results in maladaptation.
7. Conflict or inconsistency of roles results in maladaptation.
8. Conflict between internalized roles and one's values, interests, and personal causation can result in maladaptation.

These beliefs are drawn from the views of Barris et al[3] and Oakley et al.[104,105]

privileges. Roles contribute to a person's self-identity and guide one's behavior at home, work or in the community.[55,80]

The MOHO theorist believes that there should be a balance of roles and that one needs an "optimal number of appropriate roles,"[80] presumably to structure time and to ensure that purpose in life is achieved. An outline of the general characteristics of roles is provided in Table 6.1.

Three broad classes of roles generally interact: personal-sexual, familial, and occupational. Initially, the occupational role was felt to be the primary concern in occupational therapy.[3,80] More recently, however, MOHO writing acknowledges that a role may have multiple dimensions that include any combination of personal-sexual, familial and occupational roles. A taxonomy of occupational roles frequently identified in the literature is listed in Table 6.2.

MOHO theorists describe two negative roles: the sick role and the invalid role. These roles are seen as deviant roles that may be assumed when a person is ill or permanently disabled. They are in conflict with the rehabilitation goals of increasing independence and productivity in society. Persons assuming a **sick role** usually respond passively and allow health care personnel to be responsible for their well-being. When in an **invalid role**, the person is predominantly ascribed a helpless,

worthless status.[80] This status is frequently a symptom of psychosocial problems and, in particular, a symptom of depression.

Performance Subsystem

At the bottom of the hierarchy is the **performance subsystem**, which includes the skills for producing occupational (purposeful) behavior. The performance subsystem is that "most directly linked to output of the system."[80] Performance skills are placed in one of three categories: 1) perceptual-motor skills, which enable the person to receive and interpret sensory information and produce a motor response; 2) process skills used to plan and problem solve; and 3) communication skills, which are used for interaction with others.[80] Creating a treatment environment in which skills can be developed or enhanced is the treatment priority in this frame of reference. Table 6.3 provides a summary of the elements that contribute to each of the three subsystems.

Resonation

The volition, habituation and performance subsytems do not interact in a linear manner to produce a cause and effect reaction. Rather, there is a complex interaction of physical, psychosocial and environmental forces. When a change occurs in one part of any system, the whole organism is affected. For example, when a person experiences an environmental change such as losing one's job, he or she may become depressed, which can have multiple effects, in-

TABLE 6.2   OCCUPATIONAL ROLE TAXONOMY

1. Participant in an organization
2. Hobbyist/amateur
3. Friend
4. Family member
5. Care giver
6. Home maintainer
7. Student
8. Religious participant
9. Worker
10. Volunteer

The roles listed are described in Barris[3] and Kielhofner and Burke.[80]

cluding a loss of weight or a diminution of social relationships. MOHO theorists call this interaction of forces, **resonation**.[70,98] This term is probably equivalent to the dynamic interaction described by other system theorists.

According to MOHO theorists, during resonation one subsystem can be controlled or constrained by another subsystem.[70,71] For example, a person may become physically deconditioned (a deficit in the performance subsystem) when he or she stops daily jogging (a habit) because his or her depression intereferes with motivation (volition). In this example, the performance subsystem is held back by the ha-

TABLE 6.3   SUBSYSTEMS OF OPEN SYSTEM

Subsystem–Elements		Examples
V O L I T I O N	Personal Causation	Self knowledge
		Belief in personal control (internal control)
		Belief in one's abilities
		Belief in ability to succeed
		Belief in own effectiveness in environment
	Values	Beliefs (images of worth, importance, righteousness and purpose)
		Personal standards of performance
		Society's standards
		Sense and use of time
H A B I T U A T I O N	Interests	Sources of pleasure and satisfaction
		Degree of like or dislike of an activity
		A pattern of activity based on experience
	Habits	Typical (routine) behavior
		A style or pattern of behavior
		Typical use of skills and time
		Organization of skills and time
		Ability to adapt routine to environmental change
	Role	A person's position in a social group
		A person's responsibilities in a social position
		Person's belief that he/she has social position and responsibilities
		Society's expectations of a person ascribed a social position
		Personal and societal expectations that guide behavior
P E R F O R M A N C E	Perceptual-motor Skills	Reception of sensations
		Interpretation of sensations
		A motor response to sensations
	Communication- Interaction Skills	Send information to others in varied contexts
		Understand information from others (verbal and nonverbal)
		Ability to work cooperatively with others
		Ability to compete with others
	Process Skills	Ability to organize
		Ability to plan
		Ability to problem solve

Adapted from descriptions of the subsystems in Kielhofner G, Burke J: *Components and determinants of human occupation*. In Kielhofner G (Ed.): *Model of Human Occupation*, Baltimore, Williams and Wilkins, 1985, and in Kielhofner G: *FOCUS, MD*, American Occupational Therapy Association, 1988.

bituation and volition subsystems. Habituation and volition (the two higher levels) may also be constrained by the performance subsystem. For example, the person may be motivated to jog and wish to continue a daily routine of jogging but is unable to do so because of a physical disability that limits motor skills or endurance.

Person Environment Interaction

The person system may be intrinsically motivated to act but does not function within a vacuum. An important component in understanding occupation relates to recognizing the role of the environment in making available certain choices, providing boundaries, sanctioning behavior, and helping to structure the use of time. The interaction between the person and his or her environment is influenced particularly by the individual's level of arousal within the environment.

Arousal is both physical and subjective; it results from physiological output (e.g., a rapid pulse rate) as well as from feelings of excitement relative to present or past experiences. The level of arousal is influenced by the physical setting, the person's view of the environment, and the likelihood that both of these can meet a person's need for novelty. The level of arousal will determine if the person makes choices to participate in or adapt to the environment or to avoid and escape specific situations.[6]

Once the individual is aroused and involved in the environment, he or she decides if what is available is compatible with personal values and interests. The degree to which the individual senses that personal values and interests are in accord with what is offered determines the likelihood of his or her investment in activity.[6]

Feedback from the Environment as Press

Press refers to "environmental expectations for certain behavior."[6] When the individual recognizes the press of specific environments, he or she has initial information plus ongoing feedback about what behavior is expected. Press can influence the person's behavior and thereby influence the person's ability to adapt, become competent or change. Press can also influence the skills, habits, interests and values that the person acquires.[6]

The construct of press is reminiscent of the work of Murray, as presented in his personality theory, which he termed personology. As summarized by Hall and Lindzey,[52] to Murray press represented the "effective or significant determinants of behavior in the environment. In simplest terms, a press is a property or attribute of an environmental object or person which facilitates or impedes the efforts of the individual to reach a given goal."[52]

Murray, generally viewed as Freudian, placed importance on unconscious motivation in behavior. It was Murray that developed the Thematic Apperception Test (TAT), a commonly used projective instrument.

To illustrate, the lonely, cold environment of the homeless requires that these persons change or adapt typical patterns of daily living to survive. The active professional who experiences a traumatic head injury will need to evaluate the compatibility of compromised abilities and skills with those behaviors expected as a part of his or her previous lifestyle. Both the homeless person and the injured executive must first recognize the behaviors expected and then match behaviors to expectations. Both may need to meet familiar environmental demands with a compromised status (physical, psychosocial, economic or cultural).

Environmental Hierarchy

In MOHO theory, the environment consists of a hierarchy of four layers; from bottom to top these levels are materials and objects, tasks, social groups and organizations and culture.[6] See Table 6.4 for a view of the MOHO environ-

TABLE 6.4 ENVIRONMENTAL HIERARCHY

Objects	The availability, complexity, flexibility and meaningfulness of objects promotes arousal and contributes to press in the environment.
Tasks	The complexity, temporal boundaries, rules, playfulness or seriousness and social aspects of tasks influence arousal and environmental press.
Social Groups Organizations	The size, function, permeability and structural complexity of groups and organizations influence arousal and environment press.
Culture	The nature of work and play, space and time, and the transmission of knowledge and values arouse a person and influence environment press.

mental hierarchy which is adapted from Barris et al.[6]

Person-Environment Interaction

The individual typically interacts within many different environments, each having its own associated objects, tasks and social structures. While participating in these environments, the

In the social science literature, Uri Bronfenbrenner[23] describes an ecological theory that depicts the interaction between individuals and their multilevel environment. Bronfenbrenner's four levels describe 1) activities, roles and relationships in the immediate setting; 2) the person's interactions in the varied environments of home, school, work and neighborhood; 3) the governmental, health care and legal settings that influence a person's life; and 4) the cultural and subcultural factors such as attitudes, beliefs and ideologies that have environmental interaction. This theory has been used in research and clinical practice.

person practices skills, develops a sense of time, establishes a pattern of habits, and becomes aware of personal abilities and limits. Through interactions, the person learns to find and use resources in the environment and establishes standards of task performance. The use of skills, habits, time and resources promotes flexibility and effective responses to change.[6] For example, during a given day an adolescent must be flexible to be competent and comfortable in a variety of environments: interacting with peers and teachers, practicing soccer after school in the neighborhood, sharing in cleanup after dinner, doing homework, and then relaxing in front of the television.

Function and Dysfunction

Health as Performance

In contrast to the traditional view of health as the absence of illness or disease, **health** in MOHO theory is the degree to which the physical, psychosocial and environmental elements of the system work together for functioning within the boundaries of health, disease or disability. The presence of a psychiatric diagnosis or label does not tell anything about the extent of occupational function or dysfunction (although as we shall see, in discussions of patient treatment, diagnoses seem to be used to guide the process). In the face of disease and disability, the system tries to maintain a balance of occupations and maintain the well-being of the system. This process is similar to a concept in organismic theory, which suggests that the organism will do the best it can to maintain balance and equilibrium.

The person uses personal resources (such as knowledge, skills and habits) to adapt and thereby meet the expectations of the community, maintain personal integrity, participate in the culture and contribute to society. The person's ability to adapt is reflected in occupational performance.[38,72]

TABLE 6.5   FUNCTION-DYSFUNCTION CONTINUM

Achievement	Competence	Exploration	Inefficacy	Incompetence	Helplessness
Actively involved in the environment; has established standards of performance; meets standards; assumes varied roles.	Strive to improve to meet "press"; mastery of skills; formation of habits.	Search for new experiences in safe and unfamiliar environments; investigation results in new skills.	Decreased function; dissatisfaction with performance; decreased sense of control; changes in interests, values, roles and habits.	No routine; not consistently follow a routine; sense of loss of control; poor skill, habit and role performance; decreased interests and values.	Inadequate, poor or no function; few or no interests; few roles; few or disorganized habits; inadequate skills.

Adapted from Kielhofner G: *Occupational function and dysfunction.* In Kielhofner G (Ed.): *Model of Human Occupation.* Baltimore, Williams & Wilkins, 1985, pp. 63–75.

Occupational Performance Continuum

In earlier MOHO literature, a person's functional status was described as order or disorder. **Order** connotes a status of health and competent performance of daily living, work and play tasks. **Disorder** is the inability to perform occupationally, decreased or absent role performance, and inability to meet role responsibilities.[3] These dichotomies of performance have evolved into the occupational performance continuum.

The occupational function-dysfunction continuum, based on the work of Reilly, is expanded and refined to include six performance steps: achievement, competence, exploration, inefficacy, incompetence and helplessness (Table 6.5). The person may slide along this continuum throughout the life span. This mobility suggests the flexibility and changing nature of the system's performance due to the dynamic process of the person-environment interaction.

Occupational Function

Occupational function is reflected in the system's ability to take the initiative to explore, achieve and compete in the environment.† By exploring the environment, the individual becomes aware of the expectations of others and one's own abilities and learns and refines the

skills needed for competence and role fulfillment—occupational behavior flourishes. Throughout life, a person moves along this functional continuum as he or she develops and changes. It is as if there is a continuous cycle of exploring the environment, making choices, striving for competence to meet the demand of life's tasks and then achieving mastery. Then the cycle begins anew. The outcome of this cycle is a renewed sense of purpose, an enhanced system of values, a repertoire of interests, and skills and habits that support a balance of roles and responsibilities.[72]

Occupational Dysfunction

On the negative side of the continuum is **occupational dysfunction**, which is reflected in inefficient, incompetent occupational performance.† Dysfunction exists when a person is unable to meet the expectations of daily life, does not have work or leisure pursuits, is dissatisfied with his or her performance, or looses the sense of well-being and efficacy. A continued sense of inefficiency may lead to a further decrease in skill performance, a further breakdown in habits and a sense of incompetence. Continued incompetence may result in a helpless state in which skills, habits and roles may be absent or grossly inadequate for adaptation. In all levels of dysfunction, skills, habits, val-

---

[1]One assumes the openness of the system in its reaching out to the environment and remaining accessible to feedback. Openness of the system in this framework, however, is defined in terms of a continuous adequate output (performance).

[2]Although dysfunction is demonstrated in output, it certainly suggests a closing of the system, including either a breakdown in the intake and throughput processes, or in feedback or some portions of all of these.

ues, interests and roles may be disrupted to some degree. This disruption reflects the interactive nature of the elements of the human system as it grows and changes throughout the life span.[72]

In mental health settings, patients' psychosocial problems are manifested by a change in occupational function. Patients may have stopped working, ceased caring for their homes and families, lost interest in daily life, have an inbalance of work, leisure and self-care pursuits, or may express the sentiment that life has no purpose or meaning. They are often unable to identify resources for solving problems and coping, have few or no interests and may be unable to identify realistic goals. Additionally, patients may have a limited repertoire of skills and habits, or they may be unable to use their skills effectively to satisfy personal needs and role responsibilities. Table 6.6 presents an outline of occupational dysfunctions frequently seen in psychosocial settings.[6,7]

Function and Dysfunction Relative to the Life Span

As noted earlier, MOHO theory considers the development of a person as a lifetime process and one of continual adaptation, not as a process in which the personality or abilities are established during childhood or by young adulthood. The theory's position is compatible with theories of development discussed elsewhere in this text and emphasizes the system's ability to perform tasks, build habits and fulfill roles.

During the life span, occupational behavior develops as a result of physical, psychosocial, cultural, cognitive and spiritual changes. These life changes may motivate or frustrate the system and thus require the system to learn, relearn, adapt or change to achieve or maintain an adequate level of function. Occupational behavior may or may not develop in a smooth progression. However, the progression is hierarchical and the time required to ascend the hierarchy is lengthened as the person strives to achieve higher levels of occupational function.[75] In other words, it may take longer to formulate one's values and master multiple role responsibilities than to acquire perceptual motor skills or form habits.

The continuum of occupational development begins with play and expands to work, with the ideal being a balance of work and play. The emphasis on work or play/leisure

TABLE 6.6   OCCUPATIONAL DYSFUNCTION

Open System Dysfunction	Interruption of basic cycle; output shows extremes in activity or inactivity.
Decreased Intrinsic Motivation	Decreased interest and involvement in occupation. This leads to sense of failure, self-doubt, and inefficacy. Patient feels lack of control and life lacks meaning.
Decreased Decision Making	Decreased interests, interest and value conflicts, and a sense of meaninglessness, which leads to increased stress and despair, decreased performance, and diminished satisfaction in occupation.
Role Dysfunction	Loss or change in role, or role stress. These result in decreased need satisfaction, lack of skill, poor time management, or inability to meet social expectations.
Temporal Dysfunction	Poor perception and conception of time, a decreased sense of the future; being "stuck in time" and exhibiting poor management of time.
Disorder in Environmental Interactions	Conflict between the patient's ability and environmental expectations; decreased opportunity for occupation and less control over one's life. Learned helplessness as an outcome of institutionalization.
Disorder of Performance Components	Decrease or poor social, process, perceptual motor and problem solving skills; inability to anticipate consequences, organize or sequence behavior.

Adapted from Barris R, Kielhofner G, Watts J: *Psychosocial Occupational Therapy—Practice in a Pluralistic Arena.* Laurel, Maryland, Ramsco Publishing, 1983, pp. 218–226; Barris R, Kielhofner G, Neville A, et al: *Psychosocial Dysfunction.* In Kielhofner G (Ed.): *A Model of Human Occupation.* Baltimore, Williams & Wilkins, 1985, pp. 248–305.

throughout the life span is influenced by cultural expectations. This balance changes throughout the life span (e.g., the child's day is initially monopolized by play activities and later school, and the adult, world is dominated by work).

Initially, as noted by Reilly in 1974, the balance of work and play was believed to represent the norm or degree of health of the person system.[69,113] More recently, MOHO theorists suggest that the balance indicates an adaptive response in which the person is fulfilling personal needs (particularly those for exploration and mastery) and is meeting the expectations of the environment. This view of an adaptive response is more compatible with the adult developmental theory that views the person, including one with a disability, as able to develop throughout the life span.[75]

Periods of Occupational Development

As with other life span theories, the developmental periods for occupational development include childhood (early, middle and late), adolescence, early and middle adulthood and later adulthood. The occupational milestones described in the literature are influenced by the tasks described in Erickson's developmental stages. (See chapter 5 of this text for a summary of these periods.) A summary of occupational development is outlined in Table 6.7.

Childhood. During childhood, the volition, habituation and performance subsystems evolve and are differentiated through the process of play. During play and through the child's interaction with the environment, he or she gains a sense of autonomy, develops adequate skills for daily living, assumes a family role and prepares for the role of student.[102]

Adolescence. As the adolescent interacts in the environment, he or she develops a personal identity and continues to acquire and refine skills and habits. During this time, adolescents have the opportunity to increase the number of roles assumed (e.g., son/daughter,

TABLE 6.7   OCCUPATIONAL DEVELOPMENT

Period	Occupation	Outcome
Childhood Early Middle Late	Play	Subsystems evolve and differentiate Autonomy ADL skills Family role Role of student
Adolescence	Environmental Interaction	Personal identity Refine skills Acquire and refine habits Increase roles Define and develop interest, abilities and values Explore occupations Choose an occupation Begin pursuit of occupation
Adulthood Early Middle Late	Career and Work	Pursue a career Establish and maintain work skills Manage multiple responsibilities Establish and maintain a life-style with work, home and community occupations Personal achievement Economic gain Contribute to society Mentor role Change work focus to meet developmental needs

friend, student) and explore potential occupations.[4]

The adolescent's choice of occupation brings together his or her interests, capabilities and values. After making an occupational choice, the adolescent explores career options. Once his or her choice is confirmed, he or she pursues a career and ultimately specializes in a particular field. This three-step process of exploration, choice and pursuit may be repeated throughout the life span, for example, in middle or later adulthood. Each person varies in the number of times they initiate the occupational choice sequence and in the amount of time used to complete the previously described sequence.[4,14,15,48,107,125]

Adulthood. During the three periods of adulthood (early, middle and late), many changes occur that influence one's occupational life-style. This life-style is framed by the adult's career choice and work experiences. His or her lifestyle is the outcome of daily interactions in the environments of work, home and community. Through work, adults can gain a sense of personal achievement, make economic gains, and can contribute to society. Adults also become mentors to future generations.[5] The adult manages work roles and family and community responsibilities as he or she pursues interests, forms values and manages time. The pattern of occupational growth during adult life is typified by three periods: 1) an early period for establishing work skills, pursuing work goals and achieving a sense of accomplishment; 2) a middle period of evaluating one's achievements and the meaning of work in life; and 3) a late period that may bring a change in work focus as well as a continued need for stimulation and an active life-style. Thus occupational behavior may be reflected in work or leisure pursuits, depending on the individual's needs and interests.[5,116]

Summary of Occupational Development. Changing personal and societal expectations for performance are associated with the developmental stages within the life span. These expectations help to define what will be viewed as functional and dysfunctional occupational behavior.

Role of the Occupational Therapist

In the model of human occupation, the role of the occupational therapist is diverse and should complement and supplement the roles of other health professionals in the treatment setting. The therapist is primarily responsible for evaluating the occupational performance of patients and for planning interventions that provide opportunities for the individual to succeed in the environment, to strengthen needed skills, to enhance feelings of personal control and to restore the balance among occupational components.[7] Within this role, the therapist monitors occupational function and gives patients feedback regarding their performance. The therapist may confront maladaptive behavior, or relate past to current events in a safe context. In pursuit of enhancing occupational function, the occupational therapist may take on other specialized roles: role model, teacher, counselor, supervisor, coach, player, craftsman, environmental manager, and co-problem solver.

Mentor or Role Model

The therapist may be a mentor and role model and thereby encourage patients to explore the environment and play or participate in the doing experience.[7] The occupational therapist can, for instance, demonstrate new roles for patients to practice and give them feedback regarding the effectiveness of their role behavior. During therapy the therapist may demonstrate effective methods of problem-solving, which patients can practice. These as well as many other treatment experiences provide opportunities for the patient to mimic behaviors that he or she observes.

Teacher

As a teacher, the therapist may provide instruction relative to specific skills (e.g., managing stress, managing time). In giving the individual feedback regarding occupational performance or providing specific instruction, the therapist educates the patient about the effects of his or her illness on performance, how to manage symptoms, or how to cope with disability.

Counselor

The occupational therapist who endorses the MOHO may provide varied types of counseling. Occupational choice, leisure and time management counseling are described in the literature.

The goal of **occupational choice counseling** is to help the patient identify and choose activities for fulfilling occupational roles. Making occupational choices is a developmental process that follows a progression: 1) fantasy period, 2) tentative period, and 3) realistic period,[3] Through fantasy and reappraisal, the patient identifies the pleasant aspects of an occupation. Then he or she evaluates more realistically the ability of an occupation to meet personal and societal needs. Finally, the person selects an occupational role.

During **leisure counseling,** the patient and therapist identify values and leisure interests and plan time for furture leisure pursuits.[3] Usually, this counseling occurs within the context of helping the patient to establish a balance between daily living, work and leisure occupations. In some settings, the therapeutic recreation specialist assumes this role.

When counseling in the area of **time management**, the therapist focuses on the patient's view and use of time. Together the therapist and patient identify the following: 1) the amount of patient time spent in work, play, and self-care activities; 2) his or her satisfaction with the use of time; 3) the changes that need to occur in present activities; and 4) the way time will need to be used to accomplish present and future goals.[3,69]

Environmental Manager

As an **environmental manager** the therapist promotes a healthy atmosphere in which the patient can use his or her abilities and strengths and develop skills needed for successful occupation. During treatment, the therapist conveys an attitude of respect for the patient; acknowledges his or her abilities and capabilities; identifies behavioral expectations; and communicates the value of varied work, self-care and leisure activities. These activities are seen as ends within themselves and the means to elicit growth, change and learning. If necessary, the therapist may increase or decrease structure within the treatment setting and make available necessary resources.[3]

Purposeful Activity

Purposeful activity is usually identified as occupation in the human occupation framework. Occupations are used in group or individual treatment contexts. Examples of those described in the literature include daily living tasks (e.g., cooking and grooming), values clarification activities, sports, crafts, time management exercises, social skills training, problem-solving experiences, activities using creative and expressive media (e.g., art and music), community outings/visits, and work tasks. As in other frameworks, MOHO theorists suggest that activities should be graded from simple to complex, less demanding to more demanding, in order to enhance successful performance and promote feelings of competence.

Activities are often used to produce an end product and achieve a performance goal. This goal was the exclusive role of activity in earlier occupational behavior literature, which indicated that occupational therapy is "the time and place for performance where negative feelings are tolerated and controlled while the person works toward the positive feelings of accomplishment, satisfaction, control and self worth."[3] More recent MOHO literature proposes that the processing of activity with the patient can be useful in providing feedback to the patient regarding his or her occupational performance.[7]

Theoretical Assumptions

The following theoretical assumptions are adapted from the information in the model of human occupation as it relates to psychosocial occupational therapy.

1. Throughout life, the person system undergoes physical, psychosocial, cultural, cognitive and spiritual change. This change can either motivate or frustrate the person system, thereby either impeding or facilitating occupational performance.
2. This change occurs in a process that is both developmental and hierarchical.
3. Overall, a person's life moves on a path toward greater self-enhancement while maintaining a balance and meeting societal expectation.
4. The unique role for occupational therapy is derived from the occupational nature of the person system.
5. Occupational function depends on interaction of the volition, habituation and performance subsystems to maintain health and facilitate adaptation.
6. Occupational dysfunction may be expressed as any one or more of the following: change in occupational behavior (decrease, inadequate performance, cessation); participation in meaningless activities or activities inadequate in number to satisfy needs and interests; imbalance in habits, roles or activities of daily living, work and/or leisure; failure to meet role expectation or satisfy the established norm of the culture.
7. At all levels of dysfunction, there is some disruption or imbalance of skills, habits, values, interests and roles.
8. Whatever the treatment setting, the objects, tasks, social organization and culture must be considered and integrated into evaluation and treatment experiences.
9. Occupations are used to normalize function, restore balance, promote adaptation, and facilitate normal growth and development throughout the life span.

10. The treatment environment should provide clear, consistent, and functional expectations within a specific time frame. This predictable setting provides an opportunity to develop a routine and habits and to practice role behavior.
11. A group context for treatment provides an opportunity for identifying roles and assuming role responsibilities.
12. Previous interests and skills are incorporated into treatment experiences, with graded activities taking into account the existence of functional performance skills.
13. Feedback is the outcome of the person-environment interaction and maintains the system's health and integrity.
14. Occupations are used to develop skills and their constituents.
15. The case analysis method is an effective means for organizing assessment data and planning treatment interventions.

Evaluation

In the model of human occupation, the therapist evaluates occupational function to form a picture of the whole person—his or her function in daily activities, work and leisure. To establish the level of function, the therapist evaluates the interactions of the elements (subsystems) of the person system and the system's effectiveness in the environment. Analysis of these dynamic interactions can identify the multidimensional aspects of the person's disability and abilities and help to contrast the person's level of function with that which is typically considered normal for a particular stage of development.

Given the basis of system theory as a theoretical construct, it would seem that the therapist would be trying to identify the openness of the system or its ability to take from the environment what it needs, although this process is not detailed in the MOHO literature. One must also evaluate the system's flexibility or ability to respond effectively and efficiently to environmental demands (press), as well as the system's success in using feedback to maintain the system and produce a satisfactory outcome.

Occupational Analysis

Occupational analysis is a function of assessment that strives to elucidate the characteristics of a particular activity in light of the model of human occupation as presented. During occupational analysis, the therapist 1) monitors the environment to identify how individuals, groups, tasks, objects and culture produce press; 2) evaluates how a given occupation can promote a sense of purpose and help to identify one's values and interests; 3) anticipates how the occupation contributes to habit formation and the fulfillment of role responsibilities; 4) considers the performance skills required to engage in the occupation; and 5) evaluates the relationship between one's work, play and daily living tasks.[33] Occupational analysis is similar to what has formerly been referred to as activity analysis in the occupational therapy literature.[36]

Guides for Assessment of Patient Status

As in other frameworks, MOHO assessment guides suggest that the therapist use observation, interview or informal conversation and formal assessment procedures. Preferably, the assessment procedures are consistent, stable and valid. The choice of assessment approach is influenced by 1) the time available for assessment, 2) the data needed, 3) the tools available, 4) and the degree to which the assessment battery meets scientific guides.[115] See Table 6.8 for an outlined assessment guide.

The questions posed during assessment and the instruments that facilitate data collection should create a holistic picture of the patient (in so far as the focus is on occupation). The aim is to get a view that goes beyond medical diagnosis.[115] A sample of the kind of questions that the therapist would be interested in answering (adapted from those in the MOHO literature) are listed in Table 6.9.

In general, the therapist and patient cooperate to identify how the person's symptomatology bears on his or her job, interpersonal relationships, ability for self-care, safety in the community, financial status and so on. As most therapists will agree, no two persons with a compromised physical, psychosocial or cognitive status are alike. Even where two persons have an identical diagnosis, each individual's function and personal situation will diverge. This individualized perspective on occupational function should be the outcome of the occupational therapy assessment.

Assessment Instruments

Many assessment tools from occupational therapy and the social sciences have been identified with the model of human occupation. A few of those most frequently referenced are briefly described here.

Bay Area Functional Performance Evaluation (BaFPE). The BaFPE was designed by Judith Bloomer and Susan Williams to assess performance in general activities of daily living. It consists of two subtests: the Task Oriented Assessment (TAO) and the Social Interaction Scale (SIS). The assessment is based on a functionalist view and the acquisitional (behavioral), occupational behavior, adaptational,

---

TABLE 6.8   ASSESSMENT GUIDE

The occupational therapist uses interviews and tasks to identify the person's occupational function based on the following:

1. Person's sense of purpose
2. Person's value system
3. Person's goals
4. Person's interests and interest patterns
5. Balance of work, play, and self-care occupations
6. Person's roles and their compatibility with abilities and expectations
7. Person's habits and how they are used to adapt to the environment
8. Person's skills and how they are used during work, play and self-care function
9. Major body systems and how their function influences occupational performance
10. Environments in which the person functions and how they influence competence: press, values, standards and opportunities

and functional restoration frames of reference.[56] Assessment tasks, which include shell sorting, money and marketing task, drawing a house floor plan, a kinetic person drawing, and completion of a block design, are used to assess the patient's ability to paraphrase, make decisions and organize. Patient motivation, self-esteem, attention span, and ability to abstract, as well as possible evidence of mood or thought disorder, can be determined with the tasks. A

TABLE 6.9   ASSESSMENT QUESTION GUIDE

Can the person describe the following?

Personal Causation	Sense of control or locus of causality
	Personal strengths and limits; performance boundaries
	View of the past, present and future
	Compatibility of views with current medical condition and environmental situations
Values	Meaningful activities (occupations) and source of meaning
	Personal standards and how these influence his/her performance
	View of time and how this view influences performance
	Short- and long-term goals held and desired
	Value system and its compatibility with current life situation and developmental level
Interests	Specific likes and dislikes that reflect a balance of interests
	A pattern of interests (past, present and future)
	The source of interests (observe, experience or assume)
	Interest that encourage involvement in occupation
	Interests that suggest a balance of work, leisure and ADL occupations
Roles	Roles (past, present and desired)
	The compatibility of the person's roles with his/her needs and abilities; and compatibility of roles with expectations and needs of others
	The compatibility of the person's multiple roles
	His/her ability to meet the demands of multiple roles, interests and values within time constraints

Does the person demonstrate the following?

Habits	Skills and behaviors needed to fulfill his/her roles?
	Time management effective to satisfy needs of oneself and others and to meet role responsibilities
	Adaptive behavior to meet role responsibilities
	Personal flexibility to meet environmental demands
Skills	Effective communication skills during varied activities (work, self-care and leisure occupations)
	Reception, understanding and interpretation of sensory input during varied occupations
	Use of skills and sensations to problem solve in varied environments
Skill Constituents (Splinter Skills)	Cognitive boundaries (See chapters 7 and 11 on cognition for specific cognitive elements for assessment)
	An intact or compromised neurological system (consider injury, disease, development)—adequate neuromotor function
	An intact or compromised musculosketal system (consider injury, disease, development)—adequate strength, range, tone, endurance, etc.

Does the environment provide the following?

	Objects, tasks and people to present physical and social press
	Adequate press to facilitate function, challenge and/or adaptation
	A value system compatible with the person's performance standards
	Adequate support for facilitating competence and sense of control
	Opportunity for skill development, practicing habits and assuming roles

comprehensive manual and task materials for the administration of the BaFPE are available from Consulting Psychologists Press, Inc.[17,18]

Occupational Case Analysis Interview and Rating Scale (OCAIRS). The case analysis method was developed in 1982 by Cubie and Kaplan.[31,32,58] The analysis consists of 14 interview questions, ten of which are derived from the model of human occupation, and four of which give a global assessment of the system. Questions assess personal causation, goals, interests, roles, habits, output, the physical and social environment, and feedback. The global systems analysis seeks to identify the dynamics of the system; its compatibility with the environment; and past, present and future related issues.

The Occupational Role History. The Occupational Role History is an evaluation designed by Florey and Michelman,[46] and is based on the occupational behavior frame of reference and Moorehead's work on occupational role. It is used to elicit data based on the patient's occupational role history, not the patient's diagnosis. During a semistructured, one-half hour interview, 34 questions are use to determine the patient's comfort, satisfaction, and competence in work, homemaker, and school roles; to determine the areas of skill and problems; and to determine the degree of balance between work, chores and leisure. The interview also elicits demographic data, information regarding the sequence and continued development of occupational roles, and information about the patient's interests and the tasks he or she does alone or with others that lead to satisfaction or dissatisfaction with occupational roles. The data are interpreted on the basis of quality of performance in one's roles over time.[46,81,97]

The Interest Checklist. This Interest Checklist is a paper and pencil questionnaire usually used in combination with an interview designed by Matsutsuyu[93,94] to assess the patient's interests—past, present and future. The categories assessed include manual skills, physical sports, social recreation, activities of daily living, and cultural/educational interests. In addition to completing the checklist, the patient is asked to write a narrative that describes his or her interests and hobbies and to identify how he or she has used leisure time from grammar school to the present.[60,61,93,94]

Occupational Performance History Interview (OPHI). This assessment format was developed in response to a decision by the American Occupational Therapy Association to fund a project that would culminate in a standardized, generic history-taking format for use by professionals in all areas of practice.[57] Questions in the history address five content areas: environmental influences, life roles, organization of daily living routines, perceptions of ability and responsibility, and interests, values and goals.

In addition to the semistructured interview, a rating scale is provided to quantify the subject's functioning in each of the five content areas.[57] The test is available from the American Occupational Therapy Association.

Other Assessments. For a listing and descriptions of some of the social science assessments used within the MOHO framework, the reader is referred to the Instrument Library, an appendix in *A Model of Human Occupation.*[69] Other assessments continue to be developed to assess communication/interaction, motor and process skills. These developments are supported by funding from the American Occupational Therapy Association.

Treatment

The model of human occupation provides general guidelines for the application of the theory in varied treatment settings such as mental health, physical medicine, day rehabilitation and extended care. These guides describe a problem-solving process, an approach to treatment planning and a method for program development. All guides have occupation as the focus. The information that follows describes treatment in the context of mental health settings.

Occupational Function and Treatment Planning

With the exception of using system theory to organize data, MOHO theorists outline treatment guides similar to many of those of the other frames of reference described in this text. The therapist plans treatment using a five step process:

1. Having reviewed the medical documentation and following his or her initial observations, the therapist determines which clinical questions will guide assessment.
2. The therapist uses reliable and valid assessment tools to collect data pertaining to the patient and those environmental factors that influence occupational function.
3. The therapist organizes assessment findings and constructs a hypothesis to explain the patient's level of occupational function and dysfunction.
4. Using scientific information and clinical experience, the therapist identifies treatment options and selects a course of action for improving occupational function.
5. The therapist initiates a course of treatment and periodically evaluates its effectiveness.[92,115]

Within this five-step process, the therapist is sensitive to the importance of individualizing treatment and considering the patient's preferences when determining treatment goals and interventions. During this process, the therapist becomes the mediator between the patient and his/her environment, evaluating the press of the patient's environment and determining activities that will achieve the patient's goals and help the patient operate within the environment.[34,115].

Although MOHO literature asserts that diagnostic labels do not give information about occupational performance, in the actual discussion of treatment this same literature emphasizes diagnostic categories; the understanding of diagnoses seems traditionally psychodynamic in nature. Barris et al[7] provide examples of individual treatment needs for particular diagnoses. For example, the borderline patient is described as having a need to explore in a safe, interesting and playful context to develop habits and roles consistent with being an autonomous adult.[7] Bonder[19] provides similar suggestions for planning mental health treatment as well as broad guidelines for treating particular functional problems related to specific psychiatric diagnoses.

Treatment Goals

As in other frameworks, goal setting is a cooperative process, and the goals are mutually agreed on by the therapist and patient. Treatment goals, as with other theoretical approaches, may include skill development, increasing awareness of oneself and others, coping with change and enhancing adaptation, and participation in and contribution to one's environment. However, these pursuits are described within an occupational context. For example, the patient will increase social skills to increase occupational function at home and in the community. Or, the patient will participate in meaningful activities to clarify personal values and to explore the meaning of work and leisure.

Treatment Process

The therapist establishes a specific time frame for treatment (e.g., one hour a day, five times a week) and provides an organized, consistent environment with functional demands. The treatment environment is varied; for example, it may be a playful setting where the emphasis is on pleasure, not achievement. Or, a setting may be selected within the community to provide opportunities for assuming varied roles: at an employment site (e.g., at the patient's former place of employment or at a sheltered workshop) to facilitate resumption of work responsibilities; at home to reestablish daily habits and routines; or in a clinic that simulates home, work or community environments. In any of these treatment environments, the therapist conveys a message to the patient that it is safe to try new experiences and take the risks required for development and change.

During treatment, the patient's strengths, interests and values are used to identify meaningful occupations for increasing function and competence. Occupations are graded to facilitate occupational development, first providing opportunities for exploration of the environment through use of activity, and eventually establishing competency and achievement through successful activity experiences. As the patient increases his or her sense of competence, he or she achieves a feeling of internal control, a sense that achievements are an outcome of one's abilities, not a result of luck, fate or the efforts of others.

The treatment process occurs in groups or individual sessions. As noted earlier, almost any purposeful activity may be used to facilitate occupational development and role performance. Principles of restoring order (Table 6.10) are

---

TABLE 6.10   PRINCIPLES OF RESTORING ORDER

Decision Making
Provide opportunity to discover and develop interests.
Facilitate development of new interests and values to correct faulty patterns of occupational behavior.
Foster interests and values consistent with the person's everyday settings.
Enable discovery of values by providing a value system in occupational therapy.
Help people to identify ways to actualize interests, values, and goals in their lives.
Provide opportunity to identify and assess occupational choices and to pursue new choices.

Role
Provide opportunities to enter responsible active and productive roles.
Make expectations for performance clear to facilitate socialization.
Use groups as a context for performing various roles.
Use therapy to precipitate or facilitate role transition as appropriate.

Temporal Adaptation
Provide schedules that replicate time use in the larger culture.
Enable people to acquire the temporal perspective of their settings.
Guide people with maladaptive patterns of time used to identify change needs and to develop schedules of time use.
Provide opportunities to implement and practice new routines (habits) of time use.

Environment
Provide appropriate levels of arousal (challenge).
Opportunities for decision making should be present.
The atmosphere and physical environment must be consistent with expectations for performance.
Understaff settings to evoke performance.
Allow performance in a range of settings to increase flexibility of performance.

Performance Components
Provide skill training relevant to the contexts of daily life.
Follow a developmental sequence in skill training.
Acknowledge roles, interests, and values in choosing skills to be learned.
Consider the symbolic, neurological, and musculoskeletal constituents in regenerating skills.

Reprinted with permission. From Barris, Kielhofner and Watts, *Bodies of Knowledge in Psychosocial Practice* Thorofare, NJ. SLACK Inc., 1992.

discussed in earlier as well as more recent MOHO literature and can serve as a guide for using purposeful activities (occupations) during the treatment process.

Dual Function of Occupation in Treatment

The treatment principle currently acknowledged in MOHO theory but previously questioned by occupational behaviorists is the belief that activity or occupation serves a dual rather than a singular purpose. Activities previously were used solely to achieve an end product. Currently, MOHO theorists suggest that engagement in, as well as the response to, activities should be pursued. In other words, how the individual feels about what he or she has accomplished may be as important as the outcome of performance. When discussing with the patient the activity process, the therapist may identify patient values, increase the patient's awareness of occupational competence, suggest its relevance to occupational roles and future goals and increase the patient's understanding that maladaptive habits interfere with role performance. This should not suggest the feeling emphasis of other frames of reference, however, because the discussion about occupational performance remains quite focused.

Group Treatment

MOHO theorists recommend using individual and group treatment and the literature describes varied group experiences. However, these groups are not easily identified as different from other group approaches described in this text. Groups are seen as a means for developing skills and enhancing roles and habits. Activities used in groups are generally viewed as play, daily living, or work tasks. Group activities include movement exercises, games, sports, cooking and other daily living tasks, art, crafts,[59] values clarification, music, community activities, assertiveness training, social skills training[69] and others.

Kaplan[59] describes the use of the MOHO to design and implement group treatment. She sees the group as providing an environment that can arouse interest in occupational function through the introduction of meaningful activities and careful articulation of goals based on the patient's needs, goals and roles. She recommends that patients at similar functional levels be treated in three groups designed to address this level of function; achievement, competence and exploratory groups. Each group has specific goals and involves group experiences consistent with the abilities of its members.

One such group is the directive group. The **directive group** is a group experience for persons with varied problems and of various ages and diagnoses, but all are in the acute stage of illness. The group is structured and designed to support maximum participation from patients who function at a minimum level.

The group follows a consistent format:

1. Orientation—the introduction of a brief activity to inform patients about where they are and what to expect in the group;
2. Introduction of new members—approached in a manner likely to stimulate interest and mobilize the participants, for instance, throwing a ball to each member and asking each to state his or her name;
3. Warm-up exercises—usually spontaneous movement exercises;
4. Core or theme activity—motor, cognitive, social-interactive, sensory, food-centered or craft experience;
5. Wrap-up—activity is used to bring group closure, often with group or member goals and their attainment underscored;
6. Post-group—plans or directions for future groups are discussed.[69]

The reader may recognize this group sequence as similar to that of Ross and Allen. However, Kaplan sees these groups as different in nature and theory from the directive group.[69]

Of the 69 activities recommended for possible use in directive groups, the following is selected to illustrate a sample group exercise.

Facts of Three (or Five) is a cognitive game that can be used to assess cognitive skills, increase interests, build knowledge, and emphasize the cooperative and competitive nature of roles when organized as team play.

Patients are given a copy of a grid sheet, which they complete as the game ensues. (A completed sample grid appears in Figure 6.3.) When the activity portion of the group begins, participants identify a three-letter word and three categories. Then play begins. Participants take turns filling in the grid by identifying words that begin with the identified letter and satisfy a particular category. The game can be made more complex, may involve score keeping, or can require performance within time constraints. In this and other ways it can be adapted to meet patient needs.[69]

Letters / Categories	A	C	T
Occupation	Actor	Chiropractor	Therapist
Places to Visit	Austria	Catskills	Texas
Feelings	Appalled	Calm	Terrific

FIGURE 6.3   Sample Grid. From Kaplan K. (1988) *Directive Group Therapy.* Thorofare, NJ: SLACK Inc., p. 151. Reprinted with permission.

Summary

The information subsumed within this frame of reference has increased dramatically since the initial presentation of the material in the first edition of our text. Even with the cursory nature of the review, the emphases in the model of human occupation should be quite clear to the reader. Weight is placed on occupational performance as the outcome of an open system, and not on the dynamics of the open system, nor on the understanding of what might happen when the system fails to function properly. This approach gives us a starting point from which we can address both contributions and limitations of the framework at this juncture.

Contributions and Limitations of the Model of Human Occupation

Contributions

Since the initial work by Mary Reilly[110–112] and early proponents of an occupational behavior framework, diverse theoretical constructs and assumptions have been further developed and clarified. Major steps have been taken toward the creation of an integrated model of occupation. As a result of these efforts, proponents of the model have done much to return professional focus to the action aspect of the person's being, and have thereby returned attention to what is unique to occupational therapy as a helping profession. Further, they have provided a conceptual structure that can accommodate new information as it is brought into the model.

The theory is holistic insofar as it recognizes that the part affects the whole, but it does not suggest that the therapist treat every problem that a patient presents. Rather, it concerns itself solely with occupation. Therefore, the task of the therapist is not unrealistically broad. This approach can be viewed as especially important in light of the mandate in health care to limit the duration of treatment and to document the outcome of intervention.

The model of human occupation reiterates the basic tenets of occupational therapy—that the individual has power within his or her own domain to achieve purpose and well-being through active participation on one's own behalf. It presents a positive posture, emphasizing what can be, rather than what cannot be accomplished.

Because the model does not require the application of a notion of ill health, it can be seen as appropriate for medical and nonmedical settings, reactive and proactive treatment, and for addressing changes in function throughout the life cycle.

Research has been strongly emphasized in this model. Given that the pendulum often swings from a romance with quantitative to qualitative research in the social sciences and helping professions, the tenets in this framework are well suited to both research approaches. At this stage of theory development, the MOHO is in a good position to profit from a double-pronged research emphasis.

Limitations

It is in the elucidation of patient case studies that the limitations of this frame of reference become most apparent.[69] These case studies begin with a discussion of patient psychodynamics, as related to a diagnostic label. Although such a reliance on traditional psychiatric constructs is generally out of step with the MOHO, it is not surprising. This framework addresses in great detail the output of the open system, but does not give a clear picture for understanding why or how the open system closes or breaks down. If the person stops exploring and refuses to use existing skills, then what steps should be taken, and based on what theoretical assumptions? For example, withdrawal and depressive behaviors accompany many if not most psychiatric problems, as well as many physical challenges. Indicating that the environment must be sufficiently arousing is certainly sensible, but in actual practice therapists often find more is needed to prompt patients to change. Considering that the volition subsystem is ruled as the most important, it is somewhat ironic that this dilemma emerges.

Concomitantly, a great deal of assessment aims toward detailing the presence of specific interests, habits, roles and values—all considered to be components of the system's throughput; but the difficulty in changing assumptions and habits is scantily addressed.

Understandably, positive experiences beget positive experiences, but in practice we often find many persons who manage to reaffirm in each new experience that they are failures. These individuals seem unusually adept at finding ways to get others to affirm this assumption, too. Because anything that approaches unconscious motives is outside the boundaries of this model, the therapist is left to assume that this negative behavior is intentional and will change.

We found somewhat surprising the consistent emphasis given to the need to restore balance, whether among work, leisure and self-care; among roles, in habits or elsewhere. Kielhofner goes to some lengths to clarify that it is the closed, not open, system that seeks balance and tension reduction. The humanistic-existential theorists to which MOHO theorists refer, by contrast, suggest that times of imbalance while creating tension, provide the greatest opportunities for growth, learning and change. They would point out that moving quickly to restore balance might well be contrary to therapeutic goals. It is not clear why restoring balance is so important, or whose definition of balance establishes the criteria for successful function. Are persons who devote most of their time to work, perhaps to intellectual pursuits and not to physical ones, to be considered dysfunctional? Probably many students and teachers would hope not. Why are many roles necessarily better than a few? In this regard, and overall, the stress placed on conformity to some vague societal norm seems especially disconcerting, especially considering that the person is believed to be motivated by the need to achieve personal meaning and is on a "trajectory toward self-enhancement." Apparently, the path toward purpose, meaning and self-enhancement is not as wide as one might hope.

The more this framework attempts to focus on occupational therapy as performance, the more likely that the therapist practicing within the framework will need to become eclectic and draw on other bodies of knowledge when performace does not live up to skill level.

Recommended Reading List

Berlyne D: *Conflict, Arousal and Curiosity*. New York, McGrawHill Book Co., 1961.

Boulding K: General systems theory—A skeleton of science. In Buckley W (Ed.): *Modern Systems Research for the Behavioral Scientist*. Chicago, Aldine Publishing Co., 1968.

Boulding K: *The Image* Ann Arbor, University of Michigan Press, 1961.

Bruner J: On coping and defending. In *Toward A Theory of Instruction*. Cambridge, MA, The Belknap Press of Harvard University Press, 1966.

Bruner J: The skill of relevance or the relevance of skills. *Saturday Review* April 18, 1970, pp. 66–73.

Bruner J: Nature and uses of immaturity. In Bruner J, Jolly Al, Sylva K (Eds.): *Play: Its Role in Development and Evolution*. New York, Basic Books, 1976.

Caplow T: *The Sociology of Work* New York, McGraw Hill Book Co., 1954.

Erikson E: *Childhood and Society*. New York, WW Norton, 1963.

Fiebleman J: Theory of integrative levels. In Coleman J (Ed.): *Psychology and Effective Behavior*. Boston, Little Brown and Co., 1968.

Ginzberg E: *Occupational Choice: An Approach to a General Theory*. New York, Columbia University Press, 1951.

Ginzberg E: Toward a theory of occupational choice. In Peters H, Hansen J (Eds.): *Vocational Guidance and Career Development* New York, MacMillan, 1971.

Kahn R: *Organizational Stress: Studies in Role Conflict and Ambiguity*. New York, Wiley, 1964.

Kaplan A: *The Conduct of Inquiry*. New York, Thomas Crowell, 1964.

Koestler A: Beyond atomism and holism—The concept of the holon. In Koestler A, Smithies R (Eds.): *Beyond Reductionism* Boston, MA, Beacon Press, 1969.

Kluckltohn C: Values and value orientation in the theory of action: An exploration in definition and classification. In Parsons T, Shils E (Eds.): *Toward a General Theory of Action*. Cambridge, MA, Harvard University Press, 1951.

Smith M: Competence and socialization. In Clauser J (Ed.): *Socialization and Society* Boston MA, Little Brown and Co., 1968.

Super DE: *Career Development: Self Concept Theory*. New York, College Entrance Examination Board, 1963.

Super D: *The Psychology of Careers*. New York, Harper & Row, 1957.

White RW: *Competence and the Psychosocial Stages of Development*. Nebraska Symposium on Motivation, Lincoln Nebraska, University of Nebraska Press, 1960.

White RW: The urge towards competence. *Am J Occup Ther* 25:271–274, 1971.

White RW: Strategies of adaptation: An attempt at systematic description. In Colhlo G, Hamburg D, Adams J (Eds.): *Coping and Adaptation*. New York, Basic Books, 1974.

White RW: Ego and reality in psychoanalytic theory: A proposal regarding independent ego energies. *Psychosocial Issues* 3(3):1–121, 1963.

References

1. American Psychiatric Association: *Diagnostic and Statistical Manual of Mental Disorders, (DSM III)*, Washington, D.C., American Psychiatric Association, 1981.

2. Barris R: Occupational dysfunction and eating disorders: Theory and approach to treatment. *Occup Ther Mental Health* 6(1): 27–46, 1986.

3. Barris R, Kielhofner G, Watts J: *Psychosocial Occupational Therapy—Practice in a Pluralistic Arena*. Laurel, Maryland, Ramsco Publishing, 1983, pp. 218–226.

4. Barris R, Kielhofner G: Adolescence.In Kielhofner G (Ed.): *A Model of Human Occupation*. Baltimore, Williams & Wilkins, 1985.

5. Barris R, Kielhofner G: Early and middle childhood. In Kielhofner G (Ed.): *A Model of Human Occupation*. Baltimore, Williams & Wilkins, 1985.

6. Barris R, Kielhofner G, Levine R, Neville A: Occupation as interaction with the environment. In Kielhofner G (Ed.): A Model of Human Occupation. Baltimore, Williams & Wilkins, 1985, pp. 44, 45, 42, 146, 147.

7. Barris R, Kielhofner G, Neville A, et al: Psychosocial dysfunction. In Kielhofner G (Ed.): *A Model of Human Occupation*. Baltimore, Williams & Wilkins, 1985, pp. 253, 259, 258–259.

8. Barris R, Kielhofner G, Burch R, et al: Occupational function and dysfunction in three groups of adolescents. *Occup Ther J Res* 6:301–317, 1986.

9. Barris R, Dickie V, Baron K: A comparison of psychiatric patients and normal subjects based on the model of human occupation. *Occup Ther J Res* 8:3–37, 1988.

10. Barton GE: Innoculation of the bacillus of work. *Mod Hosp* 8:399–403, 1917.

11. Behnke C, Fetkovich M: Examining the reliability and validity of the Play History. *Am J Occup Ther* 38: 94–100, 1984.

12. Berelson B, Steiner G: *Human Behavior: An Inventory of Scientific Findings*. New York, Harcourt, Brace, 1964.

13. Berlyne KE: *Conflict, Arousal and Curiosity*. New York, McGraw-Hill Book Co, 1960.

14. Black M: The Adolescent Role Assessment. *Am J Occup Ther* 30:73–79, 1976.

15. Black M: The occupational career. *Am J Occup Ther* 30:225–228, 1976.

16. Bledsoe NP, Shepherd JT: A study of reliability and validity of a Preschool Play Scale. *Am J Occup Ther* 36:783–788, 1982.

17. Bloomer J, Williams S: The Bay Area Functional Performance Evaluation. In Hemphill B: *The Evaluative Process in Psychiatric Occupational Therapy*. Thorofare, N.J., SLACK Inc., pp. 255–308, 1982.

18. Bloomer J, Williams S: *Bay Area Functional Performance Evaluation (BaFPE): Task Oriented Assessment and Social Interaction Scale Manual*. San Francisco, UCSF, 1986.

19. Bonder B: *Psychopathology and Function*. Thorofare, NJ, SLACK Inc., 1991.

20. Brollier C, Watts JH, Bauer D, Schmidt W: A content validity study of the Assessment of Occupational Functioning. *Occup Ther Mental Health* 8:29–47, 1989.

21. Brollier C, Watts JH, Bauer D, Schmidt W: A concurrent validity study of two occupational therapy evaluation instruments: The AOF and OCAIRS. *Occup Ther Mental Health* 8:49–59, 1989.

22. Brokema M, Danz K, Schloemer C: Occupational therapy in a community aftercare program. *Am J Occup Ther* 29:22–27, 1975.

23. Bronfenbrenner U: *The Ecology of Human Development: Experiments by Nature and Design*. Cambridge, MA, Harvard University Press, 1979.

24. Burke J: A clinical perspective on motivation: Pawn versus origin. *Am J Occup Ther* 31(4):254–258, 1977.

25. Burke J, Kielhofner G: Defining occupation: Importing and organizing interdisciplinary knowledge. In Kielhofner G, (Ed.): *Health Through Occupation—Theory and Practice in Occupational Therapy*. Philadelphia, F.A. Davis, 1983, pp. 125–145.

26. Casanova J, Ferber J: Comprehensive evaluation of basic living skills. *Am J Occup Ther* 30:101–105, 1976.

27. Christiansen CH: Editorial: Toward resolution of crisis: Research requisites in occupational therapy. *Occup Ther J Research* 1:115–124, 1981.

28. Clark P: Theoretical frameworks in contemporary occupational therapy practice, Part I. *Am J Occup Ther* 33:505–514, 1979.

29. Clark P: Human development through occupation: A philosophy and conceptual model for practice, Part 2. *Am J Occup Ther* 33:577–585, 1979.

30. Coviensky M, Buckley V: Day activities programming: Serving the severely impaired chronic client. *Occup Ther Mental Health* 6(2):21–30, 1986.

31. Cubie S, Kaplan K: A case analysis method for the model of human occupation, *Am J Occup Ther* 36(10):645–652, 1982.

32. Cubie S, Kaplan K: A case analysis method for the model of human occupation. *Am J Occup Ther* 36(10):645–652, 1982.

33. Cubie S: Occupational analysis. In Kielhofner G (Ed.): *A Model of Human Occupation*. Baltimore, Williams & Wilkins, 1985, pp. 147–155.

34. Cubie S, Kaplan K, Kielhofner G: Program development. In Kielhofner G (Ed): *A Model of Human Occupation*. Baltimore, Williams & Wilkins, 1985.

35. Curtin C: Research on the model of human occupation. *Mental Health: Special Interest Section Newsletter* 13(2):3–5, 1990.

36. Cynkin S: *Occupational Therapy: Toward Health Through Activities*. Boston, Little, Brown and Company, 1979.

37. DeCharms R: *Personal Causation*. NY, Academic Press, 1968.

38. Dubos R: *The Mirage of Health: Utopias, Progress and Biological Change*. New York, Harper & Row. 1959.

39. Dunning H: Environmental occupational therapy. *Am J Occup Ther* 26(6):292–298, 1972.

40. Dunton WR: History of occupational therapy. *Mod Hosp* 8:380–382, 1917.

41. Dunton WR: *Reconstruction Therapy*. Philadelphia, WB Saunders, 1919.

42. Dunton WR: The "three Rs" of occupational therapy. *Occup Ther Rehabil* 7:345–348, 1928.

43. Ebb WE, Coster W, Duncombe L: Comparison of normal and psychosocially dysfunctional male adolescents. *Occup Ther Mental Health* 9:53–74, 1989.

44. Elliott M, Barris R: Occupational role performance and life satisfaction in the elderly. *Occup Ther J Res* 7:215–224, 1987.

45. Fitts H, Howe M: Use of leisure time by cardiac patients. *Am J Occup Ther* 41:583–589, 1987.

46. Florey L, Michelman S: Occupational role history: A screening tool for psychiatric occupational therapy. *Am J Occup Ther* 36(5):301–308, 1982.

47. Fuller D: The need of instruction for nurses in occupations for the sick. In Tracy S: *Studies in Invalid Occupation*. Boston, Whitcomb & Barrows, 1912.

48. Ginzberg E: Toward a theory of occupational choice. In Peters HJ, Hansen JC (Eds.): *Vocational Guidance and Career Devlopment*. Ed. 2. New York, MacMillan, 1971.

49. Gray M: Effects of hospitalization on work-play behavior *Am J Occup Ther* 26(4):180–85, 1972.

50. Gregory M, Occupational behavior and life satisfaction among retirees. *Am J Occup Ther* 37(8):548–553, 1983.

51. Gusich R: Occupational therapy for chronic pain: A clinical application of the model of human occupation. *Occup Ther Mental Health* 4(3):59–73, 1984.

52. Hall K, Lindzey G: *Theories of Personality*. New York, John Wiley and Sons, Incorporated, 1970.

53. Hall K, Lindzey G: *Theories of Personality* Ed. 2. New York, John Wiley and Sons, Inc., 1975.

54. Harrison H, Kielhofner G: Examining reliability and validity of the preschool play scale with handicapped children. *Am J Occup Ther* 40:167–173, 1986.

55. Heard C: Occupational role acquisition: A perspective on the chronically disabled. *Am J Occup Ther* 31(4):243–247, 1977.

56. Hemphill B: *The Evaluative Process in Psychiatric Occupational Therapy*. Thorofare, N.J., SLACK Inc., 1982, p. 262.

57. Hemphill B: *Mental Health Assessment in Occupational Therapy*. Thorofare, NJ, SLACK Inc., 1988, p. 65.

58. Kaplan K: A short-term assessment: The need and a response. *Occup Ther Mental Health* 4(5):29–45, 1984.

59. Kaplan K: *Directive Group Therapy*. Thorofare, NJ, SLACK Inc., 1988, pp. 135–137, 23.

60. Katz N, Giladi N, Peretz C: Cross-cultural application of occupational therapy assessments: Human occupation with psychiatric inpatients and controls in Israel. *Occup Ther Mental Health* 8:7–30, 1988.

61. Katz N, Josman N, Steinmetz N: Relationship between cognitive disability theory and the model of human occupation in the assessment of psychiatric and nonpsychiatric adolescents. *Occup Ther Mental Health* 8:31–44, 1988.

62. Kielhofner G: Temporal adaptation: A conceptual framework for occupational therapy. *Am J Occup Ther* 31(4):235–242, 1977.

63. Kielhofner G: General systems theory: Implications for theory and action in occupational therapy. *Am J Occup Ther* 32(10):637–644, 1978.

64. Kielhofner G: A model of human occupation, Part 2. Ontogenesis from the perspective of temporal adaptation. *Am J Occup Ther* 34(10):657–663, 1980.

65. Kielhofner G: A model of human occupation, part 3. Benign and vicious cycles. *Am J Occup Ther* 34(11):731–737, 1980.

66. Kielhofner G: A model of human occupation, part 1. Conceptual framework and content. *Am J Occup Ther* 34(9): 572–581, 1980.

67. Kielhofner G (Ed.): *Health Through Occupation — Theory and Practice in Occupational Therapy*. Philadelphia, F. A. Davis, 1983.

68. Kielhofner G: A paradigm for practice: The hierarchical organization of occupational therapy knowledge. In Kielhofner G: *Health Through Occupation*. Philadelphia, F.A. Davis, 1983, pp. 55–92.

69. Kielhofner G (Ed.): *A Model of Human Occupation*. Baltimore, Williams & Wilkins, 1985, p. 80.

70. Kielhofner G: The human being as an open system. In Kielhofner G (ed.): *A Model of Human Occupation*. Baltimore, Williams & Wilkins, 1985, pp. 2, 4, 9, 109.

71. Kielhofner G: The open systems dynamics of human occupation. In Kielhofner G (Ed.): *A Model of Human Occupation*. Baltimore, Williams & Wilkins, 1985, p. 41.

72. Kielhofner G: Occupational function and dysfunction. In Kielhofner G (Ed.): *A Model of Human Occupation*. Baltimore, Williams & Wilkins, 1985, pp. 63, 64–69, 69–74.

73. Kielhofner G: Model of human occupation. In Robertson SC (Ed.): *Focus*. Rockville, MD, The American Occupational Therapy Association, Inc., 1988.

74. Kielhofner G, Barris R, Bauer D, et al: A comparison of play behavior in non-hospitalized and hospitalized children. *Am J Occup Ther* 37(5):305–312, 1983.

75. Kielhofner G, Barris R: The development of occupational behavior. In Kielhofner G (Ed.): *A Model of Human Occupation*. Baltimore, Williams & Wilkins, 1985, pp. 78–81.

76. Kielhofner G, Brinson M: Development and evaluation of an aftercare program for young chronic psychiatrically disabled adults. *Occup Ther Mental Health* 9:1–25, 1989.

77. Kielhofner G, Burke J: A model of human occupation, Part 1. Conceptual framework and content. *Am J Occup Ther* 34(9):572–581, 1980.

78. Kielhofner G, Burke J, Igi C: A model of human occupation, part 4. Assessment and intervention. *Am J Occup Ther* 34(12):777–788, 1980.

79. Kielhofner G, Burke J: The evolution of knowledge and practice in occupational therapy: Past, present, and future. In Kielhofner G (Ed.): *Health Through Occupation — Theory and Practice in Occupational Therapy* Philadelphia, F.A. Davis, 1983, pp. 3–54.

80. Kielhofner G, Burke J: Components and determinants of human occupation. In Kielhofner G (Ed.): *A Model of Human Occupation*. Baltimore, Williams & Wilkins, 1985, pp. 14, 17, 18, 24–34.

81. Kielhofner G, Harlan, B, Bauer, D, Maurer P: The reliability of a historical interview with physically disabled respondents. *Am J Occup Ther* 40:551–556, 1986.

82. Kielhofner G, Henry, AD: Development and investigation of the occupational performance history interview. *Am J Occup Ther* 42:489–, 1988.

83. Kielhofner G, Miyake S: Rose colored lenses for clinical practice: From a deficit to a competency model in assessment and intervention. In Kielhofner G (Ed.): *Health Through Occupation — Theory and Practice in Occupational Therapy*. Philadelphia, F.A. Davis, 1983, pp. 257–280.

84. Kielhofner G, Takata N: A study of mentally retarded persons: Applied research in occupational therapy. *Am J Occup Ther* 34(4):252–258, 1980.

85. Khoo SW, Renwick RM: A model of human occupation perspective on the mental health of immigrant women in Canada. *Occup Ther Mental Health* 9(3):31–50, 1989.

86. Krupa T, Thornton J: Pleasure deficit in schizophrenia. *Occup Ther Mental Health* 6(2):65–78, 1986.

87. Lederer J, Kielhofner G, Watts J: Values, personal causation and skills of deliquents and nondeliquents. *Occup Ther Mental Health* 5(2):59–77, 1985.

88. Lindquist J, Mack WL, Parham D: Occupational behavior and sensory integration concepts in theory and practice, part 2. Clinical applications. *Am J Occup Ther* 36(7):433–437, 1982.

89. Linton R: *The Cultural Background of Personality.* New York, Appleton-Century-Crofts, 1945.

90. Mack W, Lindquist J, Parham D: A synthesis of occupational behavior and sensory integration concepts in theory and practice, part 1. Theoretical foundations. *Am J Occup Ther* 36(6):365–374, 1982.

91. Maddi S: *Personality Theories: A Comparative Analysis.* Ed. 5. Chicago, The Dorsey Press, 1989, pp. 355, 651, 652.

92. Mailloux Z, Mack W, Cooper C: Knowing what to do: The organization of knowledge for clinical practice. In Kielhofner G (Ed.): *Health Through Occupation—Theory and Practice in Occupational Therapy.* Philadelphia, F.A. Davis, 1983, pp. 281–294.

93. Matsutsuyu J: The interest checklist. *Am J Occup Ther* 23:323–328, 1969.

94. Matsutsuyu J: Occupational behavior approach. In Hopkins H, Smith H (Eds.): *Willard and Spackman's Occupational Therapy* Philadelphia, JB Lippincott Co., 1983, pp. 129–134.

95. Meyer A: The philosophy of occupational therapy. *Arch Occup Ther* 1:1–10, 1922.

96. Meyer A: The philosophy of occupational therapy. *Am J Occup Ther* 31: 639–642, 1977.

97. Moorehead L: The occupational history. *Am J Occup Ther* 23(4):329, 1969.

98. Moss G: *Illness, Immunity, and Social Interactions.* New York, Wiley, 1973.

99. McClelland DC: *Personality* New York, Dryden Press, 1973.

100. Newell A, Simon H: *Human Problem-Solving.* Englewood Cliffs, NJ: Prentice-Hall, 1972.

101. Neville A: Temporal adaptation: Application with short-term psychiatric patients. *Am J Occup Ther* 34: 328–331, 1980.

102. Neville P, Kielhofner G, Royeen C: Childhood. In Kielhofner G (Ed.): *A Model of Human Occupation.* Baltimore, Williams & Wilkins, 1985.

103. Oakley F: Clinical application of the model of human occupation in dementia of the alzheimers type. *Occup Ther Mental Health* 7(4):37–50, 1987.

104. Oakley F, Kielhofner G, Barris R: An occupational therapy approach to assessing psychiatric patients' adaptive functioning. *Am J Occup Ther* 39(3):147–154, 1985.

105. Oakley F, Kielhofner G, Barris R: An occupational therapy approach to assessing psychiatric patient's adaptive functioning. *Am J Occup Ther* 39:147–154, 1985.

106. Oakley F, Kielhofner G, Barris R, Reichler Rk: The role checklist: Development and empirical assessment of reliability. *Occup Ther J Res* 6:157–170, 1986.

107. Perun PJ, Del Vento Bielby D: Towards a model of female occupational behavior: A human developmental approach. *Psychol Woman Q* 6:234–252, 1981.

108. Pezzuti L: An exploration of adolescent feminine and occupational behavior development. *Am J Occup Ther* 33(2):84–91, 1979.

109. Reed K: *Models of Practice in Occupational Therapy* Baltimore, Williams & Wilkins, 1984.

110. Reilly M: A psychiatric occupational therapy program as a teaching model. *Am J Occup Ther* 20:61–67, 1966.

111. Reilly M: The educational process. *Am J Occup Ther* 23:299–307, 1969.

112. Reilly M: Occupational therapy—A historical perspective: The modernization of occupational therapy. *Am J Occup Ther* 25(5):243, 1971.

113. Reilly M (Ed.): *Play as Exploratory Learning* Beverly Hills, CA, Sage Publications, 1974.

114. Rogers J: The study of human occupation. In Kielhofner G (Ed.): *Health Through Occupation—Theory and Practice in Occupational Therapy.* Philadelphia, F.A. Davis, 1983, pp. 93–125.

115. Rogers J, Kielhofner G: Treatment planning. In Kielhofner G (Ed.): *A Model of Human Occupation* Baltimore, Williams & Wilkins, 1985.

116. Rogers J, Snow T: Later adulthood. In Kielhofner G (Ed.): *A Model of Human Occupation.* Baltimore, Williams & Wilkins, 1985.

117. Rust K, Barris R, Hooper F: Use of the model of human occupation to predict women's exercise behavior. *Occup Ther J Res* 7:23–35, 1987.

118. Shannon P: The Derailment of Occupational Therapy *Am J Occup Ther* 31 (4):229–234, 1977.

119. Slagle EC: Occupational therapy. *Trained Nurse and Hospital Review* 100:375–382, 1938.

120. Slagle EC: The training of occupational therapists for work with mental patients. *Am Assoc Adv Sci* 9: 408–415, 1938.

121. Smith N, Kielhofner G, Watts J: The relationship between volition, activity pattern and life satisfaction in the elderly. *Am J Occup Ther* 40:278–283, 1986.

122. Smyntek L, Barris R, Kielhofner G: The model of human occupation applied to psychosocially functional and dysfunctional adolescents. *Occup Ther Mental Health* 5:21–40, 1985.

123. Spranger E: *Types of men* (W. Pigors, Trans.). Halle, Germany, Niemeyer, 1928.

124. Stensrud MK, Lushbough RS: The implementation of an occupational therapy program in an alcohol and drug dependency treatment center. *Occup Ther Mental Health* 8(2):1–16, 1988.

125. Super DE: A theory of vocational development. In Peters HJ, Hansen JC (Eds.): *Vocational Guidance and Career Development*. Ed. 2. New York, MacMillan, 1971.

126. Takata N: Introduction to a series: Occupational behavior research for pediatric practice. *Am J Occup Ther* 34(1):11–12, 1980.

127. Tigges K, Sherman L: The treatment of the hospice patient: From occupational history to occupational role. *Am J Occup Ther* 37(4):235–238, 1985.

128. Tracy SE: Invalid occupation in the curriculum of the training school. *Mod Hosp* 3:56–57, 1914.

129. Tracy SE: *Studies in Invalid Occupation* Boston, Witcomb and Barrows, 1918.

130. Von Bertalanffy L: *General System Theory: Foundations, Development Application*. Rev. Ed. New York, George Braziller, 1968.

131. Watts J, Brollier C, Bauer D, Schmidt R: A comparison of two evaluation instruments used with psychiatric patients in occupational therapy. *Occup Ther Mental Health* 8:7–27, 1989.

132. Watts J, Kielhofner G, Bauer D, et al: The assessment of occupational functioning: A screening tool for use in long term care. *Am J Occup Ther* 40:231–240, 1986.

133. Weeder T: Comparison of temporal patterns and meaningfulness of the daily activities of schizophrenic and normal adults. *Occup Ther Mental Health* 6:27–45, 1986.

134. Werner H: *Comparative Psychology of Mental Development*. Chicago, Follett, 1948.

135. Werner H: The conception of development from a comparative and organismic point of view. In Harris D (Ed.): *The Concept of Development*. Minneapolis, University of Minnesota Press, 1957.

136. West WL: Nationally speaking—Perspectives on the past and future, part 2. *Am J Occup Ther* 44:9–10, 1990.

137. Wolfe R: Defining occupation. In Kielhofner G: *Health Through Occupation*. Philadelphia, F.A. Davis, 1983.

Chapter 7

OVERVIEW OF THE COGNITIVE PROCESS

Focus Questions

1. Using contemporary views, define cognition.
2. How do information processing and cognitive developmental models of cognition differ?
3. What is the sequence of operations that occurs during information processing?
4. Describe the different types of knowledge.
5. What are the underlying principles of cognitive development?
6. Describe a cognitive profile for each of the four developmental periods.
7. What are the six types of problem-solving?
8. How does the occupational therapist contribute to cognitive assessment and treatment?

Introduction

Throughout the history of psychology, cognitive studies have been influential in the research and development of the field. Prominent studies include those of Bartlett, Piaget, Jung, Koffka, Kohler, Wertheimer, Lewin, Luria, Binet, Tolman, and Rotter. After World War II, the elements of computer technology and the work in information and processing theory, as well as studies in linguistics, led to the further development of cognitive psychology. Beginning in 1960 and into the 1990s, cognitive psychology was not only influential, but also it was a focus in theoretical and applied psychology. Simultaneously, the influence of cognitive psychology and neurology has been increasingly felt in occupational therapy theory and practice. Because of this influence, the growing interest in cognitive approaches to

treatment, and the subsequent need to have a broad understanding of cognition in contemporary practice, we provide a summary of the cognitive process. This information is also a basis for understanding the cognitive approaches discussed in this text.

The applied and theoretical literature in medicine, psychology and education that addresses brain structure, organization and function is extensive and could not be adequately summarized in this chapter. We have summarized key concepts in cognitive theory to provide a basis for the application of four theoretical approaches in occupational therapy: 1) a holistic neurological approach based on the work of Aleksander Luria and elaborated in Chapter 11; 2) a cognitive-behavioral (C-B) approach, which is influenced by the work of Piaget, Bandura, and cognitive-behavioral psychologists, and exemplified in occupational therapy psychoeducational treatment programs, as discussed in Chapter 8; 3) the movement approach posed by Ross and King and described in Chapter 9; and 4) Allen's cognitive disabilities framework, summarized in Chapter 10.

The occupational therapy literature does not indicate that the profession has adopted a specific cognitive frame of reference. Luria's work is the more frequent reference in physical medicine; this neurological-holistic approach is the basis for the discussion of treatment of organic or physically based cognitive dysfunction.[1,2] In psychosocial arenas, cognitive behavioral, developmental, and neuropsychological influences are apparent. Psychoeducational programs reflect early cognitive-behavioral theory.[11] The work of Claudia Allen[3,4] addresses disruptions in normal cognitive development, and the movement approaches of Ross and and King are an outgrowth of a developing neuropsychology framework.[23,24,38,39] The theoretical approaches discussed in this text are not the only possible cognitive routes addressed in the mental health literature.

This chapter draws from several sources to provide a foundation for understanding cognition, including information processing, structural-organismic, and social learning theories. Cognition is approached more broadly than as conceived by Piagetian theory. When including some social learning tenets, we have taken the liberty of estimating when given social learning skills are most likely to emerge. Although diverse discussions abound regarding cognition, we have included Flavell, Sternberg, Bandura, and Perry and Bussey as primary references from the theoretical literature, and Kaplan and Sadock, and Lezak from the applied literature.

Theoretical Conception of Cognition

Because mental processes intrude into all aspects of human life, it is difficult to establish limits in defining cognition. Flavell[13,14] sug- gests an encompassing conceptualization of cognition that combines the traditional view of cognition with the information-processing and structural-organismic perspectives.

Traditional View

The traditional view, cognition is composed of higher mental processes that include "knowledge, consciousness, intelligence, thinking, imagining, creating, generating plans and strategies, reasoning, inferring, problem-solving, conceptualizing, classifying, relating, symbolizing and perhaps fantasizing and dreaming."[13]

In addition to the higher mental processes, the contemporary therapist understands that other components such as "organized motor movements, (especially in infant cognition), perception, imagery, memory, attention and learning . . . and social cognition" are included in a definition of cognition.[13]

Information Processing Conceptualization

Man as Machine

The information processing view of cognition began with the work of Herbert Simon, Allen Newell,[28] Walter Reitman and others.

"The information processing theorist thinks of man as a complex machine or device, in some ways analogous to a modern electronic computer, that possesses elaborate **programs** (sequences of instruction) for dealing with information in intelligent and adaptive ways. The programs consist of intricately interrelated and sequenced cognitive operations or **processes** that construct or create, receive, transform (recode, reduce, elaborate), store, retrieve, and otherwise manipulate units of information or knowledge."[13]

In this view the individual receives information or **input** from the environment through his or her sensory systems (visual, auditory, tactile, olfactory). This sensory information is processed by short-term and long-term memory components as well as other sensory buffers. It is then analyzed and transformed according to rules of the cognitive system to produce thoughts, feelings and behaviors. The rules provide the guides for constructing, monitoring and executing information. They give meaning to stimuli and produce goal-directed or planned behavior called **output** (Figure 7.1).

Although different from the structural-organismic perspective, the information processing view can complement the more traditional Piagetian perspective. Information processing theory provides an analogy for explaining the coding and organization of environmental stimuli and the role played by the person's beliefs and expectations during the process. In a sense it provides the rules for thinking and behaving. In recent years, information processing has grown from an emerging science to a dominant force in cognitive literature. Further, from information processing theory, therapists have developed multiple strategies for improving their patients' cognitive skills.

Organizing Sensation

As a person interacts in the environment, sensory input is coded and organized and represented as schema. **Schema**, as described by Rumelhart, are the tools that a person uses to acquire and retrieve knowledge.[40,41] They are unconscious mechanisms that organize prior experiences and integrate new information with that previously acquired. This organization of schema helps a person connect new experiences to existing knowledge, decreases the number of stimuli to which one must attend at any one time, and enhances the integration of experiences, thereby facilitating the retention and recall of information.[5,6,15] Tulving suggests that schema hold semantic memory.[46] Memory is discussed in more detail later in this chapter.

Knowledge Acquisition

A person acquires schema through three learning processes: 1) **accretion** (the acquisition of facts through encoding information); 2) **restructuring** (the integration of old information with new to form new schema or the acquisition of new information through repeated ex-

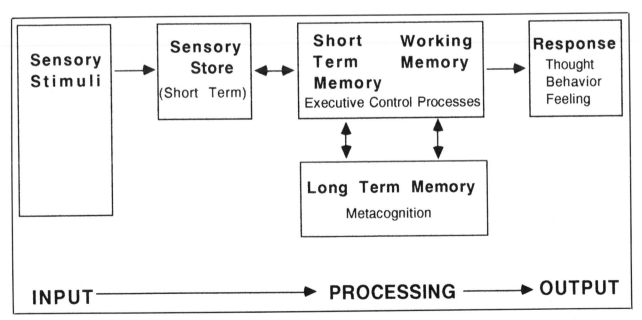

FIGURE 7.1 Information Processing Adapted from Mayer (1981). *The Promise of Cognitive Psychology*. San Francisco, CA: Freeman.

periences); and 3) **tuning** (the combination of specific facts to form general concepts and the refinement of schema as they are used in varied situations).[41,42] These three processes are similar to those that comprise Piaget's assimilation-accommodation process of knowledge acquisition.

Knowledge Content

The content of knowledge is identified as procedural or declarative. **Procedural knowledge** includes actions, decisions and processes, or knowing "how." **Declarative knowledge** consists of facts, concepts and principles, or knowing "what."[45] Table 7.1 describes and gives examples of varied types of knowledge.

Knowledge Processing: Top Down and Bottom Up

When using information, a person may use a top down or bottom up method. During **top down processing,** incoming information is analyzed through concepts that are at the top of the knowledge hierarchy. These concepts help a person make inferences, organize data, and facilitate understanding of the incoming information. During top down processing, a person encodes or retrieves information by automatically accessing general concepts at the top and then searches for the specific details or data at the bottom of the hierarchy. The details at the bottom are new data that generate or change schema and are the variables that help a person identify the specifics of the situation or the context.[29,42]

Top down and bottom up processing are evidenced in language comprehension. For example, when a person hears the word *restaurant*, his or her behavior is guided by all that the word connotes, including expectations related to using a menu and responding to the waiter, table manners and social protocol specific to the type of restaurant. Or, when a student hears the word *geometry*, he or she accesses a concept that includes the varied geometric shapes (e.g., square, triangle, circle), formulas to identify the area, radius or volume of particular shapes, and ideas for using geometric principles. This typifies top down processing.

TABLE 7.1   KNOWLEDGE CONTENT AND RELATED DIMENSIONS

Content	Definition	Examples
Declarative:		
Fact	A statement of specific data	Today is Sunday; Denver is the capital of Colo.; My name is . . . .
Concept	A definition with multiple examples that have similar criteria or features	Oranges, grapefruits & lemons are citrus fruits; France, Germany & Italy are countries of Western Europe.
Principle	The relationships among concepts; rules (if . . . then) applied in varied contexts; helps predict outcome of action or decision.	Circumference of a circle equals diameter times 3.74; If you play in the street you risk getting hit by a car; When someone does you a favor, say "thank you".
Procedural:		
Action	Step taken to accomplish a goal	The student completes the registration form; The man signs the check; He walked to school.
Decision	Select criteria or rule to make a decision to achieve a goal	The girl chose algebra for her math elective; The family decided to go to Hawaii for a vacation.
Process	Series of steps that are taken to achieve a goal	To bake a cake follow this recipe; To write your resume follow this outline; Automobile assembly.

During **bottom up processing,** attention is on specific data rather than the broad context of an experience. Sensory perceptions (e.g., sights and sounds) and attention are combined to make associations, organize perceptions, form relationships and then form concepts.[29] For example, bottom up processing gives a person specifics about a restaurant or geometry rather than the broad context. A person is aware of food odors, the decor or environmental barriers rather than being aware of the broader experience. Or, a person may focus on the length of lines when trying to identify a square or an isosceles triangle and when distinguishing how these shapes differ. Geometrical concepts would be accessed later.

Problem-Solving

Possessing the necessary information related to facts and procedures contributes to one's ability to problem-solve and function in daily life. The therapist identifies the specific knowledge content required of a task or situation to determine whether cognitive deficits exist. For example, the therapist may decide whether patients need to practice skills, learn facts about their disability, master specific procedures for self-care or otherwise build knowledge. Identifying declarative and procedural knowledge requirements allows the therapist to target strategies for learning or for remediating cognitive problems. These strategies may be used to increase motivation, support cognitive processing, or provide a means of compensation for weak or absent cognitive ability. Table 7.2 identifies learning strategies that can be used to increase knowledge content.

Transfer of Knowledge

Processed information is stored in memory and later retrieved for recognition, recall or use. Knowledge may be applied in the same or varied context. When a person does something as it is taught, in the same context, **near transfer** occurs.[17] For example, a person is taught principles of addition and subtraction and applies these principles to solve two,

TABLE 7.2 COGNITIVE STRATEGIES

Planning:	Person identifies a goal and generates activities that promote goal achievement.
Selecting:	Person identifies important and unimportant information needed to choose activities for achieving a goal.
Connecting:	Person relates new information and previous knowledge to form meaningful elaborations which facilitate learning.
Monitoring:	Person is aware of own learning and gives self feedback regarding task demands, own ability, effectiveness of one's performance, and value of the task.

Adapted from Clark (1990) Paper presented to American Educational Research Association, Boston, MA.

three, five and eight digit problems. When the individual adapts knowledge to novel situations or uses it in varied contexts, **far transfer** occurs; for example, a person can use addition and subtraction to make money transactions in the community and simultaneously manage the environmental distractions.[17] Learning strategies that support memory and use of procedural knowledge are suggested in Table 7.3.

Cognitive Strategies

We all rely on cognitive strategies to organize our everyday lives. Cognitive strategies can be used to facilitate memory and use of information as well as to monitor and direct cognitive processing. For instance, if I have several tasks I need to accomplish on a given day, I might make a list to help me remember, or, without giving it much thought, I might complete the tasks in order of their relative importance to me or my family, or even based on the geography of where these jobs take me around town. At day's end, I might reflect on what I've accomplished and make a mental note of what I need to do tomorrow.

A **cognitive strategy** is the specific mental effort invested to achieve a goal. Strategies help a person to establish a plan of action, to hypothesize the outcome of one's plan, and to anticipate the reactions of others (see Table 7.2). These strategies are also referred to as executive control functions and metacognitive strategies, but we will reserve the term metacognition for a more specialized type of cognition described next.[12]

TABLE 7.3 METACOGNITIVE/LEARNING STRATEGIES

Rehearsal Strategies–Methods which highlight the important elements of a task and which provide opportunity for practice and repetition of what is to be learned; e.g. skill practice, underlining important information in a text, repeated reading or verbal practice to memorize material, copying material, note taking, etc.

Elaboration Strategies–Methods which connect new information to previous knowledge; e.g. associating material to be remembered with images or the use of mnemonics, making an analogy between the treatment situation and current or previous community experiences, etc.

Organizational Strategies–Methods which impose a structure onto the learning task and break it down into its component parts or identify relationships; e.g. outline information or instructions, breakdown a task into component parts, draw a diagram to identify relationships between events or text, etc.

Comprehension-Monitoring Strategies–Methods which increase one's awareness of task/learning goals and progress toward accomplishment and support adapting to task demands; e.g. goal setting (long and short term), self questioning, self monitoring/checking, task adaptation, feedback, etc.

Affective Strategies–Methods which establish a safe environment for learning and risk; e.g. a supportive structure for attention and concentration, coping methods, motivation elements, time management, etc.

Problem-Solving Strategies–Methods for problem identification, solution generation, decision making, implementing a plan of action and evaluating the results; e.g. goal setting, brainstorming, increased self awareness of strengths and limits, knowledge of resources, criteria for evaluating alternatives and outcomes, group discussions, etc.

Adapted from Good & Brophy (1986). *Educational Psychology: A Realistic Approach* (3rd. Ed.) White Plains NY: Longman and Dembo MH (1988) *Applying Educational Psychology in the Classroom* (3rd Ed.) White Plains, NY: Longman.

Metacognition

Metacognition, a concept that emerged in the 1980s, has been used with increased frequency in the fields of psychology and education. It has been defined, categorized and exemplified in multiple ways. Briefly, metacognition is "cognition about cognition."[14] That is, a person is aware of what he or she does and does not know, what strategies assist that person to learn and to use current knowledge, and how and when to use this knowledge.

Metacognitive Skills. Metacognitive skills influence "oral communication of information, oral persuasion, oral comprehension, reading comprehension, writing, language acquisition, perception, attention, memory, problem solving, social cognition, and various forms of self-instruction and self-control."[14] Since the recognition of metacognitive skills, teachers and therapists have begun to teach these skills through methods such as those used in cognitive behavioral therapy, social learning programs and competency education.

Metacognitive Content. Examples of metacognition include the person's recognition of universal human qualities, such as fallibility. This information increases tolerance of errors, both personal errors and those of others. Metacognition is also the information in people's memory that tells them if they have a good or a poor memory, whether they learn best from visual or auditory stimuli, and their learning strengths (e.g., they learn social sciences more easily than biological sciences).

Metacognitive Strategies. Metacognition encompasses the strategies that a person uses to achieve a goal. For example, a student may know that making written lists is the best strategy to assist in remembering information when studying for an examination, or the individual knows how to read and learn material in a textbook versus leisurely reading a novel. Further, metacognition helps a person keep track of the progress made toward previously established goals. Overall, metacognition assists a person in learning from personal experiences, be it an increased awareness of those techniques that improved a golf score, a racquet ball game, or the outcome of a favorite recipe. The reader is referred to Table 7.3, but it must be emphasized that what one theorist or therapist might refer to as metacognitive strategy another might call a cognitive or simply a learning strategy.

Characteristics of a Good Information Processor

Possessing an adequate arsenal of cognitive and metacognitive skills plus holding adequate declarative and procedural knowledge that can be accessed in memory together enable good information processing. The successful processor seems to manage the complex interactions of personal experiences and accumulated knowledge to problem-solve and adapt to one's environment[36] (Table 7.4).

When an individual's neurological system, memory, or cognitive style are compromised, the therapist tries to identify those factors that limit cognitive processing. Information processing theory can be used to organize observation data, identify cognitive limitations, and select evaluation and treatment approaches. Those metacognitive strategies identified in

TABLE 7.4 THE GOOD INFORMATION PROCESSOR

Neurological system is intact: sensory system facilitates input into the central nervous system; large short term memory; long term memory is adequate for storage of knowledge.

Long term memory information which includes: declarative, procedural, metacognitive and motivation knowledge.

A cognitive style which includes: planning, selecting connecting, and monitoring strategies; a sense of calmness and self-efficacy; ability to selectively attend to task, control distractions, and reflect upon one's experience; motivation to become a better processor, and practice cognitive skills; and choose situations that encourage cognitive growth and develop information processing skills.

Adapted from Pressley, Borkowski, & Schneider (1989) Good information processing: What is it and how education can promote it. *International Journal of Educational Research,* 13(8):857–867, p. 863.

Table 7.3 can serve as guides for developing treatment approaches.

In summary, information processing theory has provided a way to conceptualize learning beyond stimulus response reactions. It provides a context for understanding the complex interactions of an individual's experiences, knowledge organization, learning strategies and cognitive processing.

Limits of Information Processing Theory

Recently, some cognitive theorists have suggested that information processing theory is limited because it attends to structural and surface knowledge and does not adequately address situational cognition. They question if lack of transfer is really the reason for a person's inability to use knowledge in novel and real world situations. They propose a theoretical framework called a **mental model** or situational model of cognition. In this model, knowledge is no longer viewed as something possessed by the individual. Rather, it is a relationship between the individual and a situation.[18] In any situation, knowledge acquisition and application are influenced by social and personal goals, physical and social resources, and specific features of the environment. Greeno[18] believes that if we consider these situational elements, we can increase our understanding of interactive reasoning in novel situations. This understanding can serve as a guide to structure simulated learning and facilitate learning in real world environments.

Given the occupational therapist's frequent use of simulated experiences in preparing patients to perform in real world environments, the mental model may be a viable theoretical option that could be developed within the context of occupational therapy. The model may also increase our understanding of transference and how to facilitate learning in varied contexts as well as provide a framework for research. For a detailed description of this model, the reader is referred to the original source.[18]

The Structural-Organismic Perspective

The writings of Jean Piaget[31–35] and Heinz Werner[47–49] represent the structural-organismic perspective, which identifies cognition as a complex internal system of organization that influences how the person relates in the environment. It is an assimilation-accommodation model of cognitive functioning within which one can identify stages in knowledge acquisition, symbolization and social learning.

Assimilation and Accommodation

As a person interacts every day with people and objects in the environment, he or she takes in new information. This information fits into existing cognitive structures (schemes), which will give meaning to the new event. This process gives a subjective view of the world and is called **assimilation**. During **accommodation**, the person will notice the specific properties of objects, people and events as well as the relationships among them. He or she will take in this new information and alter the existing cognitive structures (ways of interpreting information) to meet the demands of the new experience and thus develop a more objective view.[13] Assimilation and accommodation occur simultaneously throughout the process of development and if the two processes are in balance, adaptive intelligence occurs.[13]

Equilibration

The method of maintaining this balance is called equilibration. **Equilibration** is an internal self-regulatory process through which the individual controls the process of development and maturation as well as the experiences and social interactions that occur throughout life. For optimum cognitive growth to occur moderate disequilibrium is required.[13] That is, the individual must be exposed to experiences that blend both the familiar and the novel. Too much sameness is boring and fails to stimulate interest; totally novel events or experiences have nothing in them that the person can understand or relate

to. Given a moderate amount of new information, the individual will change his or her thinking as needed to achieve harmony or balance and thereby achieve a more sophisticated level of adaptability.[30]

During the assimilation and accommodation processes, schemes are developed. Structural-organismic theorists define schemes in much the same way as do information processing proponents. According to Flavell, **schemes** are the cognitive units or individual structures that house or give meaning to all experiences. Stated another way, schemes are the mental representation of experience. As the person grows and changes, more and more schemes are accumulated. They organize the person's perceptions and the events that are perceived by the person into information groups according to common characteristics.[13]

Motivation for Cognitive Development

Throughout development the basis for motivation expands and changes and several motivators can exist simultaneously. Initially, the system functions as a result of intrinsic motivation. The infant is believed to respond to its environment from birth because of an inborn mechanism that causes the child to respond to stimuli and explore the environment. As the child interacts in the environment and encounters novel experiences, he or she is also intrinsically motivated to achieve equilibration. Eventually, as the child interacts in and learns from the surroundings, a sense of personal satisfaction and competence become additional motivating forces for interaction.[13]

Development of Knowledge

Structural-organismic theory, commonly referred to as **cognitive developmental** theory, proposes that as children and adults develop they come to think about their worlds in new ways. That is, not only do they increase the quantity of their knowledge, but the nature or quality of their thinking changes also. As part of the developmental process, different kinds of knowledge come into existence. For the sake of discussion, we can group this knowledge into three kinds of information, although the reader will quickly recognize that these categories are overlapping and interdependent: physical knowledge, symbolic-representational thought, and social cognition.

Guidano and Liotti[19] integrate stage-specific and information-processing models and have identified two kinds of knowledge: tacit knowledge and explicit knowledge. **Tacit knowledge** is the original kind of knowledge and consists of information that cannot be verbalized. This information is prelogical, helps the individual focus attention and pursue a goal, communicates to the person his or her perceptions of self and the world, and eventually coordinates between experience and higher level cognitive function. **Explicit knowledge** is information that exists after language develops. This information can be verbalized, is in or has a conscious component that allows the person to explore and control the environment, and gives him or her the ability to reflect on experiences to form concepts that endure over time and that can be manipulated. The person manipulates these concepts to form reality and to consciously control the self and the environment.

Physical Knowledge. **Physical knowledge** encompasses the physical properties of objects and events (e.g., size, shape, color) and organizes this information according to principles of logic. These principles determine how the individual perceives the changes in and relationship of objects and actions over time and through space. The acquisition of physical knowledge was a primary focus of Piaget's work. Physical knowledge both provides the

basis for and depends on symbolic-representational intelligence and social cognition.

Symbolic Representational Thought. **Symbolic representational intelligence** encompasses language development, the use of language (including reading and writing), and the formation of mathematical constructs. This knowledge allows the individual to correctly name objects, communicate his or her needs, and form logical sequences of thought and action.

Social Cognition. Flavell describes **social cognitive development** as a "gradual process of differentiating self from nonself, persons from nonpersons, and one person from another."[13] These conceptions will be developed and are elaborated to form rules, laws, morals, values and ethics that assist a person during social interactions while using verbal and nonverbal communication.

Although social learning theory has not been primarily concerned with establishing age parameters for social cognition, it has contributed to the understanding of the role that imitation, modeling and observation learning play in cognitive development. Therefore, we include this information in our discussions.

Cognitive Developmental Principles

The rules of cognitive development, especially Piagetian rules, are probably quite familiar to the reader.

1. Knowledge development occurs in an invariant, sequential pattern of developmental stages characterized by the use of given cognitive structures.
2. An individual operates primarily at one stage, then, incorporating the cognitive structures identified with this stage, proceeds to the next stage, at which he or she uses new structures.
3. Progress through these stages is not automatic and is related to four enabling conditions: a) the physical maturation of the individual, especially the central nervous

system; b) physical experience with objects and sensory stimuli; c) social transmission through interaction in which people exchange increasingly complex ideas; and d) the existence of a self-regulating, internal mechanism that operates within the individual to reconcile or equilibrate maturation and experience.

4. A person may not skip a stage and jump to a higher one.
5. Persons prefer to use the highest or most complex cognitive structures of which they are capable.[35]

Although few developments challenge the general utility of cognitive-developmental principles in giving a typical picture of the progression of cognitive changes, recent literature has emphasized the following:

1. The child or adult may use cognitive structures representative of more than one stage, depending on the situation.
2. Adults and children may regress and use cognitive structures typical of stages lower than those they are capable of using, for instance, when they are under stress or have unmet emotional needs.

Therefore, a stage theory of cognitive development should not connote to the reader an all-or-nothing, acquisitional model. Further, and this point cannot be overemphasized, an adult's behavior and thoughts can be characteristic of any of the stages.

To illustrate this point, as we proceed in our review of cognitive development, we pause often to exemplify given cognitive structures as represented in adult behavior. When lower levels of cognitive reasoning predominate, however, the individual tends to be limited in the ability to effectively manage a variety of adult expectations. The reader must keep this limitation in mind when using the information from this chapter as a foundation for treatment.

Stages of Cognitive Development

The stages most frequently identified in discussions of cognitive development are organized chronologically as follows:

1. Infancy (birth to two years);
2. Early childhood (two to six years);
3. Later childhood (seven to eleven years);
4. Adolescence-adulthood (12 years and older).

As we highlight briefly how the threads of knowledge intertwine to create the fabric of cognition, we emphasize that what follows represents only a tip of the iceberg in regard to the infinite, complex and unique knowledge structure developed by each of us.

Infancy (Birth to Two Years)

Physical Knowledge

The foundation for all three kinds of cognition is laid during the period Piaget called the **sensorimotor** period of logic development. At birth the child has a biological identity and an amorphous personal-psychological identity. When developing during these first two years of life, the child is aware of and interprets bodily sensations and actively processes the information gained from exploration, body rhythms and feelings. An important part of this process in cognitive development is for the child to distinguish the sensations that come from inside from those that originate outside the self. In other words, the child establishes personal boundaries and takes a big step in the process that will continue throughout life: establishing a sense of self.

Object Permanence. The infant's beginning movements begin as random movements and initially lack goal direction. As development occurs in this period, however, movement becomes more purposeful through much **practice play** or experimentation with objects.

From this play the child makes the important discovery that objects have permanence (they exist even when temporarily out of sight) and that motor acts have predictable results (e.g., release a toy and it will fall). A key developmental accomplishment in this stage is the infant's eventual ability to hold an internal image or symbol of objects.

Egocentricity.   As the child develops, he or she becomes capable of simple imitation; that is, simple gestures and sounds can be imitated, but not coordinated, sequences of events.[30]

During infancy, the child is **egocentric**, at the center of his or her reality. All perceptions are generated from the center. Therefore, all things are as they appear to the child, and cannot be conceived in any other way. There are no alternatives. Because the child can entertain only one alternative at a time, problem-solving is rigid and limited. To problem-solve, the child uses trial and error manipulations that are tied to the obvious cues in any given dilemma. There is no sound reality testing as we think of it.

The present is the time frame that exists for the child. He or she does not have an adult conception of tomorrow or later. One result is the need to have demands met immediately, also called the need for **immediate gratification**.

Infantile Adult Behavior.   Some adult behaviors that are suggestive of this cognitive stage of development include those often described as primitive, or **regressed**. For example, a confused individual may put objects in his or her mouth or need to touch all objects in the environment to ascertain their physical properties. Or, the individual may become agitated when an important other is out of sight because of a disturbance in object permanence. These behaviors should not be confused with the continued enjoyment we all have in experiencing the sensory or sensual aspects of our world.

Symbolic Representational Knowledge

The ability to represent persons, objects and events symbolically in images becomes the ability for language. Two broad tasks related to language acquisition are considered here: learning language and learning how to use it.†

Learning Language.   How is language learned? Researchers believe that the child has both innate and acquired mechanisms that promote language development and communication. There is believed to be an innate ability to discriminate and produce speech sounds. The acquired mechanisms that promote language development and communication depend on the environment and the experiences that the person has with people and objects. For instance, the availability of models is believed to be important in speech development. The child imitates the speech he or she hears first as sounds, then words; later the child generalizes to learn the rules of grammar and syntax. Cognitive and motor development also influence language (e.g., the ability to speak depends on the ability to coordinate the mouth tongue, and facial muscles in given patterns).

Using Language.   The child talks about familiar things and experiences and uses language initially to communicate with significant others. Language in infancy begins with nonverbal gestures (the child points to and reaches for objects) and the babbling or gurgling sounds we often refer to as baby talk. These babbling sounds can be regarded as the child's experimentation with and development of all the sounds needed for later controlled, semantic speech. Near the end of this stage, many children will use one and two word structures as they learn the names of important objects and become increasingly capable of communicating their needs.

---

[1]In his discussion of communication and language, Flavell acknowledges the work of Noam Chomsky, George Miller, Roger Brown and other scientists who have made significant contributions to the study of language acquisition and development. The reader is referred to these sources. Social learning theory also provides detailed discussions of language development and related research. Chapter 11 discusses the ability to read and write as part of language development.

The infant is not only learning to talk, but is learning to use language for its private purpose and for broader purposes of social communication. The private use of language refers to its function as "any sort of aid to one's own thinking, remembering, emotional control or other non-social endeavors." The social use "refers to the use of language to send and receive messages in interpersonal situations."[13]

Social Cognition

Social cognition is knowledge about oneself and people; the relationships between people, groups, and institutions; and the rules and customs that govern these relationships.[13] Like physical knowledge, social cognition proceeds from an invariant formation to a more abstract, hypothetical form.

Attachment. The initial form of cognition is referred to as **attachment**, and is evident in the close bond between the child and primary caregivers. Whereas Freud emphasized the significance of attachment to mother, cognitive developmentalists and social learning theorists stress that attachment occurs between the infant and other consistent persons in life (e.g., father, siblings, grandparents,and babysitters); however, not all of these figures may be of equal importance to the child. That attachment exists can be seen in the infant's signs of pleasure at being with the caregiver, the distress the child displays when separated from the caregiver, and the efforts he or she makes to rejoin the caregiver.[30]

Although contact (e.g., physical, visual) is believed necessary for attachment to occur, it is not yet clear what minimum amount of contact is necessary. Certainly physical contact, play, eye contact between the caregiver and child, feeding, and other dimensions of what we think of as sensitive and affectionate caregiving do affect the attachment process.[30]

Trust and Personal Effectiveness. Through the attachment process, the child learns about the self and his or her effect on others. For example, when he or she cries, Mom responds;

when scared, the closeness of another is comforting. From successful attachment, the child gains essential cognitions related to the dependability or undependability of others, and establishes a foundation of thoughts regarding personal effectiveness and acceptability. The adult who makes frequent suicide gestures for the purpose of mobilizing a spouse or therapist may not have integrated cognitions that enable him or her to evaluate and count on the trustworthiness of others.

Summary of Infancy Period

During the infancy period, essential cognitions or awarenesses are internalized. This knowledge gives the child a sense of self as separate and powerful within his or her world. While this is by no means a conclusive list of all the information the child gains, the following is provided as the basic cognitions established by the child in the infancy period. These should be read as beliefs internalized by the child and not as literal verbalizations made by the child:

1. I am myself: I am no one else.
2. There are people who will keep me safe, fed and comfortable.
3. There are people who want to be with me.
4. I am acceptable.
5. I am powerful: I make things happen.
6. People and objects continue to exist even if I don't see them (only partially established).
7. Some objects bring pain; some bring pleasure.
8. Given motor acts have predictable consequences (only partially established).

Once the child is able to represent self, objects, and events internally (e.g., he or she knows that Mother exists even when she is not in sight), the child has the confidence and sense of safety that promotes further exploration of the environment. It is through this exploration that separation or **detachment** begins.

Early Childhood (Two to Six or Seven Years)

Physical Knowledge

During early childhood, which Piaget referred to as the **preoperational** period of development, verbal and nonverbal means of communication continue to develop, as well as behaviors that enable self-control. The child can communicate his or her desires, gains in muscle strength, and gains control in relation to the execution of purposeful action, including control over urination and defecation and control over selected aspects of the environment.

Establishing Simple Relationships. A childhood type of logic (or what Flavell calls a **semilogic**) is evident in the child's knowlege of identities and functions. An **identity** "reflects an understanding that something has remained invariant while other things have changed."[13] The classical example of an identity is seen in Piaget's experiment in which the child can identify that two identical beakers hold the same amount of water. **Functions** refer to "the child's increasing recognition of simple functional relationships and regular co-occurrences or covariations among everyday objects and events."[13]

For example, when Dad picks up his briefcase, the child knows that he is going to work; when the babysitter comes, Mom and Dad are leaving. The limited usefulness of these functions results from the child's postulates regarding **causality**. Frequently, the child at this period will conclude that if events occur together, then one must have caused the other. Or, the child inaccurately concludes that two events that often occur together must occur together.

Preoperational causal thinking is evident in the conclusions of the following young adult: Joan was brought into the hospital by her family, who verbalized concern over her behavior in the last two months. They stated that she was increasingly argumentative and irritable, that she was buying an unusual amount of goods at local stores, and spending beyond her means. When the therapist asked Joan why she thought she needed hospitalization, Joan paused and recalled the most recent event preceding her admission saying, "I think they're mad at me because I slept late this morning."

Egocentric View. The child continues to be **egocentric** and is unable to consistently entertain the views of others. For instance, the child who desires sweets for lunch may not be able to consider the stance of the parent whose primary concern is that the child have nutritious meals. Piaget's contention that children in this stage are unable to consider the views of others has not been confirmed by many people's experience or research. However, there are many limits on the child's ability to consider the views of others.

There is a magical quality in the logic of the egocentric child, for in egocentricity, he or she believes that events can be controlled by one's thoughts. An example of magical thinking is evident in the following adolescent's conclusions.

After talking to his primary therapist, John was furious. Back on the hospital unit, he told everyone that his therapist was a "jackass" and that he didn't want to see him anymore, but he said nothing of his anger to the therapist. The following day John's therapist announced that he would be going on a two-week vacation. While the therapist was gone, John was extremely depressed and noncommunicative. He finally told one of the other patients that he felt "really awful" because he had, by his anger, "made" his therapist leave.

Symbolic Representational Knowledge

The increasingly sophisticated use of language is a key development during early childhood. The child learns to use all the parts of speech (e.g., nouns, verbs, pronouns) according to most grammatical rules and builds a vast vocabulary. In addition to adequate vocabulary and sentence structure, cognitive processes will increase the effectiveness of communication: the ability to be specific in the identification of objects and people (referent, nonreferent array), the ability to be sensitive to the listener, and the ability to be sensitive to feedback.[13] As a result of improved communication, the child's ability for self-control increases, behavior becomes more purposeful, and he or she can profit from training and teaching experiences.

Referent-Nonreferent Array. First the child, as speaker, must adequately identify and describe the similarities and differences in the environment to help the listener distinguish the correct object, person or event under discussion. For example, if there is a group of children and the child wishes to tell the listener about his or her brother in the group, the child might state, "See that boy in the red shirt on the blue bicycle, with the boy in the blue shirt on a yellow bicycle; the boy on the blue bike is my brother." The child speaker has distinguished his or her brother (**referent**) within the group of children (**nonreferent**) and can now further develop the conversation.

Distinguishing Among Listeners. The second process is the child's ability, as speaker, to be sensitive to his or her listener and the communication setting. This will allow the child to adapt the vocabulary as well as the method of communication. Thus, communication can be adapted to meet the need of the child versus the adult, the stranger versus a friend, the use of the telephone versus personal contact. The adult who has not mastered this level of skill may, for instance, seem to be overly familiar with casual acquaintances or strangers.

Using Feedback. The third process is the child's ability, as speaker, to recieve and make use of feedback when speaking. **Feedback** allows the child to understand verbal and nonverbal messages conveyed by the listener and to respond to the feedback to improve the quality of the intended message. That is, he or she

can amplify or clarify communication if the listener seems confused or can modulate the message tone and delivery if the listener appears to be angry.[13] Finally, as a listener, the child becomes increasingly able to attend to one and then more than one speaker, to ask questions when needed in order to increase his or her understanding, and to respond verbally and nonverbally to the communication received.[13]

Social Cognition

During this early childhood period, the individual becomes increasingly able to separate or detach from parents. Now able to take an image of parents when he or she leaves them, and trusting they will be there upon returning, the child can leave parents for longer periods of time. Emotionally, attachment remains strong. At the same time, the child becomes capable of more complex differentiation, motives and defenses, imitation and identification.

Differentiation. **Differentiation** occurs when the child is aware of his or her own preferences for persons and objects and can separate personal feelings from the feelings of others. He or she will progress from a superficial awareness of another person's appearance and behavior to an in-depth understanding of the other's thoughts and feelings. During social cognitive development the child broadens precepts. He or she not only recognizes Mom but also can see changes in her facial expression and knows that different expressions have different meaning. The child can identify feeling in a global manner (e.g., good versus bad, and happy versus sad). A male child may break a dish for example, and then say "bad boy." Next he or she learns to identify and represent personal thoughts and opinions as well as those of others. For example, when returning home from school after a bad day you may hear the child say, "The kids think I'm stupid."

Motives and Defenses. The child begins to understand the concept of merit and blame, and can consider the significance of individual intentions or motives. Even the four or five-year-old child who has done something wrong will, upon seeing a disapproving glance from his or her mother, respond with, "I didn't mean to, Mommy," and then may follow this statement with, "I'm sorry; I won't do it again." Eventually, the child identifies the motives and system of defenses that he or she and others use. For instance, you may hear a young child or adult say to another, "Oh, you're just doing that to be my friend."

Imitation. As a part of cognitive development, the child expands on the infantile ability to imitate the behavior of others and begins to imitate complex sets of behaviors of both parents and playmates. At first, he or she tends to look at superficial qualities (e.g., those related to size and strength) and imitates parents and peers who are admired to feel important. Soon, he or she selects behaviors to imitate that are most likely to bring desired results. In this way the child becomes capable of selective imitation based on the **anticipation of consequences**.

Some theorists also believe that the child is learning about others when observing them, even when no direct imitation follows. That is, he or she can cognitively retain behaviors seen or modeled and can extrapolate rules of social behavior that can be recalled and used later.[8,9,37]

Identification. **Identification** is a type of complex imitation in which the child actively selects and retains the attitudes and beliefs of the parent or role model. In identifying with significant role models, the child may adopt their behaviors, their emotional responses, and the cognitions that he or she discerns during the observation of them. Ask a youngster in this age group what he or she thinks about the performance of our country's president or his or her thoughts about persons from other racial or ethnic groups and you will most likely learn what parents are saying at home or teachers are saying at school.

During this period, the child conceives of and describes himself or herself in terms of observable or tangible characteristics. For example, the child may identify his or her gender ("I am a boy" or "girl"), describe physical attributes (blue eyes, brown hair) and usually relates having the preferences and values of his or her parents. The child adopts the framework of others in this self-conception because it is their framework with which he or she is most familiar and because children depend on parents and significant others for self-esteem.

Summary of Childhood

During early childhood, the child interacts with the environment and continues to develop communication skills, a sense of self as different from others, and beginning skill related to self-control. Some of the key cognitions internalized during early childhood are summarized here:

1. What I want is most important, but other people have wants, too.
2. I have (specific) skills. Things I can do include (the person can name personal capabilities).
3. I can make things happen by wishing.
4. Some behaviors are rewarded; some are punished.
5. Things that look alike are alike.
6. People are not all the same.
7. Primary differences in people are in their size, strength or possessions.
8. A mistake is not as bad if it is an accident.
9. Mom (Dad, other) has predictable behaviors; these are (the person can name them).
10. Different people are treated differently.
11. My mother's (father's) face, voice and manner can tell me if she is happy, sad, angry.
12. Yesterday is over; tomorrow has not yet come.

Later Childhood (Seven to Eleven Years)

Physical Knowledge

The cognitive accomplishments of the previous period are expanded upon during the next period, which Piaget referred to as one of **concrete operational thinking**. The person becomes increasingly able to perceive the whole picture and have a balanced view. That is, he or she is able to analyze the parts in relation to the whole object or event (**decentration**) rather than focus attention on one particular stimulus (**centration**.) Now the individual is able to grasp the concepts that are needed for transformations, reversals, inversions, compensation, and reciprocity. Thinking becomes quantitative and oriented toward measurement. This development facilitates the use of number skills and knowledge that serves as the foundation for the logical thinking that occurs in conjunction with their use.[13]

Transformations. **Transformations** can be physical or temporal. For example, the person can see that amounts may remain the same even if the shape differs (**physical transformation**); for instance, when a large rock is cut into pieces, the shape changes but the weight of all the pieces is the same as that of the original large rock. **Temporal transformations** allow the person to have a firm grasp of the concept of past, present, and future time. Before this development, the person could focus only on the one aspect of time that was perceived in the present moment.[13]

When an individual's thoughts become reversible, he or she is able to "sense how one action can literally annul or negate its opposite," **inversion** and "also how one action or factor can more directly undo or make up for the effects of another, which is not its opposite" **compensation**.[13] For example, a person is shown two parallel lines of equal length, each containing ten pennies, and is asked whether the lines are equal. Then the length of one line is changed by expanding the distance between each coin. If the person identifies the change in line length and attributes this change to the broader spacing of coins, he or she is demonstrating compensation.

Number Concepts. Number knowledge and skills are evident in one's ability to perceive sets of similar objects, to count the objects, to read and write numbers, to identify the cardinal and ordinal aspects of a number (e.g., to count objects using the correct sequence and identify the last number in a series as well as to identify particular numbers before the last [e.g., the fifth of 16]), to identify similar sets of objects and compare the number and size of the objects in each set, to add and subtract objects and be able to see the reversible quality of the process.[13]

Logical Thinking. The individual functioning at this stage has a form of thinking that Flavell calls **logical**. That is, the child is able to make propositions about specific aspects of reality and then test each proposition separately to confirm the logical relationships that can exist. Flavell calls this process **interpropositional thinking**.

Interpropositional thinking uses inductive reasoning and is illustrated in psychology literature in the following experimental task. The child is given two rows of beads, equally spaced and placed parallel to each other. The child is asked to state if there are an equal number of beads in each row. Then the spacing of the beads in one line is changed, although the same number of beads still exists in each line and the lines remain parallel. The child is asked to state if the number of beads in each row is still equal. The child who confirms the response by counting the beads in each line is using interpropositional thinking. In occupational therapy there is an analogous example. The patient who is working on a tile trivet that is modeled after a sample trivet may confirm his or her decisions while working by accurately counting the tiles in each row of both trivets, the sample and the one being made.

Stage of Absolutes. Discovering the logical relationship between objects and events is a main aim of thinking in this period. However, logical relationships can be deduced only from perceptible tangible matters, not from hypothetical constructs. Whatever knowledge is discovered, information is viewed as correct or incorrect. This is a stage of **absolutes**, and there is little ability for flexibility. In children the stage of absolutes is readily seen in their interpretation of rules or laws. This stage of absolute thinking by an adult is illustrated in the following example.

An older gentleman was evaluating the benefits of a travel club and deciding whether to become a member. He based his decision to join on his desire to take a trip in the immediate future and the reimbursement of the initial fare that he would receive if he joined the club. He could not evaluate whether there were long-term benefits for joining the club. For example, in the future would the club travel to sites of interest to him? As a member of the club, would he be eligible for reduced airline fares to his desired destination? Did the majority of club benefits meet travel and social needs?

Symbolic-Representational Knowledge

The ability to use language privately as well as socially increases during this period. Vocabulary and syntax become more complex. For example, the individual can appreciate that the same word can have several meanings, that two words that sound alike can have different meanings, and that several different words can connote an identical meaning.

Empathy. The child or adult is able to use feedback in a way that was previously limited. Because the person can now **decenter** or imagine the views of someone else, he or she can also empathize with a person with whom he or she interacts. As a consequence, feedback is not restricted to taking in information in order to modify one's own performance, although it can still be used for this purpose. Feedback can now be used to better understand the needs and concerns of another.

Social Cognition

The child has come far in the process of separation from parents, and needs only occasionally to touch base with them through the day, as he or she goes about the day's many activities; however, the continuity of emotional caring continues. Although still identifying with parents, the child, in preparation for adolescence, has begun the process of distinguishing how his or her likes and preferences are, at times, different from theirs.

Peer Friendships. The child's peer friendships have become very important. More and more he or she identifies with and imitates peers, rather than parents. Being like and being accepted by peers are important and can place the child in conflict with parental ideals.

In this stage of cognitive development, the child learns to grasp the concept of personality and identifies and discusses his or her own personality as well as that of others. Whereas initial descriptions of a friend used to be, "He is nice, he has toys that I like, and we ride bikes together," descriptions become more precise than "nice," "good," or "bad" and are less tied to another's appearance and possessions. Now, the child might say, "She is my friend because she is thoughtful and considerate and listens to my problems."

Sense of Self. The child's sense of self, which comes from both the reflections and reactions of others to the child and from the increased ability to think about personal experiences, has become much firmer. It includes not only a sense of self as a physical and psychological being as he or she exists, but also has come to include an **ideal self** or thoughts about the person he or she wants to be. This ideal self develops from his or her observations of the outcome of given behaviors in others and from the incorporation of others' values. It may begin with the wish to change physical attributes ("I wish I looked like Jane; everyone likes her") and progresses to more concern about psychological traits. ("I like myself best when I'm kind and patient.")

Summary of Later Childhood

Throughout later childhood, the child builds on previous cognitive development to continue to develop a sense of self, form peer relationships, and build the foundation for logical reasoning. Key cognitions that are established during later childhood are summarized as follows:

1. Not everyone thinks and feels as I do.
2. Events have history; I have a history and a future.
3. Events have their opposites.
4. Objects and events can be organized logically.
5. I believe what I can see or prove.
6. I am mostly like my parents, but different in the following ways (person can name differences).
7. Friends are important; being like my friends is important.
8. My friend's personality is more important than what he or she possesses.
9. I have my own personality.
10. It is important to consider the feelings of others.

Adolescence and Adulthood (12 Years and Older)

Physical Knowledge

As a result of cognitive, social, and motor skill development, the adolescent begins to question how he or she has defined the self and the rules and beliefs that he or she has adopted unchallenged from parents and role models and searches for an identity that is self-defined (sometimes referred to as **autonomous identity**).

Future Orientation. Adolescents continue to use trial and error problem-solving but begin to experiment with a more scientific approach. They begin to focus on the future, raising issues such as, "Who do I want to be? What do I want to do? Whom do I wish to be with? What do I value? How will I accomplish my goals? How will I contribute to life?"

Scientific Period. Before adolescence, one's knowledge is considered prescientific. That is, the person uses trial and error learning and primarily seeks experiences that provide consistency and regularity. At about age 15 to 20 years, the individual sees the limitations of this knowledge and tries to find variety in experiences and variables in knowledge. As a result the adolescent begins to logically restructure previously acquired knowledge. This stage is referred to as the **scientific period of knowledge development**.

Formal Operational Thinking. During this period, the person forms new hypotheses about the self and the world. Experiences are designed to systematically collect data in order to validate or reconstruct previous knowledge and to amplify information. This ability to engage in hypothetic-deductive reasoning has also been called **formal operational thinking**. Now the individual can see possibilities, and not just the actual situation. He or she can anticipate future outcomes when problem-solving, is able to conceptualize an outcome after generating multiple combinations of given data, and can carry out planned, strategic problem-solving.[13] For example, the individual wishing to attend college will be able to identify personal interests, the schools that can best satisfy these interests and other resources that will help him or her to satisfy personal needs and fulfill goals.

Change in Self-Perception. During this scientific process, a cycle occurs by which one's personal identity is continuously remodeled and problem-solving is promoted. Knowledge structures maintain a basic identity of oneself and the real world and at the same time incorporates information from life's experiences to allow for growth and changes in self-perception and increasingly sophisticated problem-solving.

Symbolic-Representational Knowledge

The increased sophistication in language communication is needed for and representative of the hypothetical thinking just discussed. The individual is able to use language privately to generate and keep track of many alternatives while weighing both the obvious and more subtle differences in courses of actions. He or she is able to think through a plan and imagine its consequences without needing to physically act out behavior. The person can use language to both imagine oneself and others in the future and to reflect on oneself or others in the past in order to select the most suitable course of action.

Fantasy.   Whereas the very young child can enjoy fantasy because he or she can enter into it and lose personal boundaries within it, an adult capable of this mature level of cognition can enjoy the freedom and symbolic play comprised in fantasy, yet not lose sight of what is real and what is imagined.

Sense of Humor.   The language of the adult often includes a rich use of simile, metaphor and allegory. Words come to represent much more than the obvious or literal meaning, and they become capable of carrying a depth of private and publically shared symbolism. As a result, the adult thinking at this level can appreciate the puns and plays on words that make up sophisticated adult humor such as satire.

Social Cognition

The most characteristic changes in social cognition occur as a part of the transition into adulthood as the individual goes about establishing an identity autonomous from his or her family. To achieve autonomy the person will work to further develop and formalize self-concepts.

Self-Concept.   The mature **self-concept** includes several dimensions that relate to the following:

1. Being able to recognize and relate comfortably in a variety of different roles, which may carry different role expectations, while retaining an overall sense of wholeness;
2. Having a sense of competency to meet challenges, while being able to realistically acknowledge limitations;
3. Accepting the responsibility for one's own actions and feeling that the self has power over the outcome of personal events;
4. Being able to separate one's own ideas or ideals from those of others and to actively select those that will guide one's belief and value system.[30]

Personal Beliefs.   As a person prepares to take his or her place as a mature adult, he or she will philosophize about the world, how it should be, and how to make it better. From these philosophical ideals and from a long history of taking in and accommodating to information about the world will come an identity constructed from personal beliefs, not defined by others. He or she takes a stance and identifies thoughts, values and attitudes, many of which may differ from parental views; and he or she will behave more independently. This new self definition allows the person to separate from parents and begin a search for a partner with whom he or she can have an adult love relationship.

Having reached adulthood does not mean that cognitive development ends. Even when no new cognitive schemes develop, throughout adult life the individual will continue to take in information and accommodate to changing role expectations and learn new skills.

Not every adult achieves the so-called higher levels of cognitive function. Nor does the individual always use the most sophisticated cognitive schemes of which he or she is capable. In times of stress, for example, when motivation is diminished, when physical causes interfere with cognitive processes, or when emotional-affective needs are unmet, the person may revert to lower levels of cognitive function. Additionally, performance may represent fluctuations in cognitive levels due to factors in the environment. For example, persons with stroke, brain injury or other neurological deficits often have variable performance ability depending on the hour of the day and the environmental context in which they are functioning.

Summary of Adolescence and Young Adulthood

During adolescence and young adulthood, mature cognitions are forming. The person can fantasize and orient to the future. Logical reasoning continues to develop and influence approaches to problem-solving. Young adults change and refine their self-concept as they experience varied roles and establish a belief system. Those mature cognitions that serve as guiding structures by many, but certainly not all, young adults are the following:

1. Not everything is as it seems.
2. There are concerns (needs, causes, issues) more important than my own desires.
3. I could take many courses of action in my life; I must consider their consequences.
4. The greater welfare of humankind is my concern.
5. Most social issues are not black or white.
6. I am separate from my parents; I am responsible for my own decisions.
7. There is a world of experience beyond the verifiable.
8. I do not have to control or organize everything in my environment.

Perception, Attention, Memory and Problem-Solving as Cognitive Processes

In addition to what has been discussed regarding information and the acquisition of sensorimotor, symbolic-representational, and social knowledge, the broad definition of cognition includes perception, attention, memory and problem-solving.

Perception

In the literature, the development of perception is described as moving from a singular system during infancy and expanding to a perceptual-attentional system throughout life. The descriptions of the five senses and their development broaden to include the perception-attentional characteristics of development and descriptions of how these characteristics enable goal attainment.

Perception involves the ability to perceive space and objects, to integrate information from the multiple sensory systems (e.g., auditory, visual, tactile), to coordinate the sensory and motor systems, to remember visual images, to interpret perceptual illusions and to grasp the concept of picture perception.[13] Occupational therapy literature discusses extensively space-object perception, sensory integrative, and sensorimotor systems. The reader is referred to Chapter 9 for reading references in this area.

Attention

Selective Attention and Perceptual Learning

In the area of perception, Flavell recommends the work of Eleanor Gibson,[16] who describes the theory of perceptual learning and development. Her theory emphasizes the selective nature of perceptual processing and attentional deployment. She describes the processes through which the person comes to differentiate perceptual data and identify similarities and differences between objects and events. This perceptual sensitivity occurs as a result of abstraction, filtering and peripheral mechanisms of attention.

The infant perceives, attends to, and responds to stimuli in the environment. As the person grows, perceptions and attention become increasingly selective, focused and self-controlled or intentional. This increased control over one's perception and attention influences learning and facilitates adaptation. The person becomes able to decide *when* to attend, *what* to attend to, and the *benefits* of attending, and thereby develops an attending strategy.[20]

Attention Span

With development, attention becomes increasingly planned and strategic. As attention becomes more strategic, it also occurs over longer periods of time. The child who could only play with a toy for a few minutes grows into the adult who can enjoy a favorite book for many hours. Attention does not occur in isolation, but over time. Thus the individual screens, selects and retains the necessary data to respond and benefit from the feedback that comes from the environment and from within oneself to determine if something was missed or overlooked. The person then sets about maintaining general contact with reality as well as selectively attending to and adapting to one or more situations simultaneously.[13]

Through experience the individual becomes increasingly aware of the ability to attend and how to use attention, to direct his or her behavior and to accomplish a goal. The teacher, for example, may know that he or she can grade papers with a radio playing in the background, but not while sitting in a mall with people walking about. This ability to monitor attention and use planned attention and strategies is also a part of metacognition.

Memory

To understand memory and its development, we will examine the basic memory processes and strategies as well as knowledge and metamemory. The reader will recognize the use of information processing vocabulary in the contemporary conceptualization of memory.

Memory Hardware

The basic processes of memory are called the **hardware** of the human memory system, the fundamental operations and capabilities of the system.[13] Storage, recognition and recall are examples of basic processes. Basic memory operations influence the person's capacity to learn and know. In discussions of memory, the reader may have noticed that it is difficult to separate the definitions of memory from those for knowledge. Flavell describes this interrelationship when he states, "What a person knows influences what he learns and remembers."[13]

Types of Memory

In Flavell's discussion, two types of memory are referred to: episodic memory and semantic memory. **Episodic memory** is the knowledge that a person retains from specific, personal experiences. **Semantic memory** is acquired knowledge that comes from multiple sources. It is the knowledge that allows us to name objects, people, places and colors. For instance, when a child hears the word, bike, he or she will visualize the object that he or she knows to be a bike (semantic memory) as well as remember how he or she learned to ride the bike, the times he or she has fallen off the bike, or the friends with whom he or she rides (episodic memory).

Storing Knowledge in Memory

The process by which this knowledge is stored as memory is called **construction,** and the process by which it is retrieved is called **reconstruction**. When a person remembers something, he or she does not make an exact copy of the information that is stored. A person cannot make copies that replicate information as a tape recording or as a photograph does. Rather, he or she may add or omit information and emphasize points that are personally meaningful. As a result, people conceptually organize and reorganize data until they have a meaningful representation of the information.[13] For instance, when the child in the previous example tells someone about his or her bike and past experiences with a bike he or she reconstructs the stored information (constructions) about the bike. With each reconstruction, one will probably find some variation in the stories shared about the bike because of the difficulty in exact reproduction.

Memory Strategies

To remember information, a person may use specific conscious activities to help remember or recall information.[50] These memory activities are called **memory strategies**; in many instances they are similar to or subsumed within metacognitive learning strategies, as discussed previously. Strategies are used for storage and retrieval of information. Some examples of storage strategies include the following:

1. **Rehearsal**: The process by which a person repeats stimuli or an experience until it is remembered (e.g., a child counts from 1 to 10 until the sequence is learned perfectly).
2. **Organization**: The process by which a person organizes or categorizes information into knowledge groups with similarities. For example, the child learns that there are dogs, cats, birds and horses and then learns that they all are part of the category animal. The student organizes information into categories to be remembered for an examination.
3. **Elaboration**: The process by which the person uses visual images to create a picture or a story to remember two nonrelated items.[13] (Using these strategies in the treatment of organic brain dysfunction is discussed in more detail in Chapter 11.)

Metamemory

Metamemory refers to "knowledge about anything concerning memory." It has two distinguishing categories: sensitivity to and knowledge of person, task and strategy variables.[13] That is, the person knows when to store or retrieve knowledge as well as what will im-

prove or decrease one's memory performance. Metamemory exists when the person is able to describe his or her ability to remember or limitations in remembering, the tasks that help him or her to remember or that are more easily remembered, and the aids that are used to store and retrieve information.

Problem-Solving

Problem-solving is an active process that incorporates all of the components of cognition that have been discussed to achieve one or more of the following goals: 1) identify a dilemma (mental or physical) that requires attention, 2) identify its salient features, and 3) create a sequence of responses. The nature of the logic used in problem-solving depends on the development of cognitive structures.

Assessing Problem-Solving Ability

When investigating the ability for problem-solving, the occupational therapist has most frequently assessed the patient's ability to identify the problem, look for alternative solutions to the problem, choose one of the alternatives, make a plan of action, implement the plan and evaluate the outcome.

Categories of Problem-Solving

In addition to this general problem-solving format Bara[10] suggests that the therapist also consider categories of problem-solving. Bara identifies six types of problem-solving: 1) formal, 2) mundane, 3) physical, 4) interactive, 5) personal and 6) self. **Formal problem-solving** has limited application to clinical settings and uses mathematical and logical procedures to solve problems. **Mundane problem-solving** uses "common sense" knowledge to interact in everyday life and solve day to day problems (e.g., the person has learned not to touch fire, not to run in the street in front of a car, and not to pick up things off the ground and put them in one's mouth).

Physical problem-solving uses procedures that help us solve physical reality problems.

For example, spatial and temporal orientation help us to see interrelationships among physical events. We know to put on our boots and raincoat when it is raining; we know we need a certain amount of space to walk through a doorway without hitting our head; we know to wear lightweight clothing when it is hot.

Interactive problem-solving uses the social rules acquired from one's family and social network to understand and participate in social interaction such as the rules for interacting with one's parents, house rules that must be observed when one lives at home (e.g., times to be home, calling to notify parents that you will be late), or knowing how to greet a new acquaintance (e.g., shaking hands).

Personal problem-solving, like interactive problem-solving, uses social rules but adds a personal touch. Eventually the person learns to interpret rules using a personal frame of reference rather than just doing what one is told or expected to do, and perhaps the person has learned to manipulate social rules. Therefore, personal experience and social rules are used to interact and problem-solve in social situations.

For example, the street person, the blue collar worker, and the professional have each developed their own standards and style of interaction and method of problem-solving. All have learned from daily experiences or through observing their peers how to solve problems and the codes for interaction.

As one learns from other problem-solving experiences one learns **self-problem-solving**. The individual learns from his or her own personal experimentation. How often has a parent heard a child state, "Let me do it my way," or "I want to do this myself." Innovations may come from self-problem-solving. Self-problem-solving may reflect one's attitude toward oneself. In the previous example, the child is being assertive and seeking independence and permission to be a problem-solver. This image of independence may be accurate or may differ from what the child actually thinks and feels.

Cognition in the Context of Therapy

The cognitive system and its limits have been described within the context of therapy by the behaviorist who would "conceptualize the system as a structural network of external and internal stimulus-response connections," and by the psychoanalytically oriented therapist who would talk about the "structure and functions of the ego."[13] Rather than repeat the descriptions of these conceptualizations, which are referenced in other chapters of this text, we turn our discussion to the application of cognition in mental health from the perspective of the psychiatrist, psychologist and occupational therapist, with the emphasis on the assessment of cognition. Specific assessments and the occupational therapy interventions that incorporate cognitive theory are further addressed in subsequent chapters.

Psychiatrist's Assessment of Cognition

Through the assessment of cognitive processes, the psychiatrist strives to identify or to understand psychopathology. During the initial interview, the physician identifies the patient's motivation, needs and family experiences. The physician also identifies social and occupational experiences and interests and how they have influenced the patient's perceptions, his or her method of processing information and cognitive development. The psychiatrist then evaluates the relationship between the patient's signs and symptoms and his or her perceptual interpretation, system of information processing and developmental picture.[22]

Mental Status Examination

The psychiatrist carries out a general examination of cognitive function by using a mental status examination. The **mental status examination** is designed to establish the patient's general fund of knowledge, orientation to time, place and person; recent and remote memory; ability for behavioral control, judgment and insight; the accuracy of perceptions; thought processes; expression of affect; general behavior; speech patterns; and attitude toward self and others.[22] This information is then documented in the patient's permanent record and is used by the mental health staff as they plan and implement intervention strategies and monitor progress.

Psychologist's Assessment of Cognition

If the psychiatrist or primary therapist cannot diagnose the problem and identify a treatment plan, a psychological assessment administered by a clinical or neuropsychologist may be requested. The clinical psychologist will use skilled observation and interview in conjunction with **standardized tests** (tests that have identified validity and reliability criteria) to augument previously acquired data elicited by the psychiatrist.

Psychological Test Batteries

The test batteries most frequently used with psychiatric populations include an individual intelligence test, an association technique (e.g., person drawing or Rorschach), a story telling test (e.g., Thematic Apperception Test), completion methods (e.g., Minnesota Multiphasic Personality Inventory), and graphomotor tests (e.g., Bender-Gestalt Test).[22] The psychologist then documents the results of these tests and summarizes the patient's test behavior, intellectual ability and present functioning, capabilities and limitations, reality testing, ability for self-control, personal and interpersonal conflicts, self concept, system of defenses, symptoms, motivation and possible diagnosis and prognosis. The reader will note that tests are used to assess cognitive function as well as other areas that are influenced by cognition.[22]

Psychological Testing for Brain Damage

During the general examination, the psychiatrist may suspect that the patient has brain impairment and thus request psychological testing to validate these impressions and to provide additional information about the patient's intellectual performance and personality.[22] The data from the test will be used to describe, predict, modify or control behavior.[25]

Assessment of Functional Systems

When assessing brain damage, tests are used to analyze three functional systems: 1) intellectual functions, 2) personality/emotional variables and 3) control functions.[25] Each of these systems is briefly described. The reader is referred to the original source for a detailed description of a neuropsychological assessment approach.

Atkinson and Shiffrin[7] have classified memory into three categories based on the length of time that the information is stored: 1) sensory memory, 2) short-term working memory and 3) long-term memory. **Sensory memory** is information housed very briefly in one of the sensory systems. Examples of sensory memory are short-term visual memory or **iconic memory** and short-term auditory memory or **echoic memory**. Sensory memory is complex due to the complex nature of the sensory systems, particularly visual and auditory systems. Problems in these areas are usually described as perceptual problems rather than memory problems. **Short-term working memory** is the "system responsible for temporarily holding information while learning, reading, reasoning, or thinking."[7] It is the memory used just during the duration of dealing with a block of information. **Long-term memory** refers to facts, data, and experiences that constitute what we commonly think of as what we "know," and while typically viewed as information held for more than an hour, the long-term memory system "preserves information for anything ranging from minutes to years."[9,10]

Intellectual Function. Intelligence has four major classes of function: receptive, memory and learning, cognition-thinking, and expressive functions. **Receptive functions** include the intact sensory systems (e.g., visual, auditory, tactile) and those dimensions of perception that enable one to be aware of, register, recognize, discriminate, organize and process sensory information. The **memory functions** facilitate learning and depend on registration of information, short-term storage and long-term storage.

Thinking is a function of the entire brain. It is evident in the patient's ability to make computations, reason and make judgments, form concepts, abstract information and generalize behavior, and organize and plan. The **expressive functions** are the means by which the patient communicates and includes the ability to speak, draw, write, use physical gestures and movements, and express affect.[25]

The efficiency of these intellectual functions is influenced by the patient's ability to attend over time the level of consciousness (e.g., alert, drowsy) and his or her activity rate (e.g., the patient's speed of motor response and the speeed of the activity performed).[25]

Personality and Emotional Variables. The patient's personality can change and behavior problems can result when the patient with a neurological disability cannot meet the demands of society. Therefore, the psychologist tries to determine whether the patient's personality or emotionality are affecting his or her behavior. Often when there is brain compromise, there seems to be an exaggeration of the emotional or personality components that characterized the patient before neurological problems developed. Some personality variables are associated with changes within identified brain structures. The patient might be characterized as dull, euphoric, anxious, or depressed depending on brain structures compromised as well as on the patient's own characteristic manner of responding to stress.

Control Functions. Control functions are inferred from the patient's activity response.

Can he or she initiate and complete activities? Adapt his or her work pace as needed (e.g., work more slowly or quickly)? Shift attention to respond to the needs of the task and the environment? Are his or her solutions to problems rigid and inflexible, or too nonchalant? These variables, too, are influenced by the individual's style of relating, his or her response to stress, and the site of specific brain damage.

Alternative Assessments

Should the mental status examination and psychological testing fail to provide the depth of understanding necessary for diagnosis, problem identification and patient treatment, modern technology provides assessment alternatives such as computerized cranial tomography (CT scan).

Occupational Therapy and Cognitive Assessment

Given the previous applications of cognition and the data resources available from the mental status examination, psychological testing and modern technology, what can the occupational therapist contribute to cognitive assessment and treatment? This question is answered in part within the purview of each of the frames of reference in this text; however, an overriding emphasis in all of these frameworks lies at the heart of occupational therapy; that is, the assessment and treatment of cognitive problems within task performance.

Cognitive Assessment Through Tasks

Regardless of the theoretical framework guiding occupational therapy, Mosey[26,27] recommends that the occupational therapist use interview and individualized tasks to assess cognitive performance. Having considered the patient's age, gender, culture and ability, a task is selected. The patient is then given directions, tools and materials and asked to complete a task independently.

For instance, one assessment task proposed by Mosey is to have the patient build a specific object using Lego bricks or erector set materials. Mosey recommends tasks like this because "they can be graded . . . used repeatedly . . . (and) have the quality of play."[26,27] During the cognitive task assessment, the therapist observes current performance and identifies the level of performance required in the future when the patient returns to the community. The recommended guidelines for evaluating cognitive function during a task are adapted from Mosey and highlighted in Table 7.5.

Smith and Cognition

In a general textbook for occupational therapy education, Smith[21,43] identifies cognition as ego function and also stresses the task component of cognition. Where cognitive impairment is suspected Smith[43] proposes that the following be evaluated:

1. Ability to follow simple or complex instructions;
2. Ability to carry over learned skills from one day to the next;
3. Ability to attend to a task (attention span);
4. Ability to follow numerous steps in a process;
5. Ability to understand cause and effect;
6. Ability to problem-solve;
7. Ability to concentrate;
8. Ability to perform in a logical sequence;
9. Ability to organize parts into a meaningful whole;
10. Ability to interpret signs and symbols;
11. Ability to read;
12. Ability to compute.

Cognitive Impairment

Cognition is also defined and applied in assessment and intervention strategies in the discussions of brain injury and other disabilities that affect the patient's memory, communication and sensory, perceptual and other cognitive processes. Within this context and using an information processing analogy, Spencer[44] describes **cognition** as follows:

TABLE 7.5   COGNITIVE TASK OBSERVATION GUIDE

Physical Ability	Posture, muscle strength and endurance, gross and fine motor coordination
Initiative	Voluntarily begins tasks and maintains involvement until task completion
Organization	Arranges materials and tools and work area, and follows written, verbal or demonstrated instructions
Attention	Maintains interest in task and manages distractions to achieve goal of task completion.
Work Performance	Works efficiently and neatly, and gives adequate attention to detail; uses tools and materials appropriately; and monitors own performance
Problem Solve	Responds to the needs of the situation, manages task demands and makes choices that support task accomplishment

Adapted from Mosey A: *Psychosocial Components of Occupational Therapy.* NY, Raven Press, 1986, p. 322.

"Cognition is knowledge and understanding of the environment gained through the information processing capability of the brain. It involves the mechanisms of perception, memory storage and retrieval of information, organization, and language expression. Cognitive behavior is related to the character and effect of interpersonal relationships. Difficulty in handling input of stimuli (reception, interpretation, organization, order of importance) can hinder ability to store necessary information in the brain for retrieval, resulting in poor concentration for intellectual processing or a deficit in long-term memory. Language deficits may be evident due to lowered comprehension and thought organization. Personality changes, loss of inhibitions, distortions of judgment, and lack of abstract reasoning combine with memory loss to hinder cognitive function, problem-solving, and learning ability."

Occupational Therapist's Contributions

The discussions of head injury by Spencer[44] and others such as Abreu and Toglia[1,2] reflect a broader conceptualization of cognition than has been previously applied in occupational therapy. Beyond performance during isolated tasks and regardless of the setting, the therapist is responsible for an on-going assessment of patient functioning during activities and personal interactions in the occupational therapy and natural environment. This assessment includes noting cognition as it is reflected in daily living, work, and leisure performance. Stated another way, cognition is evaluated as the ability for the coherent, well-integrated response(s) we call **problem-solving**.

Of all the helping professionals, the occupational therapist often has the most information about the patient's ability for daily problem-solving. This ability is discerned not only through formal testing but especially through the varying treatment experiences available in the treatment setting. The occupational therapist's observations are shared with other treatment team members to increase staff understanding of patient behavior, to change and update intervention strategies, and to strengthen the consistency of treatment approaches. These observations can also be shared with patients to enhance their understanding of the gains made during the treatment process. The occupational therapist also makes referrals for testing based on observations or the results of the initial occupational therapy screening. He or she may recommend that a patient be tested by a psychologist or a technological method.

Regardless of the therapist's role in assessing cognition, multiple benefits to patient care result when the clinician has a broad understanding of cognition and its potential application in assessment and treatment. These benefits are evident in the discussions of cognitive-behavioral, holistic, movement-centered, and cognitive disabilities frameworks to which we now turn.

References

1. Abreu BC, Toglia JP: *Cognitive Rehabilitation Manual.* New York, Authors, 1984.
2. Abreu BC, Toglia JP: Cognitive rehabilitation: A model for occupational therapy. *Am J Occup Ther* 41: 439–448, 1987.
3. Allen CK: Independence through activity: The practice of occupational therapy (psychiatry). *Am J Occup Ther* 36(11):731–739, 1982.
4. Allen CK: *Occupational Therapy for Psychiatric Diseases: Measurement and Management of Cognitive Disabilities.* Boston, Little, Brown, and Company, 1985.
5. Anderson J: *Cognitive Skills and Acquisition.* Hillsdale, NJ, Lawrence Erlbaum Associates, 1981.
6. Anderson J: *The Architecture of Cognition.* Cambridge, MA, Harvard University Press.
7. Atkinson R, Shiffrin R: Human memory: A proposed system and its control processes. In Spence K, Spence J (Eds): *The Psychology of Learning and Motivation.* Vol. 2. New York, Academic Press, 1968.
8. Bandura A: *Social Learning Theory.* Englewood Cliffs, NJ, Prentice-Hall, 1972.
9. Bandura A: *Social Learning Theory.* Ed. 2. Englewood Cliffs, NJ, Prentice-Hall, 1977.
10. Bara B: Modifications of knowledge by memory processes. In Reda M, Mahoney M: *Cognitive Psychotherapies.* Cambridge, MA, Ballinger Publishing Company, 1984.
11. Crist P: Community living skills: A psychoeducational community based program. *Occup Ther Mental Health* 6:51–64, 1986.
12. Dembo MH: *Applying Educational Psychology in the Classroom.* Ed. 3. New York: Longman, 1988.
13. Flavell J: *Cognitive Development.* Englewood Cliffs, NJ, Prentice-Hall, 1977, pp. 2, 4, 5, 7, 56, 59, 98, 99, 171–174, 216–218.
14. Flavell J: *Cognitive Development* Ed. 2. Englewood Cliffs, NJ, Prentice-Hall, 1985, p. 104.
15. Gagne RM: *The Conditions of Learning.* Ed. 4. New York, Holt, Rinehart and Winston, 1985.
16. Gibson EJ: *Principles of Perceptual Learning and Development.* New York, Appleton-Century-Crofts, 1969.
17. Gick ML, Holyoak KL : The cognitive basis for transfer. In Cormier SM, Hagman JD (Eds): *Transfer of Learning: Contemporary Research and Applications.* New York, Academic Press, 1987.
18. Greeno JG: Situations, mental models and generative knowledge. In Klahr D, Kotovsky K (Eds): *Complex Information Processing: The Impact of Herbert H. Simon.* Hillsdale, NJ, Erlbaum Associates, 1989.
19. Guidano V, Liotti G: *Cognitive Processes and Emotional Disorders.* New York: The Guilford Press, 1983.
20. Hale GA, Taweel SS: Age differences in children's performance on measures of component selection

and incidental learning. *J Exp Child Psychol* 18:107–116, 1974.

21. Hopkins H, Smith H (Eds): *Willard and Spackman's Occupational Therapy.* Ed. 6. Philadelphia, J.B. Lippincott, 1983.

22. Kaplan H, Sadock B: *Comprehensive Textbook — Modern Synopsis of Psychiatry III.* Ed. 3. Baltimore, Williams & Wilkins, 1981, pp. 199, 200, 208–216.

23. King LJ: A sensory integrative approach to schizophrenia. *Am J Occup Ther* 28(9):529–536, 1974.

24. King LJ: Occupational therapy and neuropsychiatry. *Occup Ther Mental Health* 3(1):1–12, 1983.

25. Lezak M: *Neuropsychological Assessment.* New York, Oxford University Press, 1976.

26. Mosey AC: *Frames of Reference for Mental Health.* Thorofare, NJ, SLACK Inc., 1970.

27. Mosey AC: *Psychosocial Components of Occupational Therapy.* New York, Raven Press, 1986.

28. Newel A, Simon H: *Human Problem-Solving.* Englewood Cliffs, NJ, Prentice-Hall, 1972.

29. Norman DA, Gentner DR, Stevens AL: Comments on learning, schemata and memory representation. In Klahr D (Ed): *Cognition and Instruction.* Hillsdale, NJ, Lawrence Erlbaum Associates, 1976.

30. Perry D, Bussey K: *Social Development.* Englewood Cliffs, NJ, Prentice-Hall, 1984, pp. 126, 45–57.

31. Piaget J: *The Origins of Intelligence in Children.* New York, International Universities Press, 1952.

32. Piaget J: *Logic and Psychology.* New York, Basic Books, 1957.

33. Piaget J: *Plays, Dreams and Imitation in Childhood.* (Translated by Gattegno C, Hodgsen F). New York, Norton and Company, 1962.

34. Piaget J: *The Psychology of Intelligence.* Paterson, NJ, Littlefield, Adams, 1963.

35. Piaget J: *The Child and Reality.* (Translated by Rosin A). New York, Grossman Publishers, 1973, pp. 27–28.

36. Pressley M, Borkowski JG, Schneider W: Good information processing: What it is and how education can promote it. *Int J Educ Research* 13(8):857–867, 1989.

37. Rosenthal TL, Bandura A: Psychological modeling: Theory and practice. In Garfield SL, Bergin AE (Eds): *Handbook of Psychotherapy and Behavior Change.* New York, John Wiley, 1978.

38. Ross M, Burdick D: *Sensory Integration.* Thorofare, NJ, SLACK Inc., 1981.

39. Ross M: *Integrative Group Therapy: The Structured Five-Stage Approach.* Ed. 2. Thorofare, NJ, SLACK Inc., 1991.

40. Rumelhart DE: Schemata: The building blocks of cognition. In Spiro RJ, Bruce BC, Brewer WF (Eds): *Theoretical Issues in Reading Comprehension.* Hillsdale NJ, Lawrence Erlbaum Associates, 1980.

41. Rumelhart DE, Norman DA: Accretion, tuning, and restructuring: Three modes of learning. In Cotton JW, Klatzky RL (Eds): *Semantic Factors in Cognition.* Hillsdale, NJ, Lawrence Erlbaum Associates, 1978.

42. Rumelhart DE, Norman DA: Analogical processes in learning. In Anderson JR (Ed): *Cognitive Skills and Their Acquisition.* Hillsdale, NJ, Lawrence Erlbaum Associates, 1983.

43. Smith H: Assessment and evaluation—Specific evaluation procedures. In Hopkins HL, Smith HD (Eds): *Occupational Therapy.* Ed. 6. Philadelphia, J.B. Lippincott, 1983, pp. 149–174.

44. Spencer EA: Functional restoration—Theory, principles, and techniques. In Hopkins HL, Smith HD (Eds): *Occupational Therapy.* Ed. 6. Philadelphia, J.B. Lippincott, 1983, pp. 353–380.

45. Sternberg RJ, Smith EE (Eds): *The Psychology of Human Thought.* Cambridge, Cambridge University Press, 1988.

46. Tulving E: Episodic and semantic memory. In Tulving E, Donaldson W (Eds): *Organization of Memory.* New York, Academic Press, 1972.

47. Werner H: *Comparative Psychology of Mental Development.* Chicago, Follett, 1948.

48. Werner H: The conception of development from a comparative and organismic point of view. In Harris D (Ed): *The Concept of Development.* Minneapolis, University of Minnesota Press, 1957.

49. Werner H, Kaplan B: *Symbol Formation: An Organismic Developmental Approach to Language and the Expression of Thought.* New York, John Wiley, 1963.

50. Wilson B, Moffat N (Eds): *Clinical Management of Memory Problems.* Rockville, MD, Aspen Systems Corporation, 1984, pp. 9, 10.

Chapter 8

COGNITIVE-BEHAVIORAL FRAME OF REFERENCE

Focus Questions

1. How do behavioral therapy and cognitive-behavioral therapy differ?
2. How do cognitive-behavioral approaches differ from other cognitive approaches (e.g., cognitive disabilities, movement and holistic frameworks)?
3. What is the role of cognition in cognitive-behavioral assessment and treatment?
4. What is the difference between the theories of Ellis and Beck?
5. Describe Bandura's social learning paradigm.
6. Describe the roles of activities in cognitive-behavioral theory.
7. What are the differing views regarding graded activity?
8. How can occupational therapists use cognitive-behavioral theory?
9. Describe the elements of a psychoeducational course model.

Introduction

Some readers may ask if there is a difference between behavioral therapy and cognitive-behavioral therapy. Behavioral approaches give primary attention to the behaviors that need to be changed through the use of reinforcement strategies. Secondly, the behaviorist considers the thoughts that may influence behavior. Cognitive-behavioral approaches, on the other hand, primarily seek to change the thoughts believed to result in or cause specific behaviors and develop a knowledge base for problem-solving.

During the 1970s, there was a growing interest in cognitive processes and self-control within behavioral and social psychology. **Self-control** refers to the person's ability to influence his or her own growth and development rather than being controlled by outside rein-

forcers. This interest in cognitive processes and self-control conflicted with basic tenets of behavioral theory and therapy and led to a polarization between cognitive-behavior therapists and noncognitive behaviorists. This polarization caused many disputes among behavior psychologists. From this dispute was formed a special interest group for cognitive-behavioral research within the association for the Advancement of Behavioral Therapy and the Association for Behavioral Analysis. This special interest group supported cognitive research and the study of the inner person in behavioral psychology. Out of the differing opinions, the conflictual discussions, the research and the literature came cognitive-behavioral psychology.

The occupational therapy literature has not firmly distinguished between behavioral approaches and cognitive-behavioral approaches. There is a clear distinction, however, and we have chosen to identify it with psychoeducational occupational therapy programs, which exemplify cognitive-behavioral theory. The **psychoeducational** approach in occupational therapy aims to strengthen or establish a knowledge base and to change the patient's thoughts about self from "incapable" to "capable" and "competent" and prepared to respond to life's daily challenges.

Definition

The cognitive-behavioral frame of reference in psychosocial settings is an emerging frame of reference in which a person's cognitive function is believed to mediate or influence one's affect and behavior. It provides an assessment guide for determining cognitive function, affective states and generalized behaviors, which are apparent as the patient participates in the environment. It suggests that treatment include verbal and behavioral techniques to change the patient's thoughts, to bring about behavioral change and to improve function. When applying the framework, the occupational therapist uses graded activities as a means to provide progressive challenges and success experiences in order to develop cognitive abilities; to expand the knowledge and strategies that the patient can use to act upon, interact in, and gain control of the environment; to increase self-knowledge; to problem-solve; and to cope with life's challenges.

Theoretical Development

Occupational Therapy Literature

In 1982, Lillie and Armstrong[47] described a psychoeducational program for psychiatric problems. Although they did not identify it with a cognitive frame of reference, they acknowledged social learning, cognitive and behavioral theories as influential in the program development. Because of the influence of these theories, we feel that the program exemplifies a cognitive-behavioral program.

Although sporadic, references throughout the 1980s in occupational therapy literature cite educational approaches[10,33,44,61,70,76] as well as the application of cognitive-behavioral theory in occupational therapy.[13,28,47] Others suggest the compatability of other occupational therapy frameworks with cognitive-behavioral approaches.[23,34,38,68,72] This chapter discusses educational approaches and psychoeducational programming.

Cognitive-Behavioral Literature

In the 1970s, the theories of rational emotive therapists, cognitive therapists, social psychologists and some behavioral theorists merged to form cognitive-behavioral theory. The work of Ellis, Beck, and Bandura and the studies and writings of Davidson, Kanfer, Phillips, Lang, Lazarus, Mischel, Peterson, Mahoney, Meichenbaum, Goldfried, Kazdin, Wilson, and other cognitive-behavioral theorists are represented in cognitive-behavioral theory. The merger emphasized the role of cognitive processes in understanding behavior, developing self-control, planning assessment and treatment strategies, and furthering the efficacy of behavioral treatment strategies.[73] The psychologists who contributed to the cognitive framework of therapy have emphasized the importance of cognition in the mediation of behavior and interpreted classical conditioning and reinforcement in cognitive terms.

In the literature the terms cognitive therapy and cognitive-behavior therapy have been used interchangeably. We have used sources representative of both terms in our discussion of cognitive-behavioral theory and application.

Forms of Cognitive-Behavior Therapy

Mahoney and Arnkoff[48] have identified three major forms of cognitive-behavior therapy: rational psychotherapies, coping skills therapies, problem-solving therapies. The **rational psy-**

chotherapies include Ellis' rational emotive therapy (RET), Michenbaum's self-instructional training (SIT) and Beck's cognitive therapy. **Coping-skills therapies** use existing methods to facilitate coping with stressful events. Methods include covert modeling,[39] modified systematic desensitization,[29,45] anxiety management,[74] and stress inoculation.[55]

Problem-solving therapies are exemplified by Fairweather's treatment program for institutionalized adults[22] and other programs.[16,18,50,71] The therapist teaches skills that are used to find specific solutions for a presenting problem as well as strategies that can be used to solve similar problems in the future. This approach is in contrast to the problem-solving of the behavioral approach in which the therapist uses reinforcement methods to modify the patient's behavior to solve the immediate problems but does not prepare the patient for coping with future difficulties. Problem-solving therapy has the least representation in the clinically applied cognitive-behavior literature.

Because the cognitive frame of reference is in the process of development in psychosocial occupational therapy and little has been published by occupational therapists in this area, we have chosen to summarize three major contributions to cognitive-behavior theory to acquaint the reader with cognitive-behavioral principles and their potential application in occupational therapy. The three contributions are Bandura's social learning theory, Ellis' rational emotive therapy, and Beck's cognitive therapy.†

Cognitive-Behavioral Theory

Bandura's Social Learning Theory

Albert Bandura's social learning theory has had a significant impact on contemporary psychology and particularly on cognitive-behav-

---

†Many other theorists have contributed to cognitive-behavioral theory. Among them are Frank[25–27], Kelly[40], Rotter[69] and Meichenbaum.[55,56] The reader is referred to the original sources for discussion of their theories.

ior therapy. Although Bandura's work has been noted in our discussion of behavioral therapy, this chapter emphasizes its application in cognitive therapy and examines its utility in the practice of occupational therapy. Because social learning theory is comprehensive and has multiple applications in occupational therapy practice, Bandura's work should be given attention even if the reader chooses not to apply a cognitive-behavior frame of reference.[4,67]

Through an increased understanding of social learning theory, one broadens knowledge in multiple areas: the role of internal and external reinforcers, the role of cognition in mediating environment and person interactions, the role of cognition in modeling and observation learning, the role of self-control and self-regulation in learning social responses, principles of corrective learning and treatment, and the alternative sources of motivation for behavior and treatment.

Social Learning Paradigm. The cognitive-behavior therapist conceives of an interactive-interdependent paradigm of social learning. Learning is viewed as an outcome of the interaction of behavior, person, and environment. Behavior is not just the outcome of the interaction between the person in his or her environment or determined solely by the environment. Rather, behavior is seen as an **interacting determinant** of the outcome or response (Figure 8.1). How people react and their unique perceptions of the environment act on the environment as much as the environment acts on them.

For example, the occupational therapist in rehabilitation frequently encounters spinal cord injured patients with lesions at the same spinal cord level who have similiar physical abilities and limitations of function, but who vary in their response to rehabilitation and what they accomplish in treatment and in life. This difference is due in part to the patients' unique views of their disability and what each hopes to accomplish, as well as their actions in the environment. A patient's behavior can elicit empathy, sympathy, dependence, anger, acceptance, or assistance from those with whom he or she interacts. The reaction of others will affect the individual's self-image and the kinds of opportunities that become available to him or her, as well as the individual's ability to progress and cope in the future.

In the mental health setting, this interactive-interdependent paradigm can be seen in an adolescent treatment setting where several adolescents with similiar problems may participate in the same therapeutic milieu, but each will vary in his or her response to treatment as well as in personal progress. The patient's view of peers and adults, his or her beliefs about treatment, and personal values and expectations all influence the patient's behavior and his or her ability to profit from treatment. This behavior influences what parents, staff and peers expect and think of the patient; the goals they hold for him or her; the support they offer and the reactions that they have based on judgments of previous behavior. Ultimately, the adolescent influences and can control many of the current and future reactions of others through his or her behavior and can create an environment that will influence the quality of life.

From these examples we see that both environment and the person may regulate behavior and influence the outcome of interac-

tions. It is the *correlation* rather than the pairing of events that determines behavior.[4]

The Importance of Cognition in Modeling. Traditional behaviorists acknowledge that learning may occur when an individual models his/her actions after observing another individual.

Social learning theorists emphasize that cognition plays a significant intervening role in modeling. They remind us that people do not imitate or model every behavior that they observe. Rather, individuals actively think about and select those behaviors that they will try to reproduce. The behaviors they choose to imitate will depend largely on what Bandura calls **anticipated consequences**.[63] Understandably, individuals are more likely to model behavior that they believe will lead to something they want. They learn this in part by noticing the consequences that result when others engage in a particular behavior. For instance, if an adult sees another patient being praised for the care given to a craft project, the adult (our observer) may choose to imitate this behavior.

Modeling and Imitation. Modeling and imitation can play a part not only in skill building, but also in rule and attitude formation. The patient who observes another patient or staff member consistently displaying certain attitudes (sharing, concern for others) may dis-

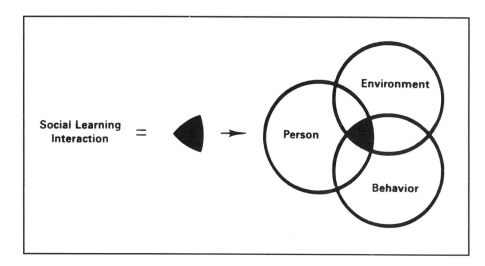

FIGURE 8.1.   Social Learning

cern the common thread that runs through diverse actions and situations and repeat a similar attitude in his or her own interactions.

As noted previously, a person is more likely to imitate someone he perceives as like the self (e.g., a male will more likely imitate a male; a member of one group will more likely imitate another group member) or someone highly regarded. However, individuals are unlikely to model behaviors that they feel incapable of (e.g., patients who believe they are incapable of mastering weaving are unlikely to model a weaver, no matter what regard they may have for the model). Bandura's work in this area is pertinent to occupational therapists. His studies suggest that if the observer (here, the patient) can see the model performing individual motor steps, while the patient imitates and practices each of these steps, the patient increases his or her own perception of self-efficacy. This process is referred to as **modeling of gradual mastery**.[4,67]

Cognition in Reinforcement. Both internal and external sources of reinforcement may stimulate and maintain behaviors and thoughts. Not only the tangible outcome or measurable reinforcement must be considered, but also the individual's expectations regarding the reinforcement. These expectations are modulated by the person's cognitive abilities, as discussed. In the social learning view, reinforcement may be an external, a vicarious, or a self-produced consequence.[4] **External reinforcers** are money, food, material goods and social approval, privileges or penalties. **Vicarious reinforcers** are symbolic (those images that a person has as a result of observing and learning from others) and include the individual's values and his or her images of success or failure.[4] For example, the student who is studying for a profession is reinforced for his or her efforts and the sacrifices that studies demand by the images held of mentors, the prestige of the profession, and the values and salary associated with the position he or she hopes to attain after graduation.

Successful performance during tasks leads

to a sense of efficacy and competence. **Competence** means that the person has internalized behaviors, which are maintained even when external reinforcers are withdrawn. When a patient succeeds and feels competent, he or she gains a sense of self-control. **Self-control** further indicates that the patient is capable of setting standards, judging personal behavior against these standards, comparing performance with previous performance, and maintaining an internal reward.

Self-produced consequences, the third type of reinforcement, come from the individual's sense of accomplishment, the sense of self-control, and his or her sense of competence that comes from success.[4] Stated simply, feeling competent and in control is a good feeling and is rewarding.

Hierarchy of Reinforcement. Social learning theory also conceptualizes a hierarchy of reinforcement based on the view that reinforcers acquire meaning and change as a result of developmental experiences. Think about how children respond to different kinds of rewards as they grow. **Initial reinforcers** are more often external, such as smiles of approval, attention from significant others, and food.[11] As cognition develops symbolic reinforcers play an important part in influencing behavior. **Symbolic reinforcers** are memories, verbalizations and internalized pictures.[4] For example, a child learns social control in part from parental discussion or reprimands that identify the laws of God, nature and society. Knowledge of these laws becomes reinforcement for social conduct. Both children and adults can control their behavior in part because they know the consequences of speeding, trespassing, or stealing. Or, a child can remember his or her mother's warnings, or perhaps recreate an image of a tragic newscast that describes a child's abduction, and thereby refuse a stranger's offer for a ride.

Next in the hierarchy is social contracting. A **social contract** is the system that identifies rewards and privileges and the punishments and censure that accompany specific behavior.[4] When an individual assumes roles and responsibilities of a job, through contractual agreement the employer provides benefits and salary. Or, when parents neglect or abuse a child, they violate the social contract for parenting and are reprimanded by society.

Personal satisfaction, the last developmental step in the reinforcement hierarchy, is an intrinsic, self-produced reward and is the best reinforcement of behavior. Because personal satisfaction is probably the reward least dependent on changing, often fickle, external circumstances, behavior based on this stage of the hierarchy is difficult to extinguish.[4] Self-satisfaction comes from self-evaluation and self-produced consequences. The person who perfects intellectual, creative or physical skills and pleases the self rather than the public and is comfortable with this pleasure has personal satisfaction.

Whatever the reinforcement, cognitive theorists emphasize that the ability to think about or anticipate reinforcement frees the individual from needing an immediate reinforcement for behavior. Traditional behaviorists state that positive reinforcement should immediately follow a desired response. Cognitive behaviorists disagree with this requirement in general, but do acknowledge that certain cognitive structures must exist for the individual to recognize and wait for a non-immediate reward.

Further Influence of Cognition in Social Learning Theory. Cognition influences motivation, goal setting and attainment, achievement of insight and acquisition, retention, and expression of behavior. Once a person has the ability to represent events symbolically, (that is, once he or she can create a mental picture of people, objects and events), then he or she is able to identify similar personal experiences or experiences of others, remember previous outcomes, and evaluate these events to anticipate possible consequences of behavior. This symbolic process allows a person to learn from vicarious experiences (e.g., those heard or read about) and to problem-solve in thought without needing trial and error learning experi-

ences. In other words, the person can imagine "what would happen if . . ." and does not have to experience everything personally to learn from it.

Goals. The ability to anticipate the likely consequences of behavior influences the person's motivation and regulates the goals that the person tries to achieve. **Goals** are statements of the general standards of conduct that regulate behavior. People use goals to evaluate their performance and their accomplishments. In the application of social learning theory, behavior is evaluated by contrasting the patient's behavior with his or her goals and by comparing present behavior with the person's previous behavior. The patient's behavior is not contrasted with that of other people or the norm.

As with traditional behavior therapy, goals should be specific enough to make identification of accomplishment possible; the conditions for behavior and the type and amount of behavior required should be stated. Consistent with the principle of creating moderate disequilibrium, the goals should be moderately difficult to maintain the person's interest and effort. If they are too easy, the patient loses interest; if they are too difficult, the patient is unable to perceive the self as attaining them. Social learning theory emphasizes that the individual's perception of self as capable of goal attainment actually increases his or her ability to accomplish goals.[63] Goals are accomplished through the satisfaction of subgoals.

Subgoals are the immediate goals that can mobilize effort and indicate what the patient is to do in the here and now. When successfully accomplished, they increase the image of self as capable and reinforce the effort needed to attain remote goals. **Remote goals** identify behaviors desired or required in the distant future to produce self-satisfaction and control. They are not incentives for the present because they are usually too far removed from the present, which has competing demands for the person's attention.

Insight. Cognition also allows the person to accurately interpret reality and develop insight. As in traditional behavioral practice, social learning theory states that when a person has **insight**, he or she is aware of the relationship between contingencies, events and what is reinforced.[4] This knowledge is believed to enhance learning, and increasing insight is a key aim of many social learning strategies. When a patient knows the reason for and benefits of treatment, he or she is more inclined to try new experiences or is more motivated to learn, provided the benefits are compatible with personal needs and interests. Insight also increases the ability for self-control.

Learning is also affected by the person's use of cognitive structures to interpret reality. A patient can misread reality, over-generalize, have false or rigid beliefs, or use faulty cognitive processing and thus misinterpret reality. Because behavior is governed by a person's beliefs and by his or her anticipation of the outcome of behavior, such misinterpretations must be corrected if adaptive learning is to take place. For example, if a patient falsely assumes that if he or she produces a well-organized resume, the first job applied for will be offered, then that assumption must be corrected.

Relevance of Bandura's Work to Occupational Therapy. Individuals within the occupational therapy profession who have supported the application of social learning theory in occupational therapy practice include Mosey and others.[14,43,59] Highlighted here is the major premise of Bandura's work, which is consistent with one of the underlying premises of occupational therapy—doing facilitates change.

In his discussion of modeling and observation learning, Bandura proposes that the efficacy of treatment is increased by actual performance or cognitive-behavioral learning rather than by relying solely on cognitive verbal methods.

Model for Success. Bandura's study provides a circular, interactive model of treatment: (1) Change a patient's thoughts from "incapable" to "capable" (to facilitate engagement in activity); (2) Use activities in which patients can experience themselves as capable.

Grade these, use physical guidance or use a model engaged in gradual mastery to ensure success while at the same time increasing patients' perceptions of themselves as capable. (3) Use verbal techniques to help patients identify their success, generalize learning, and increase their sense of self-control and competence. Success will lead to feelings of satisfaction, competence and control, which in turn helps the patient to face and cope with other day to day and future demands.†

The emphasis on actual performance during learning is similar to Jerome Bruner's concept of **enactive learning** . Bruner, often cited in education literature, emphasizes the importance of having physical experience as well as the opportunity to reflect on or talk about what one has just accomplished. This combination of enactive learning along with verbalization is thought to facilitate learning more than either action or talking alone.

Group Membership. Bandura's work on modeling raises a question about the typical grouping of patients in occupational therapy. For example, we often find that patients with similar needs and abilities are grouped together. One can consider the potential merit of pairing more functional, interactive patients with those who are perhaps less involved or less functional. If the less functional patients can identify with the more functional patients, they may profit. The patients may imitate the adaptive behaviors they observe. Therapeutic experiences of this nature have proved successful in remedying social learning problems with children.[63]

Sense of Control. Bandura's conclusions are consistent with the behavioral practice of incorporating both external and internal rein-

---

†The sense of efficacy and control that comes from success is also supported in the theory of life development intervention (LDI), which is discussed in Chapter 5.

forcement. Bandura and social learning theorists go further, however, in proposing that treatment staff actively help patients to identify properties of anticipated reinforcements and that they assist the patients to achieve a sense of control so that they can moderate their need for immediate gratification. Bandura's work also supports active intervention by the therapist to assist patients in identifying personal strengths, limitations and the cognitions used to solve problems so that patients feel in control of and responsible for their own actions.

Ellis and Rational Emotive Therapy

Of the identified cognitive therapies, rational emotive therapy (RET) introduced by Albert Ellis in 1955, may be the one best known. Ellis disagreed with the Freudian view that instincts determine behavior and the existential view that the authenticity of and the acceptance by a therapist could change a patient's beliefs and habits.

ABC Theory. Ellis was also dissatisfied with the results of his psychoanalytical practice and decided to take a cognitive approach. This approach assumes that thoughts, feelings and behaviors interact and have a reciprocal cause and effect relationship. The approach has been summarized in what is called the **ABC theory**: (A) A fact, event, behavior or attitude causes or influences the patient's belief (B), which determines the consequence (C). It is the belief not the activating event that determines the consequence. Therefore, the therapist uses interventions that dispute the patient's beliefs.

Irrational Thinking. RET strives to help the patient develop a rational basis for living through disputing those irrational views that produce neurosis or problems in living or self-defeat. These irrational views are summarized by Ellis in three statements called **musturbatory thinking**:

1. I *must* perform well and be approved by significant others. If I don't, then it is awful, I cannot stand it, and I am a rotten person.

2. You *must* treat me fairly. When you don't, it is horrible, and I cannot bear it.
3. Conditions *must* be the way I want them to be. It is terrible when they are not, and I cannot stand living in such an awful world.[15]

To counteract these irrational views and promote rational living, the rational emotive therapist does the following:

1. Gets patients to acknowledge the irrational ideas that motivate their disturbed behavior and challenges them to validate these ideas;
2. Uses logical analysis to demonstrate the illogical nature of patients' thinking and to minimize these beliefs;
3. Shows how the beliefs are ineffective and how they will lead to future emotional and behavioral disturbances;
4. Uses absurdity and humor to confront the irrationality of the patients' thinking;
5. Explains how these ideas can be replaced with more rational ideas that are empirically grounded;
6. Teaches the patients how to apply the scientific approach to thinking so that they can observe and minimize present or future irrational ideas and illogical deductions that foster self-destructive ways of feeling and behaving.[15]

RET Techniques. During individual and group treatment sessions and depending on patient need, the rational emotive therapist uses cognitive, emotive and behavioral techniques. **Cognitive methods** include disputing irrational beliefs, cognitive homework, bibliotherapy and using new self-statements.[19–21]

When disputing irrational beliefs, the therapist helps patients to see that it is their view of an event or belief about themselves that is causing the patients' symptoms or sense of defeat. The therapist then tries to get the patients to give evidence that supports their beliefs or interpretations of reality. Later during treatment, patients are asked to do the disputing themselves and to work systematically to diminish their distorted views.

Ellis' homework assignments are given to patients to demonstrate the rational or irrational nature of their thoughts and behaviors. These may include behavioral assignments, reading or specific therapeutic tasks. For example, during a public demonstration of RET for marriage and family problems, Ellis gave an assignment to a woman whom he had interviewed for 15 minutes during which they discussed her marital stress. He asked her to do the following: During the next week sit quietly, ask yourself these questions and then answer them. (1) Why must I have a perfect marriage? (2) State why it is that, "If I don't have a perfect marriage, I'm an awful person." (3) What would I change to make the marriage more perfect?

With this assignment Ellis tried to help the woman see that she had unrealistic expectations, that no marriage is perfect and that while she may have feelings about herself and her contributions to the relationship, they don't make her an "awful" person. He also asserted that she must begin to identify what she can change in the relationship or what she would like her spouse to change.

Task and reading assignments may also be used to diminish distorted thoughts and change behavior. Cognitive homework assignments are given to the patient by the therapist. These tasks are usually completed between sessions or during the treatment sessions. They are used to help the patient deal with anxiety and to help the patient dispute irrational beliefs.

For example, a person who is afraid of heights may be asked to take an elevator to the top of a building, or a person who is afraid of crowds may be asked to go to a place where a crowd of people are present. This strategy is controversial and is seldom used by occupational therapists who use graded tasks. It is also similar to implosive therapy, a classic behavioral approach in which the therapist accompanies a patient as he or she experiences a threatening situation.

Bibliotherapy is the method of cognitive treatment in which the therapist assigns the reading of literature that relates to the patient's problem. Rational emotive therapists would be inclined to have the patient read *Humanistic Psychology: The Rational Emotive Approach* or *A New Guide to Rational Living* or other similar literature.[19,20]

Emotive techniques used in RET include unconditional acceptance, rational emotive role playing, modeling, self-statements (which may be voiced aloud or said to oneself), rational-emotive imagery and shame taking. The therapist teaches patients to accept themselves. The ideas that "we all make mistakes," that "nobody is perfect," that "it's OK to be yourself," and that "one needs to learn to live with oneself" are emphasized to develop unconditional acceptance.[21]

The therapist is a model for the patient. Therefore, he or she actively participates in therapy sessions to verbalize rational thoughts and model effective task behavior, to model courage during new experiences and taking risks, and to model unconditional acceptance of oneself and the patient.

Imagery and role playing allow the patient to try out the expression of new thoughts, feelings and behaviors in thought or fantasy or in contrived (but safe) settings before risking their expression in the everyday world.

RET and Behavioral Techniques. Operant conditioning, self-management, systematic desensitization, instrumental conditioning, biofeedback, relaxation techniques and modeling are behavioral techniques used by rational emotive therapists.[17] Incorporation of these techniques into therapy reflects a broadened view of RET. Ellis has called this a second type of RET and sees it as the same as other cognitive-behavioral therapies.[17] Not all cognitive-behavioral therapists agree with Ellis. For this reason, a different presentation of cognitive-behavioral therapy as conceived by Beck is outlined, and similarities and differences between Beck's cognitive-behavioral therapy and RET are summarized and their application to occupational therapy discussed.

Beck's Cognitive Therapy

Beck has been a key contributor to cognitive-behavioral therapy.[5-9] He refers to his model as cognitive therapy (CT) and defines it as "an active, directive, time-limited, structured approach used to treat a variety of psychiatric disorders"[7] (e.g., depression, anxiety, phobias, pain and somatic problems). It is based on an underlying theoretical rationale that an individual's affect and behavior are largely determined by the way in which he or she thinks about the world.[7] Beck assumes that an individual's cognition influences how he or she perceives and experiences everyday events, that one's cognitions are based on internal and external stimuli as well as past and present experiences, that cognitions influence personal feelings and behavior, and that therapy can heighten the individual's awareness of these cognitions and how they influence his or her feelings and behaviors.[7]

Scientific Approach. The techniques of cognitive therapy incorporate a collaborative, here and now relationship in which the therapist uses behavioral techniques to elicit cognitions (help the patient to identify his or her beliefs or thoughts), to change behavior, and to discuss with the patient alternate, more healthy responses and the benefits and liabilities of changing or maintaining present beliefs and behaviors. The techniques and discussion help patients develop a scientific attitude through which they learn to recognize and monitor thoughts and behavior and systematically test their assumptions.

Cognitive Techniques. Some of the **cognitive techniques** that facilitate effective performance include graded task assignments, modeling, coaching, behavioral rehearsal, homework, stress inoculation, cognitive modeling and scripting. Patients are taught to identify irrational thoughts and cognitive distortions through rational and emotive imagery and discrimination training. Techniques develop assertive beliefs; identify personal rights; use thought-stopping, role reversal and

symbolic modeling; and incorporate educational methods.[65]

Contrast Between Rational Emotive Therapy and Beck's Cognitive Therapy

Both RET and cognitive therapy hold that behavior change comes from cognitive change; if you can change how a person views an event, you can change behavior. Differences arise in the use of terminology, the therapeutic approach, the methodology used to rethink, and the homework assignments given (Table 8.1).

Rules for Living. Beck suggests that the therapist work with the patient's **rules for living** (the patient's entire philosophy of life) and not just the "musts" in life or irrational thoughts, which are the focus of the rational emotive therapist. The rational emotive therapist has a more forceful approach in which he or she is directive in identifying, confronting and disputing irrational beliefs. Beck envisions the therapist engaged in a collaborative effort in which the patient and therapist mutually explore the patient's beliefs to identify those that lead to cognitive distortions and overgeneralizations, and then mutually negotiate behavioral assignments.

Disputing Beliefs. During treatment, the process for rethinking differs with the two therapies. The rational emotive therapist quickly identifies the "musts" in the patient's life, evaluates these thoughts and then goes about to dispute these "musts." The therapist's philosophy of life is very influential in this process. Beck supports using inductive questioning and a **Socratic dialogue method**. In this method of questioning, the therapist helps patients to identify thoughts and find the evidence needed to support their beliefs, and then works cooperatively to find the means to correct these thoughts. Later, the therapist proposes to patients that they evaluate these beliefs and, in some cases, consider changing their philosophy of life.[17]

Using Graded Tasks. Although both therapies use behavior assignments, Beck proposes that these assignments be negotiated by the patient and the therapist, and he would consider the patient's present ability and place increasing demands for performance. Tasks are graded in difficulty and work periods are increased. The rational emotive therapist does not use graded tasks, believing that they limit the patient's capabilities. Instead, the therapist usually determines the homework assignment and asks for high performance or behavior contrary to that which a patient exhibits.[17]

This difference in views poses an interesting question for the occupational therapist. Does the use of graded activities promote success? Or, does this approach convey to the patient that he or she has limitations and cannot manage a greater challenge? Is it acceptable to convey performance limitations to the patient?

ABC Theory Versus Scientific Theory. Patients engaged in rational emotive therapy undergo a logical analysis of their belief system based on the ABC theory. There is an activating event (A), which influences what a person believes (B), which in turn influences subsequent behavior or the consequence (C).

Beck's cognitive-behavioral therapy uses a scientific method to identify and test personal beliefs. The therapist helps patients make hypotheses about the reasons behind their behavior and then systematically test these hypotheses and participate in corrective experiences. These experiences will promote cognitive functioning and thereby enhance coping and problem-solving.

Based on previous discussion in this section it appears that the occupational therapist is more likely to incorporate social learning and cognitive-behavioral approaches similar to those of Beck rather than rational emotive techniques. However, all have been influential in formulating cognitive, psychoeducational interventions.

Current Practice in Occupational Therapy

The Person and Behavior

The therapist using cognitive-behavior theory sees the patient as a cognitive, psychosocial

---

TABLE 8.1   CONTRASTING RATIONAL EMOTIVE THERAPY AND COGNITIVE THERAPY

	Rational Emotive Therapy	Cognitive Therapy
Treatment Focus	Focus on "musts" and individual's irrational thoughts.	Look at individual's philosophy of life.
Nature of Therapist Interaction	Therapist is directive; challenging.	Therapist collaborates with patient in mutual exploration.
Role of the Therapist	Therapist disputes irrational beliefs; models rational behavior.	Therapist uses inductive methods; asks patient to support or dispute beliefs.
How Activities Are Determined	Therapist determines treatment activities.	Therapist and patient collaborate to select treatment activities.
Nature of Therapeutic Activities	Does not typically use graded tasks; patient confronts the task which he had been incapable of performing.	Uses tasks graded in difficulty.

being whose knowledge develops and changes throughout life. Knowledge is housed in schemes that are stored, retrieved and reorganized to produce a self-concept, a view of others, the rules for interacting with others in the environment and behaviors and skills that are used to respond to and control one's environment.

In the previous chapter we highlighted the normal or ideal progression of knowledge development. With patients in psychosocial treatment settings, however, knowledge development may be delayed or interrupted or may have resulted in maladaptive behavior. In the cognitive-behavioral frame of reference, cognition or thinking is identified as the basis for a psychiatric syndrome.

Limited or Distorted Knowledge

Dysfunction occurs due to insufficient, inflexible, or distorted knowledge. **Cognitive dysfunction** is identified by behaviors that reflect a rigid attitude, limited exploration of one's environment, a failure to establish an autonomous identity, misinterpretation of reality, and limited problem-solving skills.

Sense of Safety

A person explores and learns from the environment when he or she senses that it is safe and permissible to do so. Ideally, this sense of safety is conveyed to the child by adult role models who provide a safe and consistent environment and who communicate that they believe the child is capable of controlling the environment and can learn from exploration. In this safe, consistent, as well as appropriately stimulating environment, and from exploration, the person gains a knowledge base (tacit and explicit knowledge) that will shape the view of reality, future learning and knowledge acquisition, and one's unique approach to problem-solving. Negative experiences or limited exploration can lead to fear of the environment, distorted or limited knowledge, a rigid and defensive attitude and poor problem-solving skill.

Competence Versus Incompetence

As the person grows and interacts in the environment, he or she not only gathers information about the environment but also about the self. This self-knowldege influences emotional development. Emotional development can be seen by the individual's position on continuums that represent dependence and independence, self-interest and interest in others, personal views of reality and the ability to be empathetic, identity with others and an autonomous identity, and ability to express and control feelings. **Optimum function** reflects a balance of the two extremes for each of these continuums and is associated with a feeling of competence.

Dysfunction is usually seen when the predominant behaviors are at the extremes of the continuum or when cognitive function does not meet developmental expectations and is associated with feelings of incompetence. The person thinks he or she is incapable of being independent, lacks a sense of self, or is inhibited.

Unrealistic Reasoning

The patient with distorted self-knowledge will often use a reasoning process that tends to be dogmatic or unrealistic. This method of reasoning may be illogical, not coinciding with reality, or may involve inferences that do not have a basis.[32] For instance, when the person reasons, he or she makes inferences that may be incorrect. The patient may personalize information unnecessarily or perhaps view events from extremes (e.g., issues are judged as black or white, good or bad, possible or impossible). He or she may selectively abstract information and thus gets a distorted view or may make global generalizations (e.g., all women are bad; blonds have more fun; management doesn't care about employees). The person's thoughts are unidimensional rather than holistic with multiple perspectives, and these thoughts cannot be easily reversed or varied.[6,7,32]

Cognitive distortions and deficiencies have

also been identified within the context of specific diagnostic categories (e.g., agoraphobia, depression, eating disorders, and obsessive-compulsive disorder).[11,12] However, psychiatric labels are not necessary for the understanding and description of cognitive dysfunction.

Role of the Occupational Therapist

The role of therapist is not that of the expert and may vary from the original role of teacher to that of personal scientist. The occupational therapy literature indicates that thus far, the occupational therapist has continued in the role of a teacher. In this role, the therapist is a facilitator and participant-observer who designs and implements corrective learning experiences.

Educator-Facilitator

As an educator-facilitator, the therapist provides a structure. The educational structure in treatment is not like that in a traditional school setting. Rather, it is a structure in which patients help develop the course, identify their learning needs, and participate in determining the course content and homework assigned. The therapist designs learning experiences that occur in a classroom atmosphere and during academic and skill development groups.

During the learning experiences, the therapist-educator carefully explains the rationale behind treatment approaches and assignments and gives specific and frequent feedback regarding the patient's thoughts, behavior, and accomplishments in relation to short- and long-term goals. He or she facilitates a learning process that helps the patient gain new information and skills, knowledge that will increase self-understanding, expand resources for problem-solving and increase the person's ability for self-control and control of the environment.

Modeling a Scientific Attitude

The reader should also consider the benefits that come from modeling the attitude of a per-

sonal scientist. The **scientific attitude** requires the patient and therapist to recognize the relationship between thoughts and behaviors, to create ways to prove or disprove relationship theories, to explore life and its multiple possibilities and probabilities and to question so-called "absolute certainties."

In modeling the scientist, the occupational therapist provides a secure base for exploration and encourages patients to explore life systematically so as to hypothesize about and recognize cause and effect relationships in life. Patients then plan and carry through with experiments or learning activities to confirm or disprove hypotheses. As a personal scientist, the therapist helps patients to step back from personal beliefs, to postpone judgment of themselves and the world and to logically challenge their self theories. This scientific process can be pursued through cognitive-behavior techniques.

Questioning Generalizations

The scientist attitude is illustrated in a response to comments frequently heard in occupational therapy: "I am all thumbs," or "I'm not good with my hands." The occupational therapist replies, "What's happened to cause you to conclude that you're not good with your hands?" Or, "Does this comment refer just to occupational therapy activities, or have you had difficulties at work or home?" With these responses the occupational therapist does not accept the patient's statement as fact and asks the patient to either validate or question the generalization. Next, the therapist might ask the patient to perform specific tasks that do not relate to previous task failure and that provide the opportunity to reevaluate personal capabilities.

Participant-Observer

As a participant-observer, the therapist strives to be flexible, to individualize learning experiences and to adjust the therapeutic approach to the patient. The goal is to find a style that fits patients' needs. As a participant, the occupational therapist provides support and gives feedback to the patient in response to the thoughts and feelings that are shared, as well as his or her behavior. The therapist also shares his or her views of the problems that the patient confronts. When observing the patient, the therapist views the whole cognitive system and tries to increase the patient's awareness of the interrelationship among thoughts, feelings and behaviors, both past and present. When appropriate, the patient is helped to come to new conclusions about self and others. This can be seen in the following example.

An 18-year-old head-injured patient had multiple physical and behavioral problems as a result of her injury. She shifted from child-like, attention-seeking, dependent behavior to acting out, adolescent behavior, to appropriate expressions of concern regarding living independently, achieving an intimate relationship and being employed. (These interests were realistic provided she could gain control of her impulsive behavior.) Acting out one day, she ran away from the rehabilitation center. It was not easy for this young woman to leave given that she was wheelchair bound and had many physical limitations.

The therapist decided to share with the patient her view of the experience. Instead of again reminding the patient of the dangers of her behavior, as many other staff had done, the occupational therapist decided to focus on the tremendous amount of energy required to run away. She then challenged the patient to learn to use this energy in a positive manner rather than in the negative self-destructive manner that running away represented. This strategy helped avoid the patient's usual authority struggle that had so often sidetracked treatment.

In another example, a patient who saw himself as superior was very intolerant of what he saw as other patients' ignorance. One day the therapist chose to confront a statement the patient made to another patient, "You mean you don't know that? Everybody knows that!" The therapist suggested to the patient that he may know things that others don't but

rather than put others down for their lack of knowledge, he might see an opportunity to teach them and share his knowledge with others. She helped him to recognize that he could gain respect for his knowledge from others rather than the contempt that he seemed to elicit for being bright.

Collaborative Relationship

In summary, in the student-teacher relationship, the occupational therapist works collaboratively with the patient to identify problems and to plan and implement learning activities. The therapist provides a nonjudgmental attitude and a secure base from which the patient can reevaluate personal assumptions. The therapist communicates respect to the patient for his or her ability to learn and solve personal problems.

Function of Activities

The occupational therapist applying a cognitive-behavior frame of reference uses activities to estimate the patient's cognitive function;† to facilitate cognitive development; to increase the patient's knowledge of self, of others, and of the environment, and to help the patient to prove or disprove personally held assumptions.

Assessing Knowledge and Skill Level

The patient's current cognitive level is identified through his or her participation in activities in which beliefs and attitudes are verbalized. Activities also provide a vehicle for the patient to demonstrate the general fund of knowledge (e.g., specific information content, the ability to read and write, or use tools), as well as the skills and strategies used to apply this knowledge. In relation to knowledge, the therapist identifies strengths as well as limitations.

---

†Cognitive function includes the patient's thoughts, feelings and behaviors. This conceptualization of cognition is broader than the definition used by Allen who defines it in terms of a "voluntary motor act."[1,2]

Increasing Knowledge and Enhancing Competence

Cognitive development is facilitated through engagement in activities that provide an opportunity to develop sensory, perceptual, motor, social, academic and other knowledge. Through specific experiences that require the individual to act, knowledge can be enhanced, self-confidence increased, a sense of self-control heightened and the patient given a means to realistically assess performance.

Educational Modules. Activities are often presented within the context of an educational format, which may be identified as a program curriculum or class schedule. The occupational therapist develops course syllabi for the activities or educational modules presented. Syllabi have been developed in multiple areas including getting credit, consumer awareness, social networks and social support systems, job search, and nutrition on a budget, to name a few.[75] In general, courses have been grouped as basic living skills, community awareness, and personal growth and development.

Using Homework. Courses may include the assigning of homework. The counseling literature gives guidelines for increasing the effectiveness of homework and increasing the likelihood of its completion.[54,65] It is recommended that assignments be written and that they identify the specific tasks to be completed by the patient, or at times, by the patient and therapist together. The purpose of the assignment, instructions for the task, and other data that will enable the patient to determine when responsibilities have been fulfilled and assignments completed should be included. Assignments should be individualized to meet each patient's needs and should allow for patient input at the time tasks are initially assigned.[6,54] These guides are also applicable for many of the home programs provided by occupational therapists in the various specialty areas of treatment.

At the beginning of each treatment session, the therapist checks to see if assignments are complete and inquires regarding the patient's thoughts and feelings about the assigment. Was the task too easy? Too difficult? Was it meaningful? If the person has not completed the tasks, the therapists tries to identify why. To support the successful completion of assignments, the therapist may use follow-up reminders or calls or contingency contracts.

Theoretical Assumptions

When applying cognitive-behavior theory in occupational therapy, the therapist makes the following assumptions:

1. A person's emotions and behavior reflect cognitive function.
2. Treatment does not eliminate pathology but provides cognitive, affective and behavioral learning experiences to teach skills, strategies and methods of coping.
3. The person develops as a result of the interaction of the cognitive system, behaviors learned, and the social and physical environment.
4. Treatment is more effective when specific techniques and skills are learned (e.g., when tasks and psychoeducational experiences are used) than when only verbal methods are used.
5. The patient benefits from psychoeducational programs that integrate educational procedures and psychological techniques.
6. The patient learns skills and strategies that can be used independently to face problems and find solutions.
7. When the patient masters the use of his or her body and objects, he or she has a resource for problem-solving.
8. When a patient learns new cognitive strategies to respond to the present, he or she is preparing to confront and solve future problems.
9. When the patient changes present knowledge and skill level, he or she changes past knowledge and self-image.

10. The principles of change can be understood by the patient as a result of cognitive experiences and the therapist's feedback that describes the rationale for treatment.

11. Treatment activities can help the patient to act on and in the environment as well as help the person to monitor personal thoughts, feelings and behavior.

12. The self-monitoring process can be learned during treatment.

13. During treatment activities, a patient can change negative self-thoughts and feelings into a positive self-image.

14. The arrangement of the learning environment influences cognitive function and can facilitate cognitive development and stimulate problem-solving.

15. The patient can benefit from a structured treatment setting that controls distractions and provides repeated opportunities for skill practice and problem-solving.

16. Cognitive developmental theory can be applied when designing tasks to modify the complexity of the experience and to promote successful learning.

17. The therapeutic tasks used during educational experiences consider the patient's cognitive knowledge, level of cognitive function and personal interests.

18. Tasks with a high probability of success can stimulate cognitive development.

19. Self-regulation is the tendency toward equilibration. That is, the person can maintain a balance in which present knowledge and cognitive function are complemented by new learning and challenges, the outcome of which is growth, optimum function and quality of life.

20. Therapy should aim for the highest degree of equilibration not the highest cognitive developmental level.

21. A person has acquired self-regulation when he or she can monitor relevant data that comes from within or from the environment, use this data to choose and implement new behaviors, and practice these behaviors until they become automatic.

Evaluation

As with other therapeutic approaches in occupational therapy, the therapist applying the cognitive-behavioral framework believes that assessment is an ongoing process; "assessment and change are interdependent."[32,56] Therefore, the information that follows could be applied within the context of the initial or the ongoing evaluation process.

Targeting Change

The cognitive-behavioral framework suggests that change be targeted in terms of four prongs: In what environmental situation(s) would the patient like to feel more competent? What thoughts (or attitudes) does he or she need to reassess? What does the patient need to know more about? What skills does he or she need to learn? (See Figure 8.2.)

Automatic Thoughts

Patients may not always be aware of the information or skills needed, the thoughts to change, or even the situations in which they need to achieve competence. They may only be aware of their current feeling of discomfort. One reason for this unawareness is that many of the thoughts we have and behaviors we all engage in daily are automatic; we do not think about our own problem-solving or recognize our own internalized cognitions.

For example, when we drive a car and encounter problems suddenly presented by heavy traffic, or poor road conditions or a child running in the street, we respond without thinking about how we should react and the problem-solving process that occurs. Nor are we aware of how stimulation influences our behavior, what determines how we formulate cause and effect relationships, or the process of remembering.

This lack of awareness can again be illustrated in another automatic reaction, overeating. If you speak to people who overeat they may tell you that they will eat if food is present without thinking about whether they feel hungry or whether their bodies require nourishment. Another example is the person who automatically withdraws from social interactions without considering the potential pleasure to be gained from, need for, or benefits of responding to family, friends or new acquaintances. Finally, there is the person who expects to fail even before hearing instructions or initiating an activity.

Accessibility of Cognitive Process

An individual does not typically have immediate access to the rules of the cognitive process that influence behavior, feelings, memory and problem-solving. Because the cognitive process is not in our immediate awareness in most instances, the therapist and the patient make assumptions regarding the impact of cognition on behaviors and affect and depend on keen observation of verbal and nonverbal interactions that occur during evaluation and treatment activities to gain an understanding of how thoughts are processed and to identify situations in which change would be desirable.

Assessing Cognitive Structures

A key aim of the evaluation is to assess cognitive structures. The occupational therapist uses observation, testing and interview to determine the patient's cognitive functioning. When observing the patient the therapist tries to determine the following:

1. The patient's ability to remember, to perceive, and to attend.
2. The patient's ability to observe and accurately interpret behavior (the logic used in learning from events) including the patient's ability to identify the historical data that relate to current problems and successes, the patient's ability to identify stimuli (events, rewards) that support given behaviors, and the patient's ability to identify personal problems.
3. The adequacy of the patient's knowledge base—knowledge of information related to activities of daily living, vocational endeavors, and leisure pursuits (e.g., awareness of community resources and awareness of learning strategies).
4. The strategies the patient uses to problem-solve and their effectiveness.
5. The existence and effectiveness of specific skills needed for daily function.

Listening for a Life Theme

In addition to assessing specific cognitive structures and skills during the assessment, the therapist tries to listen for the patient's life theme and rules for living. Internalized rules for living emerge from the patient's behaviors and statements during the evaluation. Examples of rules include the following: I can take care of myself; I don't need my parents to run my life; people can't be trusted; I have to do as my spouse wants or he'll get angry.

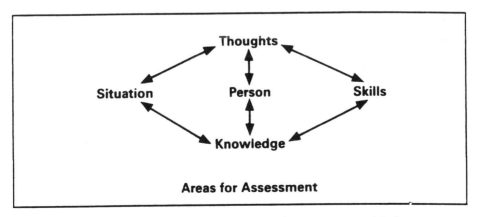

FIGURE 8.2.   Areas for Assessment: Cognitive-Behavioral Frame of Reference

Usually a theme emerges.[32] The theme is the message that underlies the rules for living and comes through consistently as the patient speaks and interacts in the interview and completes tasks. Typical life themes include the following: I am a victim of circumstance; people and life have always been against me; I am unworthy; I have never been able to use my hands; my father thinks I'm stupid; and I can't be independent. Just as a patient's thoughts convey a life theme, his or her problem-solving may reflect a lifestyle (e.g., a tendency toward patterns of behavior that are outgoing, withdrawn, intellectual, dependent, haphazard, or cautious). The therapist looks for indications of such a life-style, especially when this style tends to limit rather than enhance coping skills.

Evaluating the Person-Environment Match

The therapist also wants to assess the extent of the match between the patient and the environment. In this regard, the therapist may assess the following:

1. The patient's self-image: What are his or her interests? Personal goals? What is the patient's level of self-acceptance? Can he or she tolerate mistakes? Take risks? Can he or she exert self-control? In what areas does the patient feel capable, incapable? Do others' perceptions validate the person's self-image? Are his or her self-expectations reasonable? Is the person flexible, or does he or she respond rigidly?
2. The patient's view of the environment: Is the patient aware of and interested in the environment? Does he or she see the environment as demanding, hostile, accepting, ignoring, or rejecting? What aspects of the environment receive attention? What kinds of situations and settings are preferred? What is expected of others? What is the level of tolerance of others? Is his or her view of the environment and others realistic?
3. The patient's learning style: Does he or she initiate tasks? Does the person sit back and

observe? Who is admired? Does he or she have mentors? With whom does the person identify? Can he or she postpone gratification? Maintain diligence? What reinforcements maintain current behavior? What reinforcements might be used to build new behaviors? What strategies assist learning—verbal instruction, use of diagrams, hands-on-guidance, memory strategies? In what settings does he or she learn most easily—large group, small group, quiet, stimulating environment? Can he or she generalize learning?
4. What current and expected environmental demands is the patient preparing to meet? What knowledge and specific skills are required? What stimuli, cues, models and reinforcements are available? What demands will there be for patience, tolerance, self-control? To what degree will the patient's rules for living enhance his or her success or diminish the likelihood of success?

In summary, the occupational therapist uses the assessment to learn more about the patient's cognitive structures and the extent of information and skills he or she possesses. With this information, the therapist and the patient set priorities in each area and work to change thoughts, skills, knowledge, or specific situations. They also identify cognitive learning strategies that best match the patient's learning needs.

Assessment Instruments

Task Check List (TCL). The Task Check List designed by therapists at the Life Skills Program is an adaptation of Hewett's[3] hierarchy of educational tasks used to assess the learning needs of the adult psychiatric population. The check list itemizes key behaviors for each of the seven learning levels identified by Hewett: entry, acceptance, order, relationship, exploratory, mastery and achievement levels. The check list is used to develop an education plan for the patient[47] (See Appendix K).

Frank Hewitt[35] is an educator who has numerous publications regarding educational approaches for the exceptional learner. He identified six levels of competence that are necessary for effective learning to occur: 1) attention—"the level of competence associated with receiving and perceiving sensory stimulation, coming to and sustaining attention and retention"; 2) response—"the level of competence associated with motor responding, verbal language skills, and active participation"; 3) order—"the level of competence associated with following directions and routines"; 4) exploratory—"the level of competence associated with gaining an accurate and thorough knowledge of the environment through sensory-motor experiences"; 5) social—"the level of competence associated with gaining the approval and avoiding the disapproval of others"; and 6) mastery—"the level of competence associated with self-help skills, academic skills, and vocational and career development."

Beck Depression Inventory. In the 1960s, in an attempt to quantify psychiatric diagnosis, Aaron Beck developed the Beck Depression Inventory. Today's edition, the result of multiple revisions, is a self-report measure designed to assess the depth of an individual's depression. The patient is asked to choose from statements that describe levels of severity in depression. These choices identify the affective, cognitive, motivational and physiological symptoms of depression that the person is currently experiencing. Since its introduction, the inventory has been used by health professionals from varied disciplines. This inventory and Beck's Hopelessness Scale (1974) are cited in the occupational therapy literature. Inventory resource is Beck's *Depression: Clinical, Experimental and Theoretical Aspects* (1967).

Other Assessment Instruments. Other assessment instruments cited in the occupational therapy literature include Young's Loneliness Inventory,[77] Rotter's Internal-External Scale, and Zung's Self-Rating Depression Scale.[78]

Pre-tests and post-tests also may be used within the guides of this framework. Prior to participating in an educational group, a patient may take a **pretest** to identify current level of knowledge regarding a specific subject. After the educational experience or series of groups, the patient completes a **post-test** to evaluate the change in level of knowledge or expertise. These testing formats are also used in clinical research.

Treatment

Since the mid-1970s, multiple definitions of the therapeutic process for cognitive change have evolved. Guidano and Liotti[32] list six definitions. Of the six, two seem most applicable to occupational therapy: (1) a teaching relationship in which the therapist facilitates the development of coping strategies and self-control[30] and (2) a scientific process that helps the patient to question personal beliefs and judgments and then systematically confirm or disprove his or her thoughts, a definition first used by Kelly and later by many other cognitive theorists.[32,40,46,48,49,51,53,56,58]

Reestablishing the Cognitive System as Self-Regulating

In general, the cognitive-behavioral change process in occupational therapy encourages shared authority and responsibility in treatment by patient and therapist. The goal of treatment is to facilitate cognitive growth and improve cognitive function to reestablish the cognitive system as a self-regulating system. To be a self-regulating system the person needs a broad knowledge base, skills to function competently in the environment, knowledge of self, others and the environment, and the ability to use knowledge for problem-solving. The therapist frequently tries to improve the ability to problem-solve in a variety of daily situations, such as those proposed by Bara.[3] Refer to the discussion of problem-solving in the previous chapter.

When individuals possess adequate knowledge and skills and perceive themselves as able to cope with a range of daily problems, they experience themselves as competent. The more competent they feel, the more able they are to act flexibly and respond to a broad range of available options. As a result, they become more competent.

Treatment Goals

As with other frames of reference, the cognitive-behavioral frame of reference sets behavioral goals to bring about behavior change and uses them to evaluate treatment outcome.

Changing Behavior and Changing Thoughts. Although behavioral goals are used, it is not sufficient to have patients change just their behavior. They must also change the way they think about themselves and their experiences.[48,66] For example, the patient may learn the skills for interpersonal interaction, such as how to initiate a conversation, communicate with peers at work, and be assertive with authority figures. In addition, however, he or she must have a sense of self-competence in social situations, and must be aware of when and how to use the communication skills learned.

Desired changes in the patient's thoughts, attitudes and values may also be written as goal statements. For example, the patient can verbally identify interpersonal skills (abilities and limitations) and then identify what he or she has gained from occupational therapy.

Shared Authority. The cognitive-behavioral framework emphasizes the release of power by the occupational therapist to patients in order to increase patients' responsibility for identifying intervention goals and strategies and for evaluating the efficacy of treatment outcomes.† Therefore, authority tends to be more readily shared between patient and therapist.

Lillie and Armstrong[47] describe a unique approach to goal setting which could be replicated. The Goal Attainment through Education (GATE) group is a process of group goal setting in which each participant selects his or her psychoeducational experiences based on personal needs and interests. The group is analogous to the high school homeroom group in which students meet, learn about the available courses, and then set their goals for participation in the program.

Occupational Therapy and Cognitive-Behavioral Strategies

The occupational therapist who chooses the cognitive-behavioral approach chooses a framework with an interactive focus rather than the traditional behavioral cause and effect relationships. That is, thoughts, feelings and behaviors interact; the strategies the therapist selects emphasize this interaction.

Listening for Musts. Occupational therapy treatment does not focus extensively on "musts," nor does the therapist typically dispute the patient's beliefs in the forceful manner described by Ellis. However, the occupational therapist listens for the "must" messages in the patient's dialogue, such as might be communicated by the patient who "must" make a perfect pot the first time the potter's wheel is used and then gives up trying because he or she can't. Or, the therapist may ask the patient to identify the things he or she "must" do during a typical week at home. The therapist then helps the patient to see how these "musts" are controlling his or her life, ways to cope with the constraints and givens in life, and how to increase one's sense of success and control rather than feel defeated and apathetic.

---

†Therapists at the West Haven Veteran's Administration Hospital, West Haven, Connecticut describe the patient as being "empowered."[75]

For example, the husband who shuns responsibilities and leaves home because he feels overwhelmed by his job, his family roles, and his need to be perfect in all of these roles can be helped to modify his standards, and learn to express his feelings, and learn to ask for help from his family. (This example also applies to the woman and her role in the family.) Through behavioral and activity experiences the therapist helps the patient to gain control of his or her life through understanding the relationship between thoughts, problems and behavior.

Homework. In occupational therapy, the occupational therapist more frequently gives tasks rather than mental or verbal exercises like those of Ellis. These homework tasks typically can be accomplished quickly. For example, the patient is asked to make a draft of his or her resume before the next employment-readiness class or to make a list of the geographical areas for finding an apartment, and the benefits of each area, before the next community transition group meeting. It should be noted that "homework" need not be completed at home. The inpatient may be asked to do things on the ward or in his or her room before the next occupational therapy session.

Building Knowledge Through Reading. When using bibliotherapy, the occupational therapist is not likely to assign an entire book, as may the rational emotive therapist. Rather, the therapist in psychoeducational programs more frequently uses copied materials, short articles or brochures that could describe a budget process, nutrition and meal planning, or first aid and emergency protocol. Literature can be provided by the occupational therapist, guest lecturers, community agencies or service providers that affect the patient's life. Professionals from social service and community agencies invited to occupational therapy groups have provided literature about Medicare benefits, unemployment benefits, veterans benefits, the effects of alcohol, and weight control, to name a few.

Patients Learn Their Rights. Like the cognitive-behavioral therapist, the occupational therapist may use intervention strategies for developing assertive beliefs and identifying personal rights, may incorporate symbolic modeling and role reversal, and may use instructional models.

The occupational therapist may be responsible for running assertiveness training or social skills training groups. (The assertive group process is described with behaviorism in Chapter 4.) To develop an assertive belief system, the therapist uses lectures, therapist modeling, and role play. Patients learn that they have specific rights and that they can learn assertive behavior for effective interpersonal communication.

To identify rights, the therapist may use bibliotherapy, group discussion, or role play to help patients identify and accept their rights and to challenge such socialized messages as "think of others first." The occupational therapist helps patients learn to ask for what they need. For example, patients who sit waiting for someone to notice that they need paint or other necessary material for finishing a project are encouraged to express their needs. Or, after a cooking group, the occupational therapist may discuss the experience with patients and ask them to verbalize their thoughts about working together and how they helped each other, as well as their concerns about the work process and how it affected individuals as well as the activity outcome.

Films and Visual Media. A form of **symbolic modeling** describes the use of films and tapes to demonstrate effective interactions. During a film, a narrator explains the "rules" for the competent social interactions exhibited in the film.[31] In addition to the narrator's comments, when a film or video is used in occupational therapy, a discussion follows to heighten patients' understanding of the film's content. Further, the patient group may be given an opportunity to role play similar social encounters.

Modeling and Role Play. Three dimensions of role play include rehearsal, modeling, and coaching. When using role play, the therapist actively participates in order to portray effective methods for responding to problematic situations. The patient then rehearses the verbal and behavioral techniques demonstrated, and the therapist and patients give verbal and nonverbal feedback. Role play is used in multiple contexts in occupational therapy. Through role playing, the patient may practice job interviewing, asking for a date, personal introductions for varied social situations, registering to vote, applying for a library card, and so on.

Modeling and Physical Guidance. Modeling may be used to build task skills, such as those involved in learning an unfamiliar craft, self-care task, or sports. The therapist may act as a model or have another patient model the sequence of steps in a task, giving the patient the opportunity to practice and achieve competence in each step before attempting the next (modeling of gradual mastery).

The therapist may also use physical guidance, placing hands on the patient's hands as he or she attempts a motor act. Guidance is used to ensure success. As the patient becomes more successful, the therapist gradually removes physical support. As an important adjunct to such skill building, the therapist helps the individual acknowledge accomplishments and, when appropriate, identify the skills and reasoning used. It is hoped that through this identification of knowledge and skills, the patient increases his or her awareness of information that could be used in the future in similar situations (generalization).

Identifying Cognitive Distortions. The occupational therapist may also help the patient identify cognitive distortions and learn to test personal beliefs. Beck et al[6] suggest that the patient write down thoughts, look for underlying themes and then identify distorted thinking. To identify cognitions, the occupational therapist may use a log in which the patient writes thoughts, feelings and behaviors that occur during tasks throughout the day. For example, the patient taking a city bus for the first time might note a concern about missing his or her stop, or a personal belief that other passengers were "looking at me strangely." Log notes are then discussed with the patients to help them understand their thoughts and their consequences. The notes and discussions also influence the subsequent choice of task and treatment strategy.

Testing Cognitions. **Testing cognitions** means that the patient learns to distinguish thoughts from reality. In the previous example, the therapist may ask the patients to identify what happened or what people did that indicated people saw them as strange. In this way, the therapist helps patients to confirm or negate their thoughts. Thoughts or beliefs are treated as hypotheses to be tested by inductive analysis, not as statements of fact. If indeed the patient acted strangely, the therapist instructs or demonstrates acceptable behavior for riding the bus. Within the context of activity and the teaching relationship, the occupational therapist helps the client develop a scientific attitude and plan strategies for behavioral change.

Educational Experiences. Knowledge builds competence, and the therapist may use a classroom format to increase knowledge. Sample education experiences include money management (the patient learns to make a budget, open bank accounts, and manage a checkbook), movement and relaxation (the patient may participate in exercise or aerobic sessions, learn body mechanics, and energy conservation and relaxation techniques), and home management (the patient may learn meal planning and cooking, basic home repair, or time management).[61]

Other educational experiences include memory training (the patient may learn rehearsal strategies and how to use external aids or cueing methods), effective communication (the patient may learn to use the telephone, practice oral and written communication and interact in dyadic and group situations), understanding sexuality (the patient can learn about his or her own sexual needs as well as how to ask for a date, courting protocol, expression of sexuality and means to ensure safe sex).[70] Still other educational experiences might include anger management (the patient learns to identify angry feelings, sources of anger and alternative methods of expressing anger),[76] learning to use community resources,[47] vocational readiness (the patient can learn resume writing and job interview skills).[44] These experiences may be planned and implemented by the occupational therapist or in cooperation with other health professionals.

Educational Groups. Because of the educational and didactic nature of the therapeutic experience, groups are frequently used in treatment. Depending on the nature of the activity, class groups are usually composed of six to ten patients. Groups provide an opportunity for patients to help each other and to discuss methods of problem-solving. During class discussions the higher-level functioning patient can help the lower-level functioning patient. Patients can give each other support and support risk taking, and they can give each other feedback about their thoughts, feelings and behaviors. The groups also enable the use of role playing and modeling.

Sample Psychoeducational Group in Occupational Therapy. A comprehensive example of a psychoeducational group is represented by the program SCORE: Solving Community Obstacles and Restoring Employment designed by Kramer.[44] The SCORE program identifies the patient as a student and the therapist as a teacher and uses an educational format to establish realistic career objectives, to teach job seeking and social and interpersonal skills, and to improve self-presentation.

The program consists of 15 educational modules, which help the student (patient) assess the advantages and disadvantages of employment, evaluate work and leisure skills, practice completion of employment forms, write resumes and job inquiry letters, role play

and videotape employment interview questions and situations, and critique one's job performance and that of peers.

The modules identify learning goals and provide the teachers (co-leaders) with guidelines for task presentation, implementation and discussion. Teachers lecture on relevant topics, give instruction in employment-seeking skills, and encourage discussion of tasks and feedback to peers. Modules may be presented in a flexible schedule but Kramer recommends eight consecutive, three-hour sessions. Each student must complete the 24 hours of class work and may do so outside of class time if necessary. Modules also allow for some flexibility in presentation, which allows the course to be individualized to meet the student's needs.

The reader is referred to the original source for detailed module descriptions. Included are sample forms and a comprehensive discussion of the group format used to assist the physically and mentally disabled in the reemployment process.

Designing Educational Modules. When designing educational modules such as that described in the SCORE program, the occupational therapist uses activity analysis to develop graded learning experiences. (See Appendix G for a sample psychoeducational learning format.) The experiences are designed to develop knowledge and skills and to provide an opportunity to generalize new information and skills in different situations and settings. They provide an opportunity for the patient to recognize and correct error, as well as to identify and use personal strengths and abilities. Through these graded learning experiences, the patient masters new information and skills.

Education for Mastery. **Mastery** suggests that as a result of experience, the patient has acquired knowledge and skills, can identify a plan of action for a particular situation, is able to apply this knowledge effectively and can use experience, knowledge and skills to meet future demands. Mastery also indicates that the patient has met the goals that he or she set rather than those based on the norm or those of other patients in the group.

Treatment for Peripheral or Deep Change

The occupational therapist keeps several issues in mind as he or she plans treatment strategies designed to bring about change in the patient's pattern of behaving or thinking. The therapist and patient must decide whether the goal is to bring about peripheral or deep change.

Modifying Personal Identity. A deep change requires a remodeling of personal identity. **Remodeling** requires continuous stimulation from experiences, which allow the patient to gain knowledge and skills, form new self-statements, develop new rules for interaction, try various methods of problem-solving and then process these experiences to give data that enable a change in attitude toward self. This attitude and knowledge are integrated to modify personal identity.

To change the patient's personal identity or change deep cognitive structures, the patient and therapist have to work to bring about a change in the patient's tacit knowledge. To change tacit knowledge the therapist uses logical debate and logical challenge through the following techniques:

1. The therapist shows a patient how he or she has exaggerated an event (**decatastrophizing**).
2. The therapist challenges the patient's thoughts using logic and does not permit the patient to refuse responsibility for personal thoughts and feelings (**reattribution**).
3. The therapist substitutes a logical response for a patient's illogical reaction (**rational restructuring**).
4. The therapist uses techniques that require the patient to confront his or her self-concept and the impact this concept has on adjustment in life (**semantic techniques**).[32]

Before using these techniques, which challenge the patient's philosophies and personal identity, the therapist must assess the patient's strengths and stresses. He or she should try to answer the following questions: How much support does the patient need? Is it a good time to confront the patient? Can the patient benefit from a logical restructuring of personal knowledge? Is the patient capable of developing more adaptive thoughts, attitudes and behaviors? Not every patient should, needs, or can accomplish a deep cognitive change.[32]

Modifying Thoughts and Behavior. In most instances, the occupational therapist does not work in the realm of deep structural changes. Rather, the patient and therapist usually work to bring about a peripheral change. A **peripheral change** occurs as a result of a reorganization of attitude toward reality. This reorganization need not include a change in personal identity, but may lead to changes in behavior and thoughts, increased adaptation to the environment, decreased emotional stress and improved problem-solving.

The cognitive-behavioral literature identifies a variety of superficial change techniques: providing success experiences, role playing, assertiveness training, coping skills training, social skills training, cognitive modeling, self-instructional training, stress inoculation training, problem-solving, brainstorming and thought stopping.[32] Many of these activities have already been discussed in this chapter.

Scientific Change Process. In summary, whether the therapist seeks a superficial or a deep change, throughout the therapy experience the therapist provides a secure base for exploration and models the scientist attitude. While working toward this change of attitude, the therapist and patient should keep in mind three assumptions:

1. Cognitive change is a gradual process; to change one's knowledge base and one's attitude toward oneself takes time.

2. The therapist respects the patient's personal thoughts, feelings and views and encourages the patient to openly express them. This does not mean that the therapist has to agree with them.

3. The therapist is aware of the patient's history (thoughts, feelings, behaviors) because it will influence treatment experiences and their outcome and also the quantity, rate and manner in which new knowledge is absorbed.

Summary

The information in this chapter is based on cognitive-behavioral theory and therapy and represents the hypothesized relationship that exists between cognition and adaptive behavior. This marriage between cognitive and behavioral theories seems to be tenable for describing the relationship between thoughts, affect and behavior and the interactive process that occurs between the three elements. Although emphasizing the validity of subjective experience, the cognitive-behavioral therapist objectifies behavior change and uses such change to measure the effectiveness of psychosocial intervention. For some, this dual focus on thought as well as behavior is more comfortable than the perceived exclusivity of both psychoanalytic and behavioral therapies.

The cognitive approaches in occupational therapy are derived from emerging theoretical frameworks. As a consequence, in most instances these more recent approaches are not adequately supported by research that can specifically identify the benefits and limitations of cognitive interventions. However, we will share our initial reactions to cognitive theory and its application, and make some conjectures about the possible contributions and limitations of cognitive-behavioral theory as it is applied in occupational therapy practice as well as pose questions that have arisen as we pursued our cognitive studies.

Contributions and Limitations of the Cognitive-Behavioral Frame of Reference

Contributions

The psychology literature summarizes research that supports the use of cognitive-behavioral strategies with multiple age groups and diagnostic problems. In addition, the literature supports cognitive-behavioral approaches with children who are experiencing psychosocial and learning problems.[41,42,57] Other information supports giving patients information that would increase their awareness and understanding of the intervention strategies used by the therapist.[60] Information regarding treatment strategies may be presented to the child or adult and considers the patient's ability to understand and use the information.

The hierarchy of reinforcement, proposed by Bandura and influential in cognitive-behavioral therapy, has multiple applications in occupational therapy. These applications note the many levels of reinforcement that come into play in occupational therapy treatment and have been discussed previously in this chapter.

The application of cognitive-behavioral theory as represented by psychoeducational programs promotes an education-learning focus rather than an illness-treatment focus and is compatible with the environment of many health and community settings. In addition, an education-learning model is well suited to the area of prevention, a speciality that continues to be of interest to the occupational therapist. The occupational therapist has adopted or adapted some of the more useful components of behaviorism and combined them with cognitive developmental theory to form strategies for developing the patient's basic knowledge and skills for personal self-care, interpersonal interaction and work-leisure performance.

The psychoeducational strategies used in occupational therapy facilitate "doing" or action through activities that provide graded challenges. This approach is in accordance with the basic tenets of the profession. The classes, tasks and homework facilitate educational experiences that promote mastery of skills and competent function through individualized learning experiences and reflect the humanistic philosophy that has permeated the occupational therapy profession since its inception.

The educational model promotes treatment in groups. The group model has been recognized as both cost- and time-effective, as well as a useful vehicle for enhancing patients' ability to give to and support one and another.

The cognitive-behavioral frame of reference has the goal of promoting generalization, a goal clearly necessary if independence and reduced treatment demands are sought. Whether or not generalization is necessarily an outcome of education and treatment experiences, however, is debatable and needs to be pursued in research.

Limitations

In recent years, study in the fields of psychology, education and medicine have expanded the definition of cognition and have increased our understanding of the growth, development and function of cognition; however, much needs to be learned. We do not yet understand to what extent physiology, biology, heredity, environment and experience contribute to cognitive growth, development and performance. Although we know that cognition is a complex interactive process, we do not adequately understand the interaction of the physical and psychosocial factors previously mentioned. Therefore, one can only hypothesize about the relationship between the biopsychosocial nature of an individual and the underlying organization and function of the cognitive processes that the person uses to grow, change and adapt throughout the life span.

The ever-changing nature of the cognitive process also makes any adequate definition elusive. We do know that changes in cognition

occur slowly and in a manner similar enough to be conceived as stage specific. Most research, however, has been in the area of child development. Researchers now must ask: What factors influence cognitive development and performance during the adult years?

Given the status of theoretical development and research, the occupational therapist must acknowledge these limitations and the speculative aspect of practice. Questions that arise include: How can the therapist easily and accurately assess and identify problems of cognition? How can he or she determine what procedures and assessment tasks should be used?

To date, few cognitive assessment tools have been developed in occupational therapy. Of those available in the field of psychology, most are more appropriately given by a psychologist. Future assessment tools must be able to help determine whether a particular cognitive skill has or has not been acquired. Because skills can develop simultaneously, how can we accurately identify the cognitive developmental level? Cognitive performance may be identified with a particular developmental level but there are many degrees of function within that level. Therefore, the therapist must determine whether the patient lacks knowledge or skill, whether he or she has adequate knowledge and skills but refuses to use them, or whether the patient has knowledge and skills but uses them infrequently?

When treating a patient, the therapist continues to ask: What really influences the nature of and the growth rate of cognition? What strategies can enhance cognitive ability and performance? Because science does not know exactly what happens between the presentation of a problem and the patient's response, it is difficult to accurately assess the impact of cognitive treatment strategies used.

In addition to the previous issues that arise from the relationship between theory and practice, the occupational therapist must consider and ask: What is the cognitive demand made by a particular cognitive treatment approach? Does the patient need to function at a "high" level to benefit from a cognitive approach? If as many suggest the answer is "no," the therapist must match the particular cognitive demands made by a given treatment approach with the cognitive capabilities of the patient.

Recommended Reading List

Cotler S, Guerra J: *Assertion Training* Champaign, IL, Research Press, 1976.

Kendall P, Hollon S (Eds): *Assessment Strategies for Cognitive-Behavioral Interventions*. New York, Academic Press, 1981.

Kendall P, Hollon S (Eds): *Cognitive-Behavioral Interventions*. New York, Academic Press, 1979.

Liberman R: *Personal Effectiveness: Guiding People to Assert Themselves and Improve Their Social Skills*. Champaign, IL, Research Press, 1975.

Mahoney M: Cognitive and non-cognitive views in behavior modification. In Sjoden PO, Bates S, Dockens WS (Eds): *Trends in Behavior Therapy*. New York, Plenum Press, 1979.

Mahoney M: Psychotherapy and the structure of personal revolutions. In Mahoney M (Ed): *Psychotherapy Process: Current Issues and Future Directions*. New York, Plenum Press, 1980.

Sank L, Shaffer C: *A Therapist's Manual for Cognitive Behavior Therapy in Groups*. New York, Plenum Press, 1984.

References

1. Allen CK: Independence through activity: The practice of occupational therapy (psychiatry). *Am J Occup Ther* 36(11):731–739, 1982.
2. Allen CK: *Occupational Therapy for Psychiatric Diseases: Measurement and Management of Cognitive Disabilities*. Boston, MA, Little, Brown and Company, 1985.
3. Bara B: Modifications of knowledge by memory processes. In Reda M, Mahoney M: *Cognitive Psychotherapies*. Cambridge, MA, Ballinger Publishing Co., 1984.
4. Bandura A: *Social Learning Theory*. Englewood Cliffs, NJ, Prentice-Hall, 1977, pp. 97, 204.
5. Beck AT: *Cognitive Therapy and the Emotional Disorders*. New York, International Universities Press, 1976.
6. Beck AT, Rush A, Kovacs, M: *Individual Treatment Manual for Cognitive/Behavioral Psychotherapy of Depression*. Philadelphia, University of Pennsylvania Press, 1976.
7. Beck AT, Rush A, Shaw B, Emery G: *Cognitive Therapy of Depression*. New York, The Guilford Press, 1979, p. 3.
8. Beck AT, Ward CH, Mendelson M, et al: An inventory for measuring depression. *Arch Gen Psychiatry* 4: 561–571, 1961.
9. Beck AT, Weissman A, Lester D, et al: The measurement of pessimism: the hopelessness scale. *J Consult Clin Psychol* 42:861–865, 1974.
10. Bodenham J: Rehabilitation of long-term mentally handicapped in community housing. In Scott DW, Katz N: *Occupational Therapy in Mental Health — Principles in Practice*. London, Taylor and Francis, 1988.
11. Bowlby J: The making and breaking of affectional bonds. I. Etiology and psychopathology in the light of attachment theory. *Br J Psychiatry* 130:201–210, 1977.
12. Bowlby J: The making and breaking of affectional bonds. II. Some principles of psychotherapy. *Br J Psychiatry* 130:421–431, 1977.
13. Crist PH: Community living skills: A psychoeducational community based program. *Occup Ther Mental Health* 6(2):51–64, 1986.
14. Conte J, Conte W: The use of conceptual models in occupational therapy. *Am J Occup Ther* 31:262–265, 1977.
15. Corey G: *Theory and Practice of Counseling and Psychotherapy*. Monterey CA, Brooks/Cole Publishing Co., 1979, pp. 173, 176.
16. Davidson G: Behavior modification techniques in institutional settings. In Franks C (Ed): *Behavior Therapy: Appraisal and Status*. New York, McGraw-Hill, 1969, pp. 220–278.
17. Dryden W: Rational-emotive therapy and cognitive therapy: A critical comparison. In Reda M, Mahoney M: *Cognitive Psychotherapies*. Cambridge, MA, Ballinger Publishing Co., 1984.
18. D'Zurilla R, Goldfried M: Problem solving and behavior modification. *J Abnormal Psychol* 78:107–126, 1971.
19. Ellis A: *Humanistic Psychology: The Rational Emotive Approach*. New York: Harper and Row, 1973.
20. Ellis A: *A New Guide to Rational Living*. New York, Harper and Row, 1975.
21. Ellis A, Whiteley J: *Theoretical and Empirical Foundations of Rational-Emotive Therapy*. Monterey, CA, Brooks/Cole, 1979.
22. Fairweather B: *Social Psychology in Treating Mental Illness: An Experimental Approach*. New York, John Wiley, 1984.
23. Folts D: Social skills training. In Scott DW, Katz N: *Occupational Therapy in Mental Health-Principles in Practice*. London, Taylor and Francis, 1988.

24. Foreyt J, Rathjen D (Eds): *Cognitive Behavior Therapy.* New York: Plenum Press, 1978.

25. Frank J: *Persuasion and Healing.* Baltimore, John Hopkins University Press, 1973.

26. Frank J: Therapeutic components of psychotherapy. *J Nerv Mental Dis* 159:325–342, 1974.

27. Frank J: Psychotherapy and the sense of mastery. In Spitzer RL, Klein DF (Eds): *Evaluation of Psychological Therapies.* Baltimore, John Hopkins University Press, 1976.

28. Giles GM, Allen ME: Occupational therapy in the rehabilitation of the patient with anorexia nervosa. *Occup Ther Mental Health* 6:47–66, 1986.

29. Goldfried M: Systematic desensitization as training in self-control. *J Consult Clin Psychol* 37:228–234, 1971.

30. Goldfried M: Psychotherapy as coping skills training. In Mahoney M (Ed): *Psychotherapy Process.* New York, Plenum Press, 1980.

31. Goldstein A: *Structured Learning Therapy: Toward a Psychotherapy for the Poor.* New York, Academic Press, 1973.

32. Guidano V, Liotti G: *Cognitive Processes and Emotional Disorders.* New York, The Guilford Press, 1983, pp. 131, 150.

33. Gutterman L: Day treatment program for persons with AIDS. *Am J Occup Ther* 44:3, 1991.

34. Hayes R: Occupational therapy in the treatment of schizophrenia. *Occup Ther Mental Health* 9:51–68, 1989.

35. Hewett F, Forness S: *Education of Exceptional Learners.* Boston, Allyn and Bacon, 1984, p. 86.

36. Hewett F, Taylor F: *The Emotionally Disturbed Child in the Classroom.* Ed 2. Boston, Allyn and Bacon, 1980.

37. Kanfer F, Phillips J: *Learning Foundations of Behavior Therapy.* New York, John Wiley, 1970.

38. Kaufman CH, Daniels RD, Laverdure PA, et al: Pediatric occupational therapy within a cognitive-behavioural setting. In Scott DW, Katz N: *Occupational Therapy in Mental Health—Principles in Practice.* London, Taylor and Francis, 1988.

39. Kazdin A: Effects of covert modeling and modeling reinforcement on assertive behavior. *J Abnormal Psychol* 83:240–252, 1974.

40. Kelly G: *The Psychotherapy of Personal Constructs.* New York, Norton, 1955.

41. Kendal P: Social cognition and problem solving: A developmental and child-clinical interface. In Gholson B, Rosenthal R (Eds): *Applications of Cognitive-Developmental Theory.* New York, Academic Press Inc., 1984.

42. Kneedles R, Hallahan D: Self-monitoring as an attentional strategy for academic tasks with learning disabled children. In Gholson B, Rosenthal R (Eds): *Applications of Cognitive-Developmental Theory.* New York, Academic Press, 1984.

43. Koestler F (Ed): *Reference Handbook for Continuing Education in Occupational Therapy.* Dubuque, Iowa, Kendall/Hunt Publishing Co., 1970.

44. Kramer L: SCORE: Solving community obstacles and restoring employment. *Occup Ther Mental Health* 4(1):1–135, 1984.

45. Lang P: The mechanics of desensitization and the laboratory study of human fear. In Franks C (Ed): *Assessment and Status of the Behavior Therapies.* New York: McGraw-Hill, 1969.

46. Lazarus A: *Behavior Therapy and Beyond.* New York, McGrawHill, 1971.

47. Lillie M, Armstrong H: Contributions to the development of psychoeducation approaches to mental health service. *Am J Occup Ther* 36(7):438–443, 1982.

48. Mahoney M: *Cognition and Behavior Modification.* Cambridge, MA, Ballinger Publishing Co., 1974.

49. Mahoney M: *Scientist as Subject: The Psychological Imperative.* Cambridge, MA, Ballinger Publishing Co., 1976.

50. Mahoney M: Personal science: A cognitive learning therapy. In Ellis A, Greiger R (Eds): *Handbook of Rational Psychotherapy.* New York, Springer Verlag, 1977.

51. Mahoney M: Behaviorism, cognitivism and human change processes. In Reda M, Mahoney M: *Cognitive Psychotherapies.* Cambridge, MA, Ballinger Publishing Co., 1984.

52. Mahoney M, Arnkoff D: Cognitive and self-control therapies. In Garfield S, Bergin A (Eds): *Handbook of Psychotherapy and Behavior Change.* Ed 2. New York, Wiley, 1978.

53. Mahoney M, DeMonbreun B: Psychology of the scientist: An analysis of problem-solving biases. *Cognitive Ther Res* 1:229–238, 1977.

54. Maultsby M: Systematic written homework in psychotherapy. *Rational Living* 6:17–23, 1971.

55. Meichenbaum D: Cognitive factors in behavior modification: Modifying what clients say to themselves. In Franks C, Wilson G (Eds): *Annual Review of Behavior Therapy: Theory and Practice.* Vol 1. New York, Brunner/Mazel, 1973, pp. 416–431.

56. Meichenbaum D: *Cognitive Behavior Modification.* New York, Plenum Press, 1977, p. 259.

57. Meyers A, Craighead W: *Cognitive Behavior Therapy with Children.* New York, Plenum Press, 1984.

58. Mischel W: *Personality and Assessment.* New York, Wiley, 1968.

59. Mosey AC: An alternative: The biopsychosocial model. *Am J Occup Ther* 28:137–140, 1974.

60. Murray F: The application of theories of cognitive development. In Gholson B, Rosenthal R (Eds): *Applications of Cognitive-Developmental Theory.* New York, Academic Press, 1984.

61. Neistadt M, Marques K: An independent living skills training program. *Am J Occup Ther* 38(10):671–676, 1984.

62. Newel A, Simon H: *Human Problem Solving*. Englewood Cliffs, NJ, Prentice-Hall, 1972.

63. Perry D, Bussey K: *Social Development*. Englewood Cliffs, NJ, Prentice-Hall, 1984, p. 123.

64. Peterson D: *The Clinical Study of Social Behavior*. New York, Appleton-Century-Crofts, 1968.

65. Rathjen D, Rathjen E, Hiniker A: A cognitive analysis of social performance: Implications for assessment and treatment. In Foreyt J, Rathjen D: *Cognitive Behavior Therapy*. New York, Plenum Press, 1978.

66. Reda M, Mahoney M: *Cognitive Psychotherapies*. Cambridge, MA, Ballinger Publishing Co., 1984.

67. Rosenthal R, Bandura A: Psychological modeling: Theory and practice. In Garfield S, Bergin A (Eds): *Handbook of Psychotherapy and Behavior Change*. New York: Wiley, 1978.

68. Roth D: Treatment of the hospitalized eating disorder patient. *Occup Ther Mental Health* 6:67–87, 1986.

69. Rotter J: *Social Learning and Clinical Psychology*. Englewood Cliffs, NJ, Prentice Hall, 1954.

70. Sladyk K: Teaching safe sex practices to psychiatric patients. *Am J Occup Ther* 44(3):284–285, 1990.

71. Spivack G, Platt J, Shure M: *The Problem-Solving Approach to Adjustmentft*. San Francisco, Jossey-Bass, 1976.

72. Stockwell R, Duncan S, Levens M: Occupational therapy with eating disorders. In Scott DW, Katz N: *Occupational Therapy in Mental Health*, Principles in Practice. London, Taylor and Francis, 1988.

73. Stone G: *A Cognitive-Behavioral Approach to Counseling Psychology*. New York, Praeger Publishers, 1980.

74. Suinn R, Richardson F: Anxiety management training: A nonspecific behavior therapy program for anxiety control. *Behav Ther* 2: –510, 1971.

75. Talbot J: Methods of psychosocial education. In Ryan E, Talbot J: Preventive Psychosocial Rehabilitation Psychology for Schizophrenics: Ideology, Practice and Outcome. Paper presented at the annual convention of the American Psychological Association, Toronto, 1984.

76. Weinstein BD, DeNeff LS: Hemophilia, AIDS, and occupational therapy. *Am J Occup Ther* 44(3):228–232, 1989.

77. Young JE: Cognitive therapy and loneliness. In Emery G, Hollon S, Bedrosian RC (Eds): *New Directions in Cognitive Therapy: A Casebook. New York, Guilford Press, 1981, pp. 139–159*.

78. Zung WK, Durham NC: A self-rating depression scale. *Arch Gen Psychiatry* 12:63–70, 1965.

Chapter 9

MOVEMENT-CENTERED FRAME OF REFERENCE

Focus Questions

1. What characterizes the special population for whom this framework is intended?
2. How is adaptation defined in this frame of reference, and what is an adaptive response?
3. What two sensory systems are viewed as dysfunctional most often in this population?
4. By what criteria are activities chosen?
5. What is the therapist's role?
6. How do King's treatment goals differ from those of Ross?
7. Describe how a therapist might control sensory input.
8. What is meant by the phrase **central nervous system plasticity** and why is the assumption of plasticity important to this framework?

Introduction

In the first edition of this text, sensory-integrative therapy was identified as a special instance of developmentally based treatment, one that emphasizes sensory input, movement and noncortical activity. At that time, Lorna Jean King and Mildred Ross were cited as proponents of sensory integrative methods to be used with an adult psychiatric population. Since then, several important changes of emphasis in the area of adult sensory integrative treatment have led us to devote a separate chapter to this area of study and to describe it somewhat differently than we did in 1985. In part to differentiate this frame of reference from sensory-integration used in pediatric care and also because some have found the term **sensory integration** to be a misleading de-

scriptor of what is achieved in treatment, we have chosen the descriptor **movement-centered** frame of reference. As we turn to this framework, we see that it continues to be developmental in its basic premise, holistic, and at home with many principles of neurophysiology as described in Chapter 11. It nevertheless represents a unique contribution to occupational therapy and one we believe that can best be discussed on its own.

Definition

The movement-centered frame of reference directs itself to an adult population identified as having central nervous system (CNS) dysfunction, although often bearing psychiatric labels. This population is believed to have problems with integrating sensation into normal, fluid movement, which ultimately leads to difficulty related to body image, confidence, and task and social behavior. Activities are selected because of their neurophysiological properties and their ability to enhance the opportunity for an integrated, organized response.

Theoretical Development

Occupational therapists practicing in the area of physical dysfunction have long been concerned with motor performance and the contributory roles of sensation, muscle and joint action and, of course, nerve activity. Approaches developed by Rood and described by Stockmeyer,[56,57] work by the Bobaths,[17–19] Brunnstrom,[20,21] Knott and Voss,[40,59,60] and Ayres,[4–15] and more recently such hands-on techniques as myofascial release represent not only a part of occupational therapy's history but also its present. The principles applied in these neurophysiological approaches used in physical medicine, however, had little impact in mental health care until the early 1970s. Although earlier therapists may have recognized that when psychiatric patients engaged in hard physical labor and exercise their symptoms often improved, why and how this came about was not clear.

Ayres and Learning Disabled Children

The work of psychologist and occupational therapist Dr. A. Jean Ayres appears to have been a key impetus in bringing motor and sensory skills to the attention of therapists working in psychiatry.

Sensory Integration

Addressing what she referred to as the problem of poor sensory integration in learning disabled children, Ayres proposed that many children have difficulty moving, learning and behaving normally because their central nervous systems (CNS) have difficulty organizing sensation.[6,8] Describing a developmental scheme, Ayres wrote that higher cortical organization such as that used for conscious reasoning depends on sensory organization at lower levels. She illustrated how input from the vestibular system (e.g., inner ear), muscles and joints, and simple touch played especially significant roles in literally grounding the person and giving him or her the necessary information needed to orient the self to the environment and prepare for an adaptive response. The vestibular system, she wrote, is the "unifying system. It forms the basic relationship of a person to gravity and the physical world. All other sensations are processed in reference to this vestibular information."[12]

Adaptive Response

First, says Ayres, the brain organizes incoming sensory information. As part of this process, the brain **inhibits** (stops or slows) or **facilitates** (increases or enhances) the flow of messages across nerve junctions or synapses. This self-adjusting process, called **modulation**, may be faulty in some individuals who exhibit sensory integration problems.[12] Having sorted out information, the brain can respond adaptively. One characteristic of an **adaptive response** is that it is in itself organizing; that is, it helps the brain organize sensation and movement and in so doing leads to a more complex state of organization.[12] The repeated use of nerve pathways, including their synapses, in a specific sensorimotor function creates a kind of neural memory or map of that function. The brain can then recreate that movement easily in subsequent attempts.[12]

Development

Ayres describes the first seven years of life as primarily devoted to organizing sensations. Neural connections continue to be established until around the age of ten.[12] New connections can be established at later ages, but the process becomes much more difficult. The child who cannot adequately take in or organize sensory information fails to build nerve pathways that permit free and confident movement.[6,8,12]

Assessment

Ayres studied children of many ages but worked primarily with four- to eight-year-olds. She designed and eventually standardized assessments to identify the extent and nature of sensory integrative dysfunction. What began as individual tests in the 1960s were later combined and published as the Southern California Sensory Integration Tests (SCSIT)[7,13] and the Southern California Postrotary Nystagmus Test (SCPNT).[9,45] Since the publication of the SCSIT in 1972, this assessment has been refined and is currently available as the Sensory Integration and Praxis Test (SIPT).[14]

Therapeutic Intervention

Ayres believed that because a child's CNS undergoes much development through age ten, sensory integrative skills not developed at the earlier or typical developmental period might still be developed during childhood, given appropriate therapeutic intervention.[12] The central idea of sensory integrative therapy is to provide controlled sensory input in a manner that the child can effectively integrate, thereby enabling the development of an adaptive response.[12] If the child is older, therapy may help him or her "learn how to facilitate certain messages and inhibit others, to direct information to the proper places in his or her brain and body, and to put all the messages together into useful perceptions and behaviors."[12]

Although Ayres devoted the bulk of her study to children with learning disabilities, she has observed:

"It always comes as a surprise to me when the theory of sensory integrative dysfunction and its treatment is identified primarily with learning disorders. It surprises me because I see this theory as a way of looking at one aspect of development in human beings and some of the malfunctions that befall those beings. Most of the concepts derive from basic research on the vertebrate brain, a science that knows virtually nothing of educational handicaps . . . My interest in perceptual disorders arose when treating the overtly brain damaged such as stroke and cerebral palsied patients. It then extended to children 'brain damaged' (a term freely used at that time) but without upper motor neuron disorder, and then on to the child with minimal brain dysfunction." (As quoted by King,[39] but not otherwise documented for source).

King and Adult Schizophrenia

Occupational therapist Lorna Jean King, like Ayres, views **sensory integration** as the ability of the human organism to perceive, process and use sensory data in a way that permits fluid, purposeful movement. The integrative process depends on the constant interaction of all systems within the organism, and is believed to be governed by the CNS, and especially the noncortical or subcortical portions of the CNS—those housed in the cerebellum and brain stem. You can easily illustrate subcortical movement to yourself. Think for a moment of arising from a chair to select a favorite television program. You are (most likely) able to do this without having to think about how to get up; nor do you experience a loss of balance. Perhaps you daydreamed about an earlier phone call or an unfinished conversation. Because you did not have to concentrate on the process of moving or keeping your balance, one could say that your actions were accomplished subcortically. For adequate subcortical regulation to occur, the necessary input must occur from all of the senses, plus proper arousal. That is, the person cannot be overstimulated or understimulated.

Characteristics of Process Schizophrenia

L. J. King treated chronically disabled psychiatric patients, many of whom had a diagnosis of process schizophrenia. King observed that in addition to experiencing sensory distortions (e.g., loss of visual form and size constancy) many of these patients exhibited physical characteristics similar to those described by Ayres. These included poor muscle tone, a dislike of movement, and a lack of response to vestibular input. Generally, this pattern included the following:

1. Limited mobility of the head;
2. "S" curvature of the spine (lordosis);
3. Shuffling gait;
4. Tendency to hold arms and legs in a flexed, adducted and internally rotated position;
5. Dominance confusion;
6. Atrophy of the thenar eminence and weak grip strength;
7. Poor balance;
8. Lessened responsiveness to vestibular stimulation (e.g., lack of nystagmus with spinning).[34,35]

King cites the categories discussed by Sullivan regarding schizophrenia.[58] **Process schizophrenia** is the diagnosis given to a person who began having problems early in childhood, necessitating treatment in contrast to reactive schizophrenia, which suggests that he or she functioned at least marginally well until a breakdown occurred during a period of recognizable stress.[34] This classification of process versus reactive schizophrenia is not used in the current nomenclature, and it can be noted that by definition, in the *Diagnostic and Statistical Manual of Mental Disorders (DSMIIIR)*, the label schizophrenia implies some degree of chronicity.

It should be noted that the physical posturing and movement described by King in relation to process schizophrenia is similar to the extrapyramidal or Parkinsonian-like effects that follow the long-term use of antipsychotic medications. It has been difficult to determine the extent to which medication may be responsible for physical problems.

Underactive Vestibular System

King postulated that persons with process schizophrenia, like learning disabled children, are unable to move fluidly because they have an ineffective proprioceptive feedback mechanism, the most important component of which is an underactive or underreactive vestibular regulating system.[34] That is, the person with process schizophrenia cannot, at a subcortical level, effectively use sensory information regarding his or her own position in space. This inability leads to restrictive, protective movement. By limiting movement, the individual tends to exacerbate the problem by decreasing vestibular and proprioceptive input. Having to think about moving slows the person, and movement loses its fluidity. This tends to interfere with the individual's ability to engage in normal physical activity, ultimately lessens his or her comfort in social situations and increases withdrawal.

Decreased Sense of Pleasure

In what would appear to be a related characteristic, many persons with process schizophrenia have difficulty experiencing events as pleasurable, a symptom referred to as **anhedonia**. King wanted to reverse what she described as a downward spiral of decreased movement and decreased social involvement. She introduced activities designed to increase proprioceptive and especially vestibular sensory input, and to increase the likelihood of movement regulated subcortically. Interestingly, she observed that patients with anhedonia seemed to enjoy vestibular input. Once her patients began to enjoy moving, motivation became less of a problem, and patients' interaction with each other became more spontaneous.

Noncortical Activities

Activities, said King, were to be first and foremost noncortical and pleasurable,[34] as opposed to many exercise and dance routines in which the participants' attention is brought to their own movement patterns. Activities were also chosen for their ability to normalize movement patterns, strengthen upper trunk stability and increase flexibility. It was believed that these motor changes would improve body image and self-confidence, improve attentional and social response, and lay the necessary foundation for building skills related to cognition and daily tasks.

Treatment of the Adult Population

Following King's 1974 publication, interest grew in sensory integration treatment for an adult population. Studies were developed to better demonstrate physical characteristics specific to process or chronic schizophrenia.[23,32,42,43] A link between sensory integration treatment and patient improvement was studied in relation to changes in verbalization,[16] ward behavior,[50] physical changes,[36,50] and changes in body image.[22,41,50] One problem that became evident in these early studies was that there was no standardized assessments to evaluate sensory integration in adults. Therefore, researchers used tests such as the SCSIT to evaluate adult function. This approach was criticized, as was the premise that an approach developed with and for children with learning disabilities could be applied to an adult population.

In 1983, King responded to some of these criticisms. She first emphasized that evidence increasingly pointed to psychiatric disorder as being primarily neurological, not social, in origin. She reviewed the studies that had been done to verify the findings described in her earlier publication and found them inconclusive. She suggested, however, that as the profession of occupational therapy becomes better at research, the efficacy of sensory integration techniques would be more evident.[38] Work has been done to standardize portions or adaptations of the SCSIT for use with adults.[24,31,33,48,49] Perhaps King's pivotal point is that process schizophrenics traditionally have not responded well to medication or verbal therapies; therefore, anything that can bring about improvement is worth exploring.

Ross and Burdick and the Expansion of Movement Treatment

In 1981 Mildred Ross, an occupational therapist, and Dona Burdick, a recreation therapist collaborated to write *Sensory Integration: A Training Manual for Therapists and Teachers for Regressed, Psychiatric and Geriatric Patient Groups*.[52] These therapists saw in their long-term and regressed patients some postures and movement patterns similar, but not necessarily identical, to those identified with process schizophrenia, as well as similar problems with motivation, short attention span, and disorganized behavior.

Movement Activities

Believing that these patients, too, had sensory integration deficits, Ross and Burdick articulated an approach that could be used in treatment groups. Activities were selected that would involve "full body movement for a total body adaptive response."[52] As with King's approach, activities were chosen for their neurophysiological properties, and many either gave strong sensory input (especially vestibular or proprioceptive) or required patients to physically move.

In addition, these therapists envisioned a developmental process within the treatment group. The first stages of the group were designed to alert and evoke interest, provide sensory input and demand a movement response. These activities were thought to be organizing and believed to pave the way for activity more cognitive in nature. Later group stages were designed to elicit a response that involved verbalization, reflection or reasoning.

Movement-Centered Approach

In 1991, Ross revised the original Ross and Burdick publication. This second book, *Integrative Group Therapy: The Structured Five-Stage Approach*,[51] was renamed to reflect its somewhat altered content. Ross identifies the sensory integrative theories of Ayres and King as only an incomplete part of the rationale for her movement-centered approach, or what she refers to as "motor rehabilitation."[52] The work of Dr. Karol Bobath and Mrs. Berta Bobath, known as neurodevelopmental theory (NDT), is credited for its usefulness in helping the therapist to look at movement, for its emphasis on balance, posture and movement patterns, and for the permission it gives the therapist to handle and guide the patient.[17–19,51]

Ross recommends the study of other neurodevelopmental approaches so that the therapist might expand his or her knowledge of movement. Those cited included spatiotemporal adaptation,[27] proprioceptive neuromuscular facilitation (PNF),[40,59] and the functional integration of Feldenkrais.[25,26] Ross suggests that movement is the key for it produces "immediate and profound physiological changes that can influence behavior."[51]

Expanding to Include Cognitive Goals

In contrast to King's focus on noncortical treatment activities, Ross moves beyond these activities to include cognitive behavior change as a treatment goal. She proposes that the organization achieved by the sensory and motor phases of treatment paves the way for the patient to then think about what was accomplished, to give feedback to other group members, and to learn or modify problem-solving strategies. Toward this end, the author discusses the application of Abreu and Toglia's cognitive rehabilitation model.[1,2] As described in Chapter 11, Abreu and Toglia's work is with persons with traumatic brain injury. They use a holistic approach in which they assume that the brain injured individual is still capable of learning but needs assistance with maximizing existing problem-solving stategies and learning new cognitive strategies that will better compensate for existing limitations.

Identifying a Patient Population

Ross defines her patient population and that considered suited for integrative therapy some-

what more broadly in her 1991 text. In this book, she describes her patients as part of a special population or "those groups of individuals who require more than the usual amount of cues and assists for their CNS to become organized sufficiently to make an appropriate and sustained response. Their nervous systems require assistance from the environment and their caretakers to perform adaptively."[51] Such special populations might include persons in geriatric centers, those with developmental disability, or hemiparesis, or chronic psychiatric problems, plus any others who are judged to have neurological impairment.

Comparing Ross and King

Ross' population expands beyond that discussed by King, and her theoretical base goes beyond that of sensory integration to include several movement-centered theories traditionally associated with treatment in the area of physical dysfunction. Ross also expands her treatment goals to include cognitive or cortical activity, in contrast to King's emphasis on the noncortical. However, several similar themes exist in both authors' writing, including an emphasis on movement and sensory stimulation, with special attention afforded the proprioceptive and vestibular systems; a belief in the need for sensory information to be given in a controlled manner by the therapist; a belief in the organizing role of movement; a focus on the pleasurable nature of activity; a developmental view of the way movement patterns evolve; a reliance on the body-mind relationship; and an understanding of many, if not all, psychiatric processes as neurological at their base. This final emphasis is consistent with the position taken by Claudia Allen and discussed in Chapter 10. In contrast to Allen, however, King and Ross express the view that neurologically compromised persons can learn and improve as a result of therapeutic intervention.

Current Practice in Occupational Therapy

The Person and Behavior

Normal Human Function

The person is, above all, a single, unified organism or whole; anything that affects the body will influence thinking and emotion, and ultimately behavior. This view is consistent with other holistic frames of reference detailed in this book, but the emphasis in intervention in this framework is on the physiological side of a person's being.

Adaptation. It is the nature of the person to organize and adapt and thereby to become more complex. **Adaptation** is an active process by which the person meets the challenges of his or her environment, while at the same time fulfilling personal needs and desires. The adaptive process is in itself self-satisfying and self-perpetuating. Adaptation is often accomplished most efficiently when it is organized subcortically, or unconsciously.[37] Stated another way, a great deal of what each of us does daily we do without special attention. This frees our attention and energy to be focused on more cognitively demanding tasks. When a person perceives himself or herself adapting successfully, he or she feels a sense of mastery, which acts as a powerful internal motivator for future adaptation.

Developmental Process. Adaptation is a developmental process within the organism, one that is governed by the laws of growth and development evidenced within the phylogenetic history of the species. Activity governed by phylogenetically older parts of the CNS (e.g., the brain stem) form the foundation for adaptive activity governed by phylogenetically newer portions (e.g., the cerebral cortex). Likewise, sensory and motor skills developed in early childhood do so in an invariant order and form the basis for skills that will emerge in later childhood and adulthood. The CNS retains some plasticity in that changes can occur within the CNS in late childhood and adulthood, but these are more difficult to bring about than would be expected in early life.

The brain is "primarily a sensory processing machine" and sensory input is the raw material upon which all adaptation is based at any age.[12] In other words, the brain needs information before it can direct the person how to act. Sensation and its accurate perception also lays the foundation for an accurate and positive body concept. Good movement promotes body scheme, stimulates better posture, and is organizing to the CNS.[51]

Dysfunction

Dysfunction is an impairment in the ability for successful adaptation. As defined in this frame of reference, the dysfunctional person is one who has neurological or CNS damage. This damage may result from disease processes considered clearly organic in their genesis, such as mental retardation and Alzheimer's disease; from so-called functional disorders, such as schizophrenia and depression; or when aging, neglect or social factors have created a personal environment devoid of adequate sensory stimulation. Those children who have untreated sensory integration problems may adapt relatively well and exhibit only minor impairments as adults; or, they may, at the extreme, go on to develop severe perceptual disturbances, very low self-esteem and disorganized behavior, as is seen in schizophrenia.[37,51]

Characteristics of Dysfunction. Whatever the origin of the sensory and motor deficits, characteristics often shared in common by persons with **sensorimotor dysfunction** include mood disorders (agitation, confusion or apathy), poor social and communication skills, a dislike of movement, an inability to sustain interest and attention, a rigid or flexed body posture, a lessened ability to ignore unpleasant sensation, poor body image and low self-esteem. This population also has limitations of higher cognitive function.

Role of Stress. The contributory role of stress in psychiatric dysfunction is referred to by proponents of movement therapy. Because of the reciprocity between physical and emotional states, psychological stress—the stress of everyday life can be expected to exact a physical toll. In this respect, states of **dis-ease** are often conceptualized as ones in which the body or mind have broken down from stress overload. Many schizophrenic individuals have, for example, described an increase in hallucinations and distortions in time perception during periods of increased stress.[29]

Stress as an etiological component of dysfunction is cited here because physically demanding activity such as that used in movement-centered approaches has also been used as a means to reduce stress. It has been postulated that movement contributes to the normalization of function in the schizophrenic patient because of its ability to reduce stress.[38]

Role of the Occupational Therapist

Spontaneity

Movement-centered therapy is a poor choice for therapists who want to stay seated or distant from their patients. Picture therapists making hands-on contact with patients, perhaps giving them vestibular stimulation through spinning them in a desk chair, playing Simon Says, or tossing a ball, and you get a feel for the very active role taken by the therapist. King states that the role of the therapist is to have fun and be spontaneous.[34] The therapist's enthusiasm and active participation not only serve as a model for the patients, but they become a part of the sensory environment, acting to alert and energize. In a similar vein, Ross describes the therapist's role in group treatment as being "an interactive facilitator and part of the environment who must move about, provide appropriate touching, use a calm voice and make eye contact to obtain membership involvement."[51] This technique also contributes to what Ross refers to as the therapist's "special role in making members feel wanted, safe and expectant."[51]

Controlling Sensory Input

The therapist has an equally vital role in controlling the environment, not just creating excitement and stimulation. Because many patients for whom this treatment is appropriate have difficulty modulating sensory input, the therapist creates an environment in which sensory messages are neither too intense, too rapid nor too subdued to be effectively integrated, and an environment that provides an opportunity for movement at the level at which the patient can succeed.

Praising

The therapist also recognizes the importance of his or her role in bringing the patient's attention to successes. Many dysfunctional persons have been reluctant to move about and tend to see themselves as failures. Frequent and clear praise for involvement acts not only as a behavioral reward but may be necessary if the patient is to recognize his or her own accomplishments or improvement.

Hands-on Contact

As with other frames of reference, the therapist has a continuing role in observing patients, thereby being able to respond to them and modulate environmental stimuli. The therapist may use hands-on guidance to reposition the patient during an activity.

Of all the therapeutic frames of reference discussed in this text, this approach makes most emphasizes the value of acceptable touch. That is, in his or her touch the therapist has a means to supply proprioceptive and tactile input, to calm, to alert, to reassure, and to recognize. If we recall the patients described by Ross—often older, or tending to regress and withdraw—we realize this population is often left alone and receives little appropriate touch from others. A hug for a job well done, an arm around the shoulder, or taking a person's hands and guiding them through the process of mixing a cake batter are examples of useful and appropriate touch. Not incidentally, this touch can communicate nonverbally caring and support.

Responsibilities of the Patient

Because many of the persons participating in movement-centered therapy tend to regress, at least initially, there is not the expectation that they will enter into a contract with the therapist. This does not mean, however, that all the responsibility for treatment is the therapist's alone. As Ross writes, the therapist must hold two fundamental beliefs: 1) that each participant can learn and 2) that each participant has some wisdom that needs to be shared. According to Ross, "Even though the group is composed of people who find it difficult to express their needs in an organized manner; even when they are enslaved to emotions that they cannot effectively harness ... they know something others do not know ... They have experience and possess a wisdom that they can share and, in return, receive from other members."[51]

The Function of Activity

Elicit an Adaptive Response

Activities used in movement-centered approaches are analyzed and selected primarily for their physiological properties and their ability to elicit an adaptive response. That is, the activity involves the participant in enjoyable, goal-directed behavior. The patient does not come to treatment to engage in aimless, repetitive reaching or bending, but will reach for blocks in a relay game or bend to plant a garden. Thus, the activities used in occupational therapy will be parts of life which, when accomplished, can help the patient to feel a more effective person within his or her own world.

Provide Sensory Input

The therapist is especially interested in the ability of the activity to alert or calm the CNS.

Vestibular input given slowly, as occurs in gentle rocking, and heavy proprioceptive pressure are calming and may be used, for example, with an agitated patient. Softer touch can be stimulating, as are cold temperatures, strong odors, and so on. Tables 9.1 and 9.2 provide other examples of alerting and soothing stimuli.

It is not only the ability of the sensation to calm or alert, but the very fact that sensory information is entering the CNS that provides the patient with something to which he or she can respond. Using activity that will stimulate many or even all of the senses is encouraged. Because many patients seem to have problems related to the vestibular and proprioceptive systems, activity is chosen especially for its in-

TABLE 9.1   ALERTING AND CALMING THROUGH SENSORY STIMULATION

Senses	Methods Used to Stimulate	Behaviors
Touch		
Protopathic	Rubbing/different textures, self touch	Alerting
Epicritic	Self touch	Calming
Vestibular	Rotation	
	—Fast	Alerting
	—Slow	Calming
Proprioception	Pressure—Light	Alerting
	—Moderate	Calming
Vision	Bright colors—Light	Alerting
	Pastels—Low Intensity	Calming
Hearing	Contrast Sounds— Loud	Alerting
	Repetitive changes— Slow	Calming
	Melodious and soft sounds	Calming
Smell	Pungent Smells	Alerting
	Potpourri of sweet smells	Calming
Taste	Strong Flowers— Crunchy	Alerting
	Smooth texture—tepid temperatures	Calming

Ross M : *Integrative Group Therapy.* Thorofare NJ, SLACK Inc., 1991, p. 151. Reprinted with permission.

TABLE 9.2 ALERTING AND CALMING THROUGH MUSIC AND MOVEMENT

Alerting	Calming
Increased muscle activity with increased muscle tension	Decreased motor activity, relaxed muscle fibers.
Head up, chest out, general extension pattern.	Head down, torso bent (forward flexion) deep breathing.
Light touch, patting, whisking, brushing movements.	Heavy pressure touch, massage.
Percusive movements	Swinging or sustained movements.
Non-repetitive or uneven rhythmic patterns. Uneven locomotor movements (skip, gallow, slide)	Slow, repetitive movements, axial or locomotor.
Fast, loud music of variable intensity, sharp sounds	Slow, dreamy, lyrical music: Adagio.
Linear acceleration and deceleration in locomotor patterns	Linear movement consistency.
Defy gravity, up and down	Give in to gravity, body hanging, collapse or ragdoll movements.
Fast spinning or twirling	Slow turning

Ross R: *Integrative Group Therapy* Thorofare NJ, SLACK Inc., 1991, p. 152. Reprinted with permission.

corporation of vestibular stimulation (e.g., movement of the head through many planes); because it incorporates deep pressure touch; and because of its ability to give proprioceptive feedback to joints and tendons (e.g., clapping and jumping).[34,35]

Normalize Movement

King, Ross and Ayres all pay particular attention to the posture and movement patterns used in the treatment activity. Ross refers to her desire to ultimately reach a level of "full-body" movement for a "total-body adaptive response."[52] We are assuming that this goal would not always be achieved within one activity, but several activities might be used within one treatment session in order to use a broad range of muscle groups and stimulate many senses.

In accord with the dysfunctional posture and movement that King identified as characteristic of process schizophrenia, she proposed that therapeutic activity could counter abnormal movement or normalized patterns of excessive body flexion, adduction and internal rotation, and increase joint range of motion.[34] Playing volleyball would exemplify this kind of activity. In an effort to normalize tone, activity should include the bilateral use of tonic muscles against resistance, as occurs in digging a garden or playing tug-of-war. These embody the **heavy work patterns** to which Rood refers.[57]

Citing the work of Bobath and Bobath, Ross also discusses the importance of proper positioning in seated activities and the use of activities that demand shifting, reaching and bending and that thereby stimulate balance responses, and counter the collapse into flexion and extension.[51]

Provide a Vehicle for Pleasant Experiences

Ayres, King and Ross all emphasize that activities experienced as pleasurable by the patient are more likely to be repeated and, therefore, more likely to lead to a habituated, adaptive response. As Ross says, "whatever is pleasurable" to the patient can be a potential treatment activity. She adds that when therapists get too concerned about the age appropriateness of tasks, they might be confusing their personal values with the patient's own preferences.[51] In addition to emphasizing that the activity be pleasant (pleasure of course being a subjective state), King writes that activity be **noncortical**, or that patients have their minds on the fun that they are having and not on how their bodies are moving.[34] Perhaps slightly different in tone, King suggests, too, that if the activity does not "induce smiles and pleasure" as from recreation, it should bring about a feeling of mastery, as from a work-oriented task. In either case, the participant feels a sense of satisfaction.

Provide a Vehicle for Socialization

Movement treatment can be carried individually, but often occurs in a group context. Activities are then selected in part for their ability to engage patients with each other. Not only does the therapist provide sensory stimulation, but patients may be asked to pass materials to each other, to pat each other, apply textured materials to each other's arms, to sing together, stamp their feet in unison or give each other verbal feedback. In this way, the adaptive response(s) being built include those of normal social behavior. As patients become less physically withdrawn and more at ease, they often become more willing to risk social spontaneity. The adaptive response spiral then moves forward as success and fulfilling social contact lead to further engagement and self-confidence.

Facilitate Cognitive Skill Building

As discussed, King proposes staying with non-cortical activities, whereas Ross uses a movement-centered base to prepare for eventual developmental of cognitive strategies. Activities are evaluated and selected in relation to cognitive retraining (see Chapter 11). In the example of group treatment that follows later in this chapter, both cognitive and noncortical activities are used in one group session.

Theoretical Assumptions

The following theoretical assumptions are based on the theoretical views of Ross and King:

1. The person is best viewed as a "single organism, highly complex and completely unified."[34]
2. "Anything that affects the body will inexorably affect the mind and vice versa."[34]
3. The same principles of neurophysiology are applicable and adaptable to persons of all ages.[52]
4. It is the nature of the person to organize through adaptive response.
5. It is self-satisfying for the person to engage in purposeful, goal-directed activity.
6. Higher cortical organization depends on organization at lower levels.
7. The CNS becomes more complex in a sequential manner.

8. The CNS is "plastic" and remains capable of change even in adulthood.
9. The person (child and adult) often selects just the activity that he or she needs for healthy development.
10. The vestibular system is the unifying system, as it forms the framework for organizing experience.
11. Good movement promotes body scheme and is organizing.
12. Movement produces "immediate and profound physiological changes that can influence behavior."[51]
13. Much so-called "mental" illness is physiological in origin.
14. Persons with CNS damage have more difficulty integrating relevant sensation and ignoring irrelevant stimuli.
15. Persons with CNS problems are capable of learning.
16. "Treatment which provides controlled sensory input, within the context of meaningful activity, and which results in an adaptive response (or behavior) will enhance sensory integration and improve behavior."[52,54]

Evaluation

An accurate assessment of the patient's functional abilities, especially as related to movement and body-scheme, serves several related purposes:

1. It suggests the activities at which the patient can succeed and helps the therapist know where to begin.
2. It may shed light on the reason(s) for poor function.
3. It allows the therapist to establish a baseline of function, state goals and subsequently measure progress.
4. It may give useful information about the cues and environmental structure that help the patient to succeed and can point to a need for future testing.[55]

Assessment instruments are selected for their utility in screening for neurological deficits, often those identified as **neurological soft signs** deviations that do not localize within the CNS, but lead to problems with learning, motor, sensory and integration functions.[24]

Assessment Instruments

Southern California Sensory Integration Tests (SCSIT) and the Sensory Integration and Praxis Tests (SIPT). Although these tests have been standardized for children age 4 to 10, selected subtests have been used with adults, and some work has established normative test scores for adults.[7,14] Table 9.3 lists the subtests within the SIPT, available from Western Psychological Services, Los Angeles, California.

Schroeder-Block-Campbell Adult Psychiatric Sensory Integration Evaluation (SBC). The SBC was developed to provide a standardized, comprehensive evaluation tool for use by occupational therapists working with an adult psychiatric population. It consists of three subscales, and takes about 75 minutes to complete, but does not have to be completed at one sitting. The Physical Assessment subscale evaluates neurophysical abilities needed for

TABLE 9.3   AREAS OF FUNCTION

1. Space visualization
2. Figure-ground perception
3. Manual form perception
4. Kinesthesia
5. Finger identification
6. Graphesthesia
7. Localization of tactile stimuli
8. Praxis on verbal command
9. Design copying
10. Constructional praxis
11. Postural praxis
12. Oral praxis
13. Sequencing praxis
14. Bilateral motor coordination
15. Standing and walking balance
16. Motor accuracy
17. Postrotary nystagmus

Areas of Function identified by the Sensory Integration and Praxis Tests (Ayres, 1989)

everyday tasks, for example, those related to balance, coordination and hand function. The Abnormal Movements subscale measures abnormal movements such a hypokinetic and hyperkinetic movement, in addition to such extrapyramidal symptoms as akathesia and tardive dyskinesia. The Childhood History section asks the patient about early growth and development, and looks for indications of developmental delays or other neurological soft signs. A nonstandardized use of the person-drawing elicits information pertaining to body image.[28,53]

Parachek Geriatric Behavior Rating Scale. This quick screening tool consists of ten multiple choice items, three related to physical condition, four to self-care and three to social behavior. Scores are designed in part to help designate functional levels (level one through three), the lowest level indicating a need for substantial nursing care, and the person rated at the highest level capable of most self-care. A treatment manual has been designed for use with the Parachek scale and suggests possible occupational therapy treatment activities.[46,47]

Smaga and Ross Integrated Battery (SARIB). Said to be based on clinical experience, this battery "evaluate[s] clients with low functional ability for placement in similar ability groups."[55] An extensive test, this battery could conceivably be performed in several sittings. Its subtests include the Llorens-Rubin Motor Control Test, the Elizur Test of Psycho-organicity (in itself a standardized test available from Western Psychological Services), Schilder's Arm Extension Test, and a request for a person-drawing.[44] Overall, test items relate to range of motion, posture, gait, balance, strength, visual performance, coordination, motor planning, sensory perception, stereognosis, proprioception, judgment, memory and "other behaviors that influence performance." The test is described in detail, with scoring sheets, in Ross' *Integrative Group Therapy: The Structured Five-Stage Approach.*[51]

Many other standardized and nonstandardized tests have been cited in the literature for use with this frame of reference. These tests include portions of the Frostig and Purdue perceptual tests, various versions of the draw-a-person, the Nurses Observation Scale for Inpatient Evaluation (NOSIE),[30] and the Allen Cognitive Level Test.[3]

Treatment

Just as the object relations frame of reference assumes that if the patient feels differently and perceives his or her problem-solving as having improved, one could expect this individual's appearance to reflect this in a brighter affect, the movement-centered framework believes that if one moves with more confidence, his or her feelings about the self can be expected to improve. The stage is then set for social skill building and for tackling cognitive problems. Thus it is perhaps prudent to remind ourselves that while therapeutic intervention is movement-centered, the goals go beyond enhanced movement.

Goals

The ultimate aim of treatment is to bring about an organized, adaptive, whole-person response. Treatment goals are written as changes in functional, demonstrable behaviors in the area(s) of movement, sensorimotor skill acquisition, posture, affect, social interaction (including verbalization), body-image, self-esteem, and cognition. More specifically, these goals might begin with one or more of the following.

Patient exhibits:

1. Increased awareness or use of both sides of body;
2. Normalized whole-body flexor-extensor tone;
3. Improved balance and posture during activity;
4. Increased voluntary movement of the head through more than one plane during activity;
5. Improved motor planning;
6. Increased range of motion during activity;
7. Normalized gait;
8. Normalized patterns of adduction and internal rotation;
9. Increased spontaneous movement during activity;
10. Increased tolerance of touch.

Subsequent to, or at times along with these movement-centered goals, goals might include those related to normalized affect, clarity of thinking, and socialization. Typifying these goals, but not to be considered as inclusive are the following.

Patient exhibits:

1. Signs of increased spontaneity (e.g., smiling, initiating conversation);
2. Lengthened attention to a task;
3. Appropriate assertive behavior (e.g., asking for assistance);
4. Signs of increased confidence and improved self-image (e.g., improved hygiene, willingness to take appropriate risks);
5. Ability to share materials, space, and ideas with others during activity;
6. Increased ability to stay calm, alert and effectively in control.

Treatment Process

King limits her description of the actual process of treatment to a somewhat general discussion of the characteristics of activities to be used, and the exhortation to the therapist to keep the treatment session fun. Journal articles that address this framework also tend to discuss treatment briefly. Ross goes into much greater detail, but her application of this model is exclusively with groups, and as noted, includes a strongly cognitive component. Therefore, the therapist choosing this treatment approach has a good deal of leeway when envisioning the specifics of a treatment program to be used with an individual or group of patients.

Both King and Ross believe there is an advantage to treating in groups, in part because a group enhances the fun and available energy, and because group treatment is more efficient. This does not imply that movement-centered intervention has to be carried out within a group. In fact, the therapist may use a one-to-one format with the patient who cannot yet tolerate the group.[34]

Beginning Treatment

The stage is set when the therapist takes control of the treatment environment. The therapist pays special attention to the sensory stimulation within the setting, striving to maintain the optimum necessary level of arousal and creating a sense of safety.

King writes that, in general, activities are either recreation or games. They are selected according to the physical demands that they make. Task-oriented activities, states King, "will usually be effective after a patient's level of functioning has been raised to a certain level."[34] This relates to the need to begin by alerting the participant and selecting an activity at a level at which the patient can succeed. The goal is to alert pleasure centers and build confidence.

Using the Vibrator

When a participant is agitated, apathetic or confused, Ross advises the therapist to give proprioceptive input.[51] One way to supply this input is through the use of a hand-held vibrator. Ross writes, "Persons who may reject other kinds of touch or are suffering from sensory deprivation for any reason can demonstrate immediate pleasure after the vibrator is offered, often resulting in a relaxing effect that can last from minutes to a few hours."[51] It is recommended "not as a treatment tool in itself," but as a tool that encourages participation in treatment.[51]

The kind of vibrator to which Ross refers is one with a low amplitude and a frequency range (Hz) of 100 or higher. It is used only if the patient indicates his or her desire, and only

for two or three minutes. Used in this way the vibrator may be moved along the chin, on the back, arms or other areas as described by Ross.

Using Motor Activity

The literature describes treatment sessions from one-half hour to one hour long, typically, having one or more gross activities that are introduced after sensory input has been supplied, as indicated. These motor activities in themselves continue to supply heightened, controlled sensory stimulation. For example, a typical treatment session might have an individual begin with two or so minutes, with the therapist supplying input with the vibrator. Then the patient might be asked to stand against a piece of large paper on the wall, while the therapist traces around the arms and upper torso. Finally, the two might toss about a beach ball, or use some other activity in which the patient has to reach above the head.

Throughout treatment, the patient is encouraged to explore and enjoy the media offered, and the therapist remains flexible, observing the patient's reactions to activity, and modifying treatment as needed.

Therapeutic Group

By far, the most extensive development of a movement-centered group is found in Ross's *Integrative Group Therapy*.[51] Following a five-stage model, Ross uses neurodevelopmental principles to sequence the presentation of motor, perceptual and cognitive activities, as well as to establish guidelines for therapist intervention and expected participant behavior. Each of these stages occurs within the individual group session. Outlined very briefly, these five stages are as follows.

Stage 1. In stage 1, members are acknowledged, and the purpose of the group is stated. The goal is to get participants' attention, and to help members to feel "wanted, safe, and expectant."[51] The therapist tries to arouse the members' alerting and pleasure centers through the use of activity involving sensory input and by encouraging touching and handling of interesting media. For example, simple musical instruments might be passed around, textured items rubbed on arms and faces, or scented soaps passed around the group.

Stage 2. Here, movement is emphasized. Movement activities can be selected to be arousing (e.g., blowing and chasing soap bubbles, ripping newspaper in preparation for later use) or calming, as when rolling a patient in a parachute. Whatever the movement selected, the therapist is careful to choose activities at the level at which members can succeed.

Stage 3. In this stage, tasks are offered that require "less physical and more thoughtful action."[51] Having been able to attend and succeed at a task, the participant has more available energy and ability to perform. Games, including those that are competitive, might be introduced to emphasize perceptual motor accuracy. These games include safe darts, identifying and naming objects in the room, touch-discrimination activities, Simon-Says, the hokey-pokey, and games of pantomime.

Stage 4. Members are asked to focus on a cognitive task. They are encouraged to be thoughtful and creative and to share verbally with each other. For example, participants might be asked to share how they felt about themselves or the activity in which they participated. Poetry, creative storytelling, reminiscence, show and tell, and brief slide presentations could be used to stimulate dialogue.

Stage 5. This stage closes the day's session. The therapist informs the group before closing so that they might mentally prepare. The therapist determines an appropriate closure, given the group's mood and the session theme.

Summary

It seems reasonable to suggest that every psychiatric condition brings with it some physical, often observable manifestation. Whether the downcast eyes of the person depressed, or the determined face of the compulsively preoccupied, the nail-biting of the anxious, or the rapid speech of the person in a manic phase, we often see in the dysfunctional population as well as ourselves, signs of what is experienced internally. For some individuals, this physical evidence is far more striking that problems involve the whole person. It is to this group of persons, many with symptoms that have been unresponsive to the traditional arsenal of psychiatry, that movement-centered therapy is directed.

In this frame of reference, the mandate is to get up and get moving, and to touch those things that for some reason lie outside of everyday experience. Proponents use theories of growth and development to support the contention that in making contact and moving the body, adaptation occurs first at the unconscious level within the CNS. The conscious decision to act then becomes more an available option, and learning is facilitated. Movement-centered approaches stand out as an instance in occupational therapy where sensation and movement, not the psyche or thinking self, are the focus in a holistic framework.

Contributions and Limitations of the Movement-Centered Frame of Reference

Contributions

A significant contribution of this frame of reference lies in its outreach to a group or special population that has tended to be managed in some kind of residential care but whose quality of life has often been compromised. Both King and Ross assert that in their experience, patients involved in this kind of treatment do improve, and that improvements carry over even after treatment has been terminated. This framework identifies a classical use of occupational therapy, wherein activity is used to elicit a total-person, adaptive response.

Although holistic in its ideology, this framework is quite focused on movement and sensation and does not attempt to be all things to all persons as holism is sometimes accused.

While one should not confuse writing style with content, both King and Ross are upbeat in their writing, which fits with the optimistic tenor of the framework. It is not that cures are promised, but one is given a way of looking at dysfunction and remediation that recognizes some health, even in the very disturbed, as well as a belief that intervention is worth pursuing.

It is perhaps ironic that professionals again need permission to touch their patients, but with the abuse of touch that has come to light in our society it is helpful to be reminded of the healing quality of appropriate and caring touch. This permission fits with the overall theme of therapist involvment within the treatment process. Ross' writing implies that the therapist takes a nurturing role with patients, not a position outside of what many would see as implicit in all therapy, but perhaps outside of what therapists consider comfortable.

Limitations

Gaps within this framework need to be addressed. These are well articulated by King when she writes, "The first question to ask about any treatment for any condition is 'Does it work?' If the answer is negative, one need go no further. If the answer is positive, then one needs to narrow the question to, 'For which patients is it most successful?' The answer to that question, by helping to define the characteristics of a certain group, will assist with answering the third question, 'Why does it work?'"[39]

Although some limited research was conducted in an effort to support King's initial findings the results were, in King's own words, "meager" and inconclusive.[39] Ross' approach goes far beyond sensory integration practice, but is not guided by any specific research findings. Part of the problem is that relatively few persons are involved in research in occupational therapy, and certainly not all of those are interested in movement approaches. King or Ross are not being discounted when

they say that their patients have improved, but the influence of many other variables is unclear. For example, to what extent might their own enthusiasm influence treatment outcomes?

If one assumes for a moment that movement approaches do work, many unanswered questions remain. For whom and why do they work? King's reference to the suitability of this framework to process (versus reactive or paranoid) schizophrenia has created some confusion. How chronic in terms of years need one be to be considered a suitable candidate for treatment? If, as both Ross and King propose, this framework is suited to many geriatric patients, what are the criteria for its use? Schizophrenia is a medical diagnosis; older age, even regression, is not.

Medication's role in the physical symptoms of many of those special populations treated has not been clearly separated from other possible causes of CNS dysfunction. It may not be possible to determine this role because it is difficult to find a population in long-term care that has not received medication.

In terms of very practical questions and based on anecdotal information given by King and Ross, it is not evident how long movement-centered therapy is best carried out with a patient. Days? Weeks? Months? Is there a point of diminishing returns, and to what time frame do Ross and King refer when they write that improvement persists even after treatment is terminated? What steps, if any, are needed to keep participants from regressing if they live within an environment in which little is going on?

As with other frames of reference discussed in this text, there are caveats specific to this framework. Ross' suggestion to her readers that they become well informed in the area of neurophysiological approaches needs to be underscored. The potential for random or reckless spinning, misuse of a vibrator, or other overstimulation or noxious stimulation exists, especially when a therapist is not keenly aware of potential physical and emotional responses to sensation.

With the return emphasis in psychiatry on neurological function, and the expanded ability to see how the CNS really operates, it would seem that much that could be learned within this framework that would contribute to humankind's understanding of function and dysfunction. Many professionals with a great deal of commitment will need to work toward this goal.

References

1. Abreu B, Toglia J: Cognitive rehabilitation: A model for occupational therapy. *Am J Occup Ther* 41:439–448, 1987.

2. Abreu B, Toglia J: *Cognitive Rehabilitation Manual.* New York, Authors, 1984.

3. Allen CK: *Occupational Therapy for Psychiatric Diseases: Measurement and Management of Cognitive Disabilities.* Boston, Little, Brown and Company, 1985.

4. Ayres AJ: Deficits in sensory integration in educationally handicapped children. *J Learning Disabilities* 2:68–71, 1969.

5. Ayres AJ: Improving academic scores through sensory integration. *J Learning Disabilities* 5:24–28, 1972.

6. Ayres AJ: *Sensory Integration and Learning Disorders.* Los Angeles, Western Psychological Services, 1972.

7. Ayres AJ: *Southern California Sensory Integration Tests: Manual.* Los Angeles, Western Psychological Services, 1972.

8. Ayres AJ: An interpretation of the role of the brainstem in intersensory integration. In Coryell H (Ed): *The Body Senses and Perceptual Deficit.* Boston, Boston University Press, 1973.

9. Ayres AJ: *Southern California Postrotary and Nystagmus Test Manual.* Los Angeles, Western Psychological Services, 1975.

10. Ayres AJ: Cluster analyses of measures of sensory integration. *Am J Occup Ther* 31:362–366, 1977.

11. Ayres AJ: Learning disabilities and the vestibular system. *J Learning Disabilities* 11:30–41, 1978.

12. Ayres AJ: *Sensory Integration and the Child.* Los Angeles, Western Psychological Services, 1979.

13. Ayres AJ: *Southern California Sensory Integration Test: Manual.* Rev ed. Los Angeles, Western Psychological Services, 1980.

14. Ayres AJ: *Sensory Integration and Praxis Tests.* Los Angeles, Western Psychological Services, 1989.

15. Ayres AJ, Heskett WM: Sensory integrative dysfunction in a young schizophrenic girl. *J Autism Child Schizophr* 2:174–181, 1972.

16. Bailey D: The effects of vestibular stimulation on verbalization in chronic schizophrenics. *Am J Occup Ther* 32(7):445–450, 1978.

17. Bobath B: *Adult Hemiplegia: Evaluation and Treatment.* Ed 2. London, W. Heinemann Medical Books, 1978.

18. Bobath B, Bobath K: *Motor Development in the Different Types of Cerebral Palsy.* London, W. Heinemann Medical Books, 1975.

19. Bobath K: *A Neurophysiological Basis for the Treatment of Cerebral Palsy.* Ed 2. London, Heinemann Medical Books Ltd; Philadelphia, JB Lippincott, 1980.

20. Brunnstrom S: Motor behavior of adult hemiplegic patients. *Am J Occup Ther* 25:6–12, 1961.

21. Brunnstrom S: *Movement Therapy in Hemiplegia: A Neurophysiological Approach.* New York, Harper and Row, 1970.

22. Crist P: Body image changes in chronic non-paranoid schizophrenics. *Can J Occup Ther* 46(2):61–65, 1979.

23. Endler P, Eiman M: Postural and reflex integration in schizophrenic patients. *Am J Occup Ther* 32(7):456–459, 1978.

24. Falk-Kessler J, Quittman M, Moore R: The SCSIT: A potential tool for assessing neurological impairment in adult psychiatric outpatients. *Occup Ther J Res* 8(3):131–146, 1988.

25. Feldenkrais M: *Body and Mature Behavior—Anxiety, Sex, Gravitation and Learning.* New York, International Universities Press, 1966.

26. Feldenkrais M: *Awareness Through Movement: Health Exercises for Personal Growth.* New York, Harper and Row, 1977.

27. Gilfoyle EM, Grady AP, Moore JC: *Children Adapt.* Ed 2. Thorofare, NJ, SLACK Inc., 1980.

28. Hamada R, Schroeder C: Schroeder-Block-Campbell Adult Psychiatric Sensory Integration Evaluation: Concurrent validity and clinical utility. *Occup Ther J Res* 8(2):75–88, 1988.

29. Hatfield A: Patients' accounts of stress and coping in schizophrenia. *Hosp Community Psychiatry* 40(11):1141–1145, 1989.

30. Honigfield G, Gillis R: NOSIE-30, a treatment-sensitive ward behavior scale. *Psychol Rep* 19:180–182, 1966.

31. Hsu Y, Nelson D: Adult performance on the Southern California Kinesthetic and Tactile Perceptual Tests. *Am J Occup Ther* 35:788–791, 1981.

32. Huddleston C: Differentiation between process and reactive schizophrenia based on vestibular reactivity, grasp strength, and posture. *Am J Occup Ther* 32(7):438–444, 1978.

33. Jongbloed L, Collins J, Jones W: A sensorimotor integration test battery for CVA clients: Preliminary evidence of reliability and validity. *Occup Ther J Res* 6(3):131–150, 1986.

34. King LJ: A sensory integrative approach to schizophrenia. *Am J Occup Ther* 28(9):529–536, 1974.

35. King LJ: Information from author's notes taken dur-

ing a workshop given by Ms. King at Colorado State University, Ft. Collins, Colorado, May 19, 1974.

36. King LJ: *The Objects Manipulation Test.* Scottsdale, AZ, Greenroom Publications, 1977.

37. King LJ: Toward a science of adaptive responses. *Am J Occup Ther* 32(7):429–437, 1978.

38. King LJ: Occupational therapy and neuropsychiatry. *Occup Ther Mental Health* 3(1):1–12, 1983.

39. King LJ: Occupational therapy and neuropsychiatry. In Robertson S (Ed): *Mental Health Focus: Skills for Assessment and Treatment.* Rockville, MD, American Occupational Therapy Association, 1988, pp. 3.52, 3.59.

40. Knott M, Voss DE: *Proprioceptive Neuromuscular Facilitation.* Ed 2. New York, Harper and Row, 1968.

41. Levine I, O'Connor H, Stacey B: Sensory integration with chronic schizophrenics: A pilot study. *Can J Occup Ther* 44:17–21, 1977.

42. Levy D, Holzman P, Proctor L: Vestibular responses in schizophrenia. *Arch Gen Psychiatry* 35:972–981, 1978.

43. Lindquist J: Activity and vestibular function in chronic schizophrenia. *Occup Ther J Res* 1(1):56–78, 1981.

44. Llorens L : An evaluation procedure for children 6–10 years of age. *Am J Occup Ther* 21(2):64–67, 1967.

45. Mailloux Z: An overview of the Sensory Integration and Praxis Tests. *Am J Occup Ther* 44(7):589–594, 1990.

46. Miller E, Parachek J: *Parachek Geriatric Behavior Rating Scale: Revised and Expanded Treatment Manual.* Phoenix, AZ, Center for Neurodevelopmental Studies, Inc., 1989.

47. Parachek J, King LJ: *Parachek Geriatric Rating Scale and Treatment Manual.* Phoenix, AZ, Center for Neurodevelopmental Studies, Inc., 1986.

48. Petersen P, Goar D, Van Deusen J: Performance of female adults on the Southern California Figure-Ground Visual Perception test. *Am J Occup Ther* 37:525–530, 1985.

49. Petersen P, Wikoff R: The performance of adult males on the Southern California Figure-Ground Visual Perception test. *Am J Occup Ther* 37:554–560, 1983.

50. Rider B: Sensorimotor treatment of chronic schizophrenia. *Am J Occup Ther* 32(7):451–455, 1978.

51. Ross M: *Integrative Group Therapy: The Structured Five-Stage Approach.* Ed 2. Thorofare, NJ, SLACK Inc., 1991.

52. Ross M, Burdick D: *Sensory Integration: A Training Manual for Therapists and Teachers for Regressed, Psychiatric and Geriatric Patient Groups.* Thorofare, NJ, SLACK Inc., 1981.

53. Schroeder C, Block M, Trottier E, et al: *SBC Adult Psychiatric Sensory Integration Evaluation.* Ed. 3. Kailua, HI, Schroeder, 1983.

54. Sensory Integration International, 1988: Neurobiological Foundation for Sensory Integration. Document, seminar presented in September at Boston University, Boston, MA, 1988.

55. Smaga B, Ross M: Assessment: The Smaga and Ross Integrated Battery (SARIB) assessment. In Ross M: *Integrative Group Therapy: The Structured Five-Stage Approach.* Thorofare, NJ, SLACK Inc., 1991, pp. 107–142.

56. Stockmeyer S: An interpretation of the approach of Rood to the treatment of neuromuscular dysfunction. *Am J Physical Med* 46:900–956, 1967.

57. Stockmeyer S: A sensorimotor approach to treatment. In Pearson P, Williams C (Eds): *Physical Therapy Services in the Developmental Disabilities.* Springfield, IL, Charles C. Thomas, 1972.

58. Sullivan H: *The Conceptions of Modern Psychiatry.* Washington, DC, William Allen White Foundation, 1947.

59. Voss DE: Proprioceptive neuromuscular facilitation: The PNF method. In Pearson P, Williams C (Eds): *Physical Therapy Services in Developmental Disabilities.* Springfield, IL, Charles C. Thoms, 1972, pp. 223–281.

60. Voss DE, Ionta M, Myers B: *Proprioceptive Neuromuscular Facilitation: Patterns and Techniques.* Ed. 3. New York, Harper and Row, 1985.

Chapter 10

COGNITIVE DISABILITY FRAME OF REFERENCE

Focus Questions

1. According to Allen, what is wrong with a holistic or generalist position in occupational therapy?
2. What constitutes a cognitive disability?
3. How does Allen's definition of cognition compare to that used by other frames of reference in this text?
4. Compare and contrast Allen's six cognitive levels with the behaviors subsumed in Piaget's sensorimotor period.
5. Why are persons with a cognitive disability not expected to learn or improve as a result of occupational intervention?
6. What is the key role of the occupational therapist?
7. What behavior(s) might one expect from a patient presented a task beyond his or her cognitive ability?
8. How can a therapist manage patient behavior?

Introduction

In the first edition of this text, Claudia Allen's theoretical approach to date (1985) was discussed as one example of a developmental frame of reference. At that time, Allen's work was predicated on Piaget's sensorimotor period. In subsequent literature, Allen states that her work is no longer based on Piaget's principles, but rather on those of Soviet psychology.[3,4,6,23] More recently, she credits Piaget and information processing theory as influences.[5] This evolution suggests a varied commitment to a developmental framework and exemplifies a theoretical framework that evolves from practice and searches for a theory base. Because Allen's work has been increasingly cited and applied in occupational therapy, this chapter describes Allen's cognitive disabilities frame of reference.

Definition

The cognitive disabilities frame of reference assumes that the majority of psychiatric patients with functional as well as organic disorders have some degree of cognitive impairment. This impairment is debilitating, especially for those who have major affective disorders. The impairment is reflected as a change in task behavior, which results from changes in brain structure or function. The emphasis in this frame of reference is assessment of the reduction in task behavior. As an alternative to expecting improvement, the therapist's primary goals are to assess patient cognitive level, monitor task performance and make environmental recommendations compatible with functional level. Once the cognitive level is identified, the therapist selects activities at which the patient can succeed to maximize the patient's task performance. The therapist may also use assessment data to recommend community placement or suitable environmental adaptations. Unlike in other frameworks, activities are not expected to bring about change but are used to monitor the patient's response to medication as evidenced during task functioning.

Theoretical Development

Beginning with written material circulated but not published in the 1970s, Allen expressed dissatisfaction with the prevailing psychodynamic, behavioral, sociological and sensory-integrative models in use in mental health. Basing her conclusions on observations made with her own patients, she proposed an intervention model that would make better use of the activity focus basic to occupational therapy. The model would be primarily concerned with patients' cognitive skills, especially as these skills influenced the ability to learn.

Questioning the Generalist Approach

In this earliest material and in later publications the author is highly critical of a holistic or what she terms a "generalist" approach taken by occupational therapists who work in mental health care.[1,2]

"I have been frustrated by our generalist approach to identify the parameters of practice. The difficulty is that the generalist approach fails to establish an important problem. As a result, our professional discussions contain the implicit assumption that a therapist needs to read every book in the library and offer services to every person in the community . . . We need a better method of identifying our population."[2]

Compounding the problems of a generalist approach, Allen suggests that most psychiatric patients fit into one of these two categories: 1) They are unlikely to show improvement, or 2) if they do improve, it is not likely to be due to their involvement in activity. In Allen's early work, the patient population is specifically identified as either "schizophrenic" or "psychotic."

Sensorimotor Stage and Cognitive Impairment

Piaget's first developmental stage, known as the sensorimotor stage and typically used to describe the development of knowledge in infants age 0 to 2 years, is selected to describe adult patient problem-solving as used in task behavior. These patients, he concludes, have a cognitive impairment and are unable rather than unwilling to perform adequately in many of the tasks they face.

Cognitive Disability in a Medical Model

In 1982 and 1985 publications, the population of patients judged to have a potential performance deficit subsequent to cognitive impairment is expanded to include most of the psychiatric population. Allen supports the view that the cognitive and behavior changes of mental illness result from biological changes in the brain. Seeking to define cognitive impairment in a way that will be objective and verifiable, Allen identifies **cognitive disability** as a "restriction in voluntary motor action originating in the physical or chemical structures of the brain and producing observable limitations in routine task behavior."[2] A cognitive disability inhibits task performance, prevents goal achievement, and promotes idle behavior. These problems result in a poor adaptive response and limit independent function in the community.[1]

Organic Cause of Disability

In a 1985 publication, Allen uses professional data to conclude that roughly 80% of the patients treated by occupational therapists have "disorders with potential for a cognitive impairment," and by definition are attributable to an organic cause.[2] These disorders include developmental, mood, behavior, anxiety, organic mental, personality, substance use, and personality disorders and schizophrenia.

Criteria for Treatment

In developing her framework, Allen distinguishes between those illnesses with an **acute component** (e.g., manic depression and depressive psychosis), in which cognitive disability is more likely to resolve with the use of medication, and **chronically disabling disorders** (e.g., chronic schizophrenia), in which patients will need help in compensating for residual disability. Psychiatric patients with a cognitive disability are treated by occupational therapists using this frame of reference. Other mental health professionals treat those patients who do not have a cognitive disability.

Assessing Voluntary Motor Behavior

To objectify the extent of cognitive disability, Allen proposes using guided observation of the patient engaged in a specified motor task. (The Allen Cognitive Level Test has the patient imitate the therapist doing leather lacing; the Lower Cognitive Level Test asks the patient to imitate the therapist clapping hands. These tests are discussed in more detail in the section Assessment Instruments.) The patient's performance in one or more of these tests determines his or her level of cognitive function and in turn predicts the ability to do familiar activities and learn new ones. It also helps caretakers to anticipate the most suitable post-treatment placement for the patient.[3]

Cognitive ability and disability are specific to the ability to act on a sensory cue and make an effective motor response. Cognition is viewed, as much as possible, apart from verbal facility or the ability to think about what one thinks about and consequently is not used in the broader sense described in other chapters in this text.

Cognitive Hierarchy

Cognitive function is classified on a scale of six levels ranging from severe disability at the first level to normal ability at level six (Table 10.1). These levels are described as "an ordinal description of functional states as delineated by the sensorimotor association used to guide voluntary motor actions."[3] When the therapist observes the patient in task behavior and is determining where on the scale his or her performance would place the patient, the therapist pays attention to the attributes of motor behavior. These attributes are grouped as presented in Table 10.2.

Allen provides an overview of these levels by describing what is typically seen in the individual patient at each level.[3,6] We have summarized this in Table 10.3.

Movement Away from Piaget and Developmental Precepts

As previously indicated, in her earliest work Allen writes that Piaget's sensorimotor period is the basis for identifying her cognitive hierarchy. One can see important points of departure, however, as many of the behaviors described by Allen in case examples are adult behaviors not yet learned by the child, and as many of the affective postures of the cognitively disabled as noted by Allen are not the healthy, exuberant faces or postures of a normal child. Perhaps more fundamentally problematic, although not discussed in her work, is that the behaviors that span Allen's "sensorimotor" hierarchy (specifically the higher levels) are not consistent with Piaget's "sensorimotor" period, but rather are indicative of much higher developmental levels (Table 10.4).

In 1985, Allen elaborates about her dissat-

[handwritten in margin: Maturational Process]

isfaction with Piaget's and general developmental postulates regarding the manner in which cognitive skills are built. Citing and in apparent agreement with Mounoud, Allen states that the development of cognitive abilities is a "maturational process that depends only very indirectly on the interactions of the child with the environment . . . and that . . . it is strongly determined by genetic regulation."[2,20]

Allen says that she also wonders to what extent the rules of normal cognitive development can be applied to understanding cognitive disability and its remediation. The conclusion drawn is that the rules are not the same.

TABLE 10.1   OVERVIEW OF COGNITIVE LEVELS

Level 1	The patient is conscious but responding to internal stimuli. He or she does not experience self as separate from the environment. Behavior appears to be instinctive and/or habitual, and the patient can be engaged only to a minimum extent in his or her own care. Grooming, dressing, bathing and other nursing care must be provided, and the person is often restricted to bed. Level 1 functioning may be seen in patients having head trauma, stroke, and severe dementia.
Level 2	The patient is motivated to maintain a state of comfort, and at times becomes involved in bizarre posturing. He or she appears to have a primitive sense of self as separate within the environment. The patient may be able to assist the care-giver in some nursing tasks, but may also become suddenly distressed and resistive. The patient may follow others in walking to a destination, but may also engage in aimless pacing and wandering. Twenty-four hour nursing care is still required. Diagnoses often associated with Level 2 function include severe psychosis, head trauma, CVA, and dementia.
Level 3	The patient can respond to tactile cues with manual actions in order to produce an interesting result. Often he or she engages in repetitive, seemingly pointless or inappropriate actions. Long term repetitive training may enable a limited function of routine tasks. Patients may need much reminding in order to see a task to completion, and twenty-four hour supervision is suggested. Level 3 functioning is commonly seen in patients with dementia, acute mania, toxic psychosis, and acute schizophrenic episode.
Level 4	The patient relies on visual cues and tends to comply with the actions needed to achieve a short-term goal. Established daily routines can be followed, and attention to projects can be sustained for about an hour, but no new learning is involved. Reliance on visible cues allows for misinterpretation of reality, especially when visible cues are not obvious or are ambiguous. Training can be used successfully with this person if it is situation specific. Level 4 is commonly ascribed to patients with mild dementia, acute manic episodes, and chronic schizophrenia. It is important to note that patients at this level who have a well established routine may appear to cope well day-to-day, but they can not anticipate and adequately cope with unexpected events, thus requiring caregiver assistance.
Level 5	The patient can use overt trial and error and experimentation to problem solve. New learning is occuring, and inductive reasoning is being used. Because he or she has to see the results of his or her actions on the environment, problems may occur when the need to anticipate or plan is required for performance. Vital tasks such as dressing, eating, etc. are accomplished without difficulty but in such chores as those related to cooking, money management, shopping or traveling, problems with planning ahead may be evidenced. Level 5 may be "the usual level of function" for some (about "20% of a control population") and a "distressing disability for others (about 80%)" (Allen, 1987) Level 5 function has been given to persons with remitting affective disorders, personality disorders and "good prognosis schizophrenic disorders" (Allen, 1987, 188.)
Level 6	Level 6 describes the absence of disability. Symbolic cues guide motor action. The person can think of hypothetical situations or do mental trial and error. Future events can therefore be planned well in advance. Behavior is organized; verbal and written instructions can be followed and the therapist need not demonstrate. If a psychiatric illness had existed Level 6 would indicate full recompensation to normal ability.

TABLE 10.2   ATTRIBUTES OF MOTOR BEHAVIOR

Attention to Sensory Cues	The cues to which the patient attends (e.g. internal or visceral cues as opposed to touchable or visible ones) and the ability to ignore irrelevent stimuli.
Motor Actions	The extent to which motor behavior appears consciously planned and executed, and the extent of imitation.
Conscious Awareness	The motives that compel behavior, the sensations produced, and the kind of reasoning employed in problem-solving (e.g. inductive as opposed to deductive; covert versus trial and error), as well as the ability to attend to a task over time.

Is Skill Building a Reasonable Goal?

Staying with this line of reasoning, Allen proposes that skill-building is not a reasonable goal for adult patients who have a cognitive disability. As she writes, "Changes in cognitive level are observed in acute conditions. (These changes) do not seem to be explained by the patient's experiences in the occupational therapy clinic . . . (these) changes have

alternative explanations . . . such as the effectiveness of psychotropic drugs, the natural healing process, and the natural course of the disease . . . Although cognitive level changes in many acute conditions . . . it is remarkably stable in most chronic conditions."[2] The role of treatment by the occupational therapist is to assess cognitive level, observe for behavior changes that would suggest that medications are working to clear the condition, and identify and make available activities and environmental conditions in which the patient can succeed.

Task Analysis

In order for the therapist to provide those activities in which the patient can be expected to succeed, he or she must be able to analyze the cognitive demands of the activities in which the patient will be involved. Only then can activities be matched to the patient's cognitive level. According to Allen, task analysis also allows the establishment of criteria that can be used to demonstrate that one activity is the cognitive equivalent of another. In other words, if a patient is involved in putting together a tossed salad on one day, and doing a copper tooling the next day, the therapist

TABLE 10.3   COGNITIVE LEVELS

As delineated by the Sensorimotor Association used to guide Motor Action						
Attribute	**Level 1: Automatic Actions**	**Level 2: Postural Actions**	**Level 3: Manual Actions**	**Level 4: Goal-Directed Actions**	**Level 5: Exploratory Actions**	**Level 6: Planned Actions**
Attention to sensory cues	Subliminal cues	Proprioceptive cues	Tactile cues	Visible cues	Related cues	Symbolic cues
Motor Actions						
Spontaneous Limited	Automatic None	Postural Approximations	Manual Manipulations	Goal-directed Replications	Exploratory Novelty	Planned Unnecessary
Conscious awareness						
Purpose Experience	Arousal Indistinct	Comfort Moving	Interest Touching	Compliance Seeing	Self-control Inductive reasoning	Reflection Deductive reasoning
Process	Habitual or reflexive	Effect on body	Effect on environment	Several actions	Overt trial and error	Covert trial and error
Time	Seconds	Minutes	Half hours	Hours	Weeks	Past and future

Allen C *Occupational Therapy for Psychiatric Diseases: Measurement and Management of Cognitive Disabilities.* Boston, MA, Little Brown & Co., p. 34. Reprinted with permission.

Summary of Piaget's Periods of Cognitive Development

Period	Characteristics of Period
Sensorimotor (0-2 yrs)	
Stage 1 (0-1 month)	Reflex activity; can't differentiate self from other objects
Stage 2 (1-4 months)	Hand-mouth coordination; minimum differentiation self from others
Stage 3 (4-8 months)	Hand-eye coordination; repeats interesting events
Stage 4 (8-12 months)	Coordination of two simple motor schemes; Searches for hidden object (object permanence); Starting to deduce that events outside self make things happen
Stage 5 (12-18 months)	Further experimentation with objects
Stage 6 (18-24 months)	Can imagine absent objects; can imagine movements not seen (but language not necessary in this imagining; time frame is the 'now'
Preoperational (2-7 yrs)	Language-mediated problem solving; semi-logical problem solving; Thinking is inflexible; things are not as they appear and this is not questioned by the child
Concrete Operational (7-11 yrs)	Can solve problems regarding tangible objects and events. Applies logic to problem solving; uses physical trial and error; inductive reasoning
Formal Operational (12 years and older)	Can think about a problem and anticipate "what would happen if"; covert trial and error; deductive reasoning; reflection on past events and future plans

Symbolic thinking

Allen's Sensorimotor States of Cognitive Development

Attribute	Level 1: Automatic Actions	Level 2: Postural Actions	Level 3: Manual Actions	Level 4: Goal-directed Actions	Level 5: Exploratory Actions	Level 6: Planned Actions
Attention to sensory cues	Subliminal cues	Proprioceptive cues	Tactile cues	Visible cues	Related cues	Symbolic cues
Motor actions						
Spontaneous	Automatic	Postural	Manual	Goal-directed	Exploratory	Planned
Imitated	None	Approximations	Manipulations	Replications	Novelty	Unnecessary
Conscious awareness						
Purpose	Arousal	Comfort	Interest	Compliance	Self-control	Reflection
Experience	Indistinct	Moving	Touching	Seeing	Inductive reasoning	Deductive reasoning
Process	Habitual or reflexive	Effect on body	Effect on environment	Several actions	Over trial and error	Covert trial and error
Time	Seconds	Minutes	Half hours	Hours	Weeks	Past and future

TABLE 10.4. Comparing Piaget's and Allen's descriptions of the sensorimotor period of development (age 0-2 years).

Allen's sensorimotor states of cognitive development is reproduced from Allen C. (1985) *Occupational Therapy for Psychiatric Diseases: Measurement and Management of Cognitive Disabilities*, Boston, MA: Little, Brown and Co. The summary of Piaget's period of cognitive development is adapted from Wadsworth, B. *Piaget's Theory of Cognitive Development* NY; David McKay Company, Inc. 1971.

would have a means to judge if differences in that patient's performance on those two days was due to changes within the patient, or due to the inherent differences in the tasks at hand.

The same attributes that specify the cognitive levels for patients are used to describe task equivalence, although slightly regrouped in their presentation (Table 10.5). As with cognitive performance level, the **task analysis** addresses 1) the sensory cues used in the activity and 2) the nature of the motor actions, including the number of steps involved, the extent and type of tool used and the nature and relative use of verbal and demonstrated instruction. Allen also suggests that the therapist con-

sider patient preferences and the role of past experiences in the patient's performance on said tasks, but this is not currently specifically included in the task analysis.

New Theoretical Directions

In the late 1980s, Allen further disavowed Piaget:

The search for measurable treatment objectives turned up Piaget's sensori-motor period which was modified for clinical purposes... Unhappily, an extensive critical analysis of Piaget's work suggested that Pia-

TABLE 10.5   TASK ANALYSIS

	As delineated by the Sensorimotor Association, Required for Motor Action					
Attributes	Level 1: Automatic Actions	Level 2: Postural Actions	Level 3: Manual Actions	Level 4: Goal-Directed Actions	Level 5: Exploratory Actions	Level 6: Planned Actions
Matter						
Sensory cue	Threshold of consciousness	Proprioceptive cues	Tactile cues	Visible cues	Related cues	Symbolic cues
Perceptibility	Penetrates subliminal state	Own body furniture and clothing	Exterior surfaces	Color and shape	Space and depth	Intangible
Setting	Internal	Range of motion	Arms reach	Visual field	Task environment	Potential task environment
Sample	Alerting stimuli	Demonstrated action	Material object	Exact match	Tangible possibilities	Hypothetical ideas
Behavior						
Motor actions Number	Automatic One action	Postural One action	Manual One action	Goal-directed One step at a time	Exploratory Several steps at a time	Planned Infinite
Tool use	Stimulated use of body parts	Spontaneous use of body parts	Change use of found objects	Hand tools used as a means to an end	Hand tools used to vary means and end	Tool making Power tools
Other people	Shouting Touching	Moving	Manipulating objects	Sharing goals	Sharing explorations	Sharing plans and recognizing autonomous plans
Direction	Verbs	Pronouns	Names of material objects	Adjectives	Prepositions	Conjunctions
Verbal	Introjections	Names of body parts		Adverbs	Explanations	Conjectures
Demonstrated	Physical contact	Gross motor and guided movements	Action on an object	Each step in a series	Each step and precautions for potential errors	Not required

Allen C. *Occupational Therapy for Psychiatric Diseases: Measurement and Management of Cognitive Disabilities.* Boston, Little, Brown and Company, p.82. Reproduced with permission.

get was cooking his own theoretical soup in the form of equilibrium, adaptation, assimilation and accommodation. The results of the critical analysis left measurable treatment objectives twisting in the wind ... A decade of analyzing Western philosophy, as well as behavioral and social science literature was not particularly productive. Finally, an examination of the concept of activity developed in Soviet psychology supported a theoretical base that seems plausible.[4]

Allen underscores, however, that a "strict adherence" to her references is "not essential nor even beneficial," because the "detection of tautologies and the special needs of occupational therapy's patient population justify departures from the original sources."[3]

Activity Analysis in a New Light

While modifying her theoretical base and continuing to refer to the sensorimotor nature of cognitive skills used for voluntary behavior, and while retaining the task analysis presented in Table 10.5, Allen adds a new hierarchy in describing activity. She bases her hierarchy on that of Soviet psychologist Leontyev and uses his definition of activity as the "units of life that orient people to the world of objects."[3,18,19] The "world of objects," says Allen, must be adjusted for and by disabled people.[3]

Three Levels of the Activity Hierarchy

The most recent activity hierarchy has three levels (Table 10.6). These levels become clearer if we look at how Allen proposes using the hierarchy in day-to-day treatment of the disabled. Allen tells the therapist to begin at the bottom of the hierarchy. The therapist should examine the activity and determine the sequence of steps, the level of coordination, the cognitive skills and the materials and tools the activity requires. Then, decide if the patient is capable of successfully accomplishing the activity.[3]

Activity Results

The therapist next asks questions pertaining to the middle of the hierarchy in order to objectively answer the query, "What result does this activity bring?" Allen advocates a focus on results because, as she says, these can be objectively described and thereby used to develop performance standards.[3] Using the work of another Soviet psychologist, Kotarbinski,[14] Allen identifies four types of activity results: 1) constructive, 2) destructive, 3) preventive, and 4) preservative. Table 10.7 provides brief descriptions of each of these activity results.

Allen views most arts and crafts activities, activities of daily living and prevocational tasks as typically having **constructive** or **destructive** results. If the therapist had standards of performance for these activities (if, for example, there were objective standards for specific craft projects), he or she could make recommendations about the patient's ability to function outside of the clinic. These recom-

TABLE 10.6   ACTIVITY HIERARCHY

Level 1	This includes the social/personal meaning of the activity to the patient. Understanding this level means having an understanding of the reasons the patient chooses to participate in this activity, and the special meaning it has for the person in the context of one's social values.
Level 2	The second level of the hierarchy refers to the outcome of the activity, or what is actually done plus the associated results. Allen calls this level "satisfactory results".[3]
Level 3	This level is referred to as that of "feasible operations." This includes information related to how, when, where, and under what conditions the activity is carried out.

TABLE 10.7   ACTIVITY RESULTS

Constructive	Adding a property to an object, as occurs with nailing, typing, glueing, painting, adding decorative features.
Destructive	Subtracting a property from an object, as with sanding, chipping, and filing.
Preventative	Actions aimed at avoiding injury to self or other, as in coming in from a windstorm to avoid being hit by flying debris.
Preservative	Actions aimed at maintaining the property of objects, as with activities done to maintain body temperature, protecting furniture with wax, etc.[3]

mendations, then, are based on the assumptions that the person's skills for craft completion are transferable and that the person can successfully use these skills in varied environments.

Activities that bring about **preservative** and **preventive** results relate more directly to patients' ability to protect themselves and their children from harm. Standards of performance in these activities would help establish whether patients could live independently in the community and care for their families.[3]

Desirable Activities

Finally, the therapist addresses the top of the hierarchy, desirability of proposed patient activities. **Desirable activities** are those that "provide a sense of belonging" and relate not only to personal choice but also to social and historical conditions.[3] According to Allen, cognitive disabilities often cut dramatically into the patient's social sphere, affecting both role choice and the scope of activities that can feasibly be accomplished. Those activities that are feasible may be reflected by the patient, family or social group. The therapist must then draw on a "tremendous amount of ingenuity to identify activities that are both desirable and feasible."[3]

Research

Research using a cognitive disabilities framework has been conducted with a depressed population,[12] patients with senile dementia,[11,24] adolescents,[13] a schizophrenic population,[2,22] chemical dependency,[21] and a broader psychiatric population.[7,10,15] Research continues to refine the descriptions of cognitive levels and the analysis of activities. It also evaluates the application of the model with populations in and outside of mental health settings.

Current Practice in Occupational Therapy

The Person and Behavior

Because Allen consistently applies the term *normal human function* when she refers to the activity of nondisabled persons, this term is used in this text. The focus in this frame of reference is not on normal human function; therefore, our discussion of this dimension can be developed only briefly.

Cognitive Function is Central

As conceptualized by Allen, the person is one in whom all activity appears clustered about cognitive function. Cognitive capacity as a brain-regulated process responds to chemical and structural brain changes and is not significantly affected by the person's interaction with the environment. The success and breadth of human function depends on the level of cognitive function and the compatibility of cognitive parameters within the environment. **Normal human function** is defined as the observable "process of engaging in purposeful motor actions within a context of material objects and people."[3] If this description of human function is contrasted with others, it becomes apparent that personality, feeling states, self-concept and social skills are not directly addressed. Normal cognitive function is quantitatively designated at a cognitive level six in Allen's cognitive hierarchy and is characterized as the ability to use symbols to think about, anticipate and plan action.

Motivation

In agreement with what she refers to as an "organismic world view," Allen proposes that people regulate their own behavior and will do the best they can, given their situation.[2] One's best or what a person is capable of is referred to as their **capacity** and includes their present abilities as well as their potential to develop new abilities.[4] Capacity is divided into two operational abilities: physical and cognitive ability.[4] Although social feelings and skills are not cited as a part of capacity, Allen acknowledges that the ability to carry out acceptable social roles is influenced by cognitive and physical capacity.

Normal human function produces results that affect material objects and people. These results are achieved within the context of the person's history and social group, and the person's ultimate satisfaction with what he or she has accomplished in activity may depend on the extent to which this activity fits with the social group's values. Seeing his or her own success can be expected to carry over as a positive motivator for continued task performance.

Dysfunction

Dysfunction is described as an "impairment in sensorimotor information processing"[4] that occurs within the brain. When other explanations are given for dysfunction (i.e., a patient's lack of motivation, the role of feelings), they are considered secondary, and by implication are the domain of concern of psychology, not occupational therapy.

Dysfunction assumes that a biological abnormality results in impairment, disability or handicap.[5] Dysfunctional behavior is represented within the cognitive hierarchal scale from level one through five. Persons with cognitive disability are regarded as limited in their ability to learn.

Role of the Therapist

Therapist as Assessor

In all of the frames of reference discussed in this book, the role of the therapist is, of course, to assess, plan treatment, and carry out treatment objectives. In the cognitive disabilities framework, however, the role of therapist as assessor is so central that we identify it as the dominant therapist mission. As articulated by Allen, the "ideal role of the therapist is to evaluate the disability with accuracy and precision in order to specify areas where change in capacity or community support can be realistically achieved."[3] The therapist is an observer-assessor throughout the patient's tenure, documenting changes in function and cognitive level when they occur.

Therapist as Expert

The therapist is the expert who knows the cognitive demands of activities as well as the patient's capabilities. Therefore, the therapist knows which activities are feasible for the patient. Although patients are not expected to know which activities are feasible, their input is elicited to identify activities that they enjoy.

Therapist as Environmental Manager

Using his or her expertise, the therapist selects or modifies tasks in the environment so to enhance patient success. Allen refers to this task as **environmental compensation** and writes, "Compensation is done by (the therapist) matching the complexity of the task to the patient's cognitive ability so that the patient has the opportunity to experience the successful manipulation of material objects."[2] Simplifying the task is in contrast to what she refers to as **biological compensation** (changing a person's biological make-up) and **psychological compensation** (teaching a skill).[2] As a behavior manager, the therapist maintains a treatment environment in which the patient will be safe, and the aim is to foster pleasant experiences.[2]

Therapist as Consultant

If it is determined that a life-long cognitive disability exists, the therapist helps identify the extent of community and caretaker support that is required. By reporting to social service or legal agencies regarding the patient's cognitive level, the therapist contributes to the process of establishing legal competency, if needed.

According to Allen, "The therapist can offer an opportunity for positive experience in the task environment; the patient decides whether or not to accept that opportunity."[2]

Function of Activities

Measurement

Activities consist of voluntary motor actions that can be analyzed according to their level of cognitive demand (Table 10.5). Activities provide a vehicle for patient observation so that sensorimotor function can be measured and cognitive change objectively demonstrated.

Success Experience

Therapeutic activities are activities within the limits of the patient's cognitive capacity. Although Allen asserts that any voluntary motor actions that a person wants to do "as long as they are legal" are within the scope of therapeutic activity, those activities described consistently in Allen's work are those commonly referred to as activities of daily living and crafts. In fact, Allen strongly recommends and supports the use of crafts with the cognitively disabled. Through the use and grading of craft activities, the therapist can control the required standards of performance, present varied problems for patients to solve, and facilitate concrete evidence that identifies patient function (ability to replicate a sample, repair an error, etc.).[5] Contrasting psychiatric patients with those who have physical limits, Allen writes, "Given a choice, people who do not have physical disabilities may prefer crafts . . ."

and she adds that she has been "struck by a consistent clinical pattern: at levels 3, 4, and 5 the most popular tasks are crafts."†

Environmental Compensation

As part of the task environment, a therapeutic activity is said to compensate for a patient's cognitive disability by using his or her remaining abilities in a way that enables the individual to achieve results that are personally satisfying and socially acceptable. In this way a therapeutic activity can be viewed like a piece of adaptive equipment.[2]

Activities that are appropriately matched to the patient's cognitive level may reduce anxiety and discomfort associated with the disease. For example, if a patient experiences hallucinations or disturbing thoughts, the focus on a task may help to interrupt and redirect disturbing stimuli.

Although admitting that references that credit occupational therapy for its ability to "keep the patients busy" can be slightly annoying, Allen purports that the statement is true because activity involvement helps the patient to wait it out until medications take effect.[2]

Theoretical Assumptions

The following theoretical assumptions are based on Allen's works:

1. Cognition is observable as a voluntary action that is regulated by sensorimotor associations in the brain.
2. A cognitive disability is caused by a biological defect.
3. Abnormalities of the brain characterize the majority of occupational therapy's patients.
4. The observed routine task behavior of dis-

---

†This should not suggest to the reader that a preference for crafts is endogenous to cognitive limitations. Such a preference, for example, may reflect Allen's own enthusiasm for craft activities. Additionally, we do not know what other choices that these patients have been offered.

abled persons is different from the behavior of nondisabled persons.

5. Persons with cognitive disability are limited in their ability to learn.

6. Involvement in activity does not change cognitive level.

7. Limitations in task behavior can be described hierarchically by cognitive levels that parallel Piaget's first, or sensorimotor, period of cognitive development.

8. The level of function of persons with cognitive disability improves only if psychotropic intervention or the course of the disease process brings about a change in brain function.

9. Skill building is not a tenable goal when working with a majority of occupational therapy's psychiatric population.

10. The task environment may have a positive or negative effect on a patient's ability to function.

11. Patients will do the best they can, given their situation.

12. Patients with cognitive disability attend to those aspects of the task environment that are within their range of ability.

13. Therapists can select and modify a task so that it is within the patient's cognitive ability through the application of task analysis, also referred to as environmental compensation.

14. Successful task completion and a pleasant task experience are primary positive outcomes of occupational therapy service.

15. Task choice is influenced by the diagnosis and the disability.

16. Steps in a task that require abilities beyond the patients cognitive level will be either ignored or refused.

17. An objective standard of performance for occupational therapy tasks would allow for an objective statement regarding the patient's ability to function outside the treatment facility.

18. For patients with a cognitive dysfunction, and therefore for the majority of occupational therapy psychiatric patients, measurement and management of cognitive disability are more tenable goals than improvement or change of cognitive level of function as outcomes of occupational therapy intervention.

19. A generalist approach is not constructive for occupational therapy as a profession.

20. The assessment of cognitive level can contribute to the decision-making process that determines legal competency.

Evaluation

Assessment is a here-and-now process of identifying a person's level of cognitive function, including assets and limitations.

Preliminary Assessment

According to Allen, assessment should begin with a review of the patient's medical chart to identify the reason for admission and to establish initial occupational therapy goals. The therapist needs to be knowledgeable about psychiatric diagnoses (their symptoms, treatment and probable course) so that he or she might contribute to establishing a diagnosis, if it is in question, and to recognize and document changes in the disease process.

Role of Diagnoses

Diagnoses also give information about the expected level of cognitive function, and Allen goes to some lengths in her 1985 text to correlate her cognitive levels with diagnostic categories, as described in the *Diagnostic and Statistical Manual of Mental Disorders (DSM III)*. It is not that any particular diagnosis presents at only one cognitive level, but Allen predicts a certain range of levels specific to the various diagnoses. For example, if a patient identified as having dementia begins to exhibit task function at a level 5, Allen proposes that the diagnosis is depression not dementia.[2]

Chart Review

Chart review acts as an initial screening tool in determining who is eligible for clinic attendance. Patients at level 1 would not attend the clinic, nor would patients who might behave unpredictably, present an elopement or suicide risk, are refusing, are in restraints, or are mute.[2] The therapist then uses one or both of two performance tests designed to give an initial estimate of cognitive function: the Allen Cognitive Level Test and the Lower Cognitive Level Test.

> Similarly, Allen challenges the belief that anorexia nervosa includes a component of thought disorder, as she counters, "I have not (with anorexia nervosa)... been able to detect a cognitive disability unless there was another diagnosis to explain it."[2] By implication, if an individual performs well on the motor tasks Allen uses, it is assumed that a thought disorder does not exist. In our experience, however, this is not always true. Persons diagnosed as paranoid schizophrenia, for example, typically display blatant thought disorder as related to their persecutory system, but often perform very well on voluntary motor tasks.

Interview

As in other frames of reference, Allen proposes using a semistructured interview to gain performance information in the areas outlined in Figure 10.1. If needed, the interview can be postponed until the patient can provide an accurate self-appraisal. Allen suggests that the therapist take notes during the interview and show the patient these notes if he or she requests.[2]

Assessment Instruments

Allen Cognitive Level Test. Developed by Allen and refined by Moore, this assessment is based on the complexity of the leather lacing stitch that a patient is able to imitate and incorporates judgments made by the therapist

---

> **Semistructured Interview Guide**
>
> Past history
> Recent living situation
> Current social support system
> Responsibility for self-care tasks
> Work and educational history
> Interests (past and present)
> Patient's perception of abilities
> Patient's perception of limitations
> Patient's goals

FIGURE 10.1.   Interview Guide

about the thought process that the patient uses when completing the task. The therapist prepares the leather strips to be used, demonstrates and describes how a given stitch is made, then asks the patient to complete two stitches. Given the performance, a level of 1 to 6 is applied.[2] She does not recommend using this test with patients at levels 1, 2, or 6.[5] The assessment kit and score sheets are available from various crafts stores.

Allen Cognitive Levels Test (Expanded). Allen's Cognitive Level Test described previously has been expanded, some instructions modified, and patients asked to complete three, rather than two, leather lacing stitches. The scoring for this assessment has been elaborated to provide subscores or points within each of the major cognitive levels to better indicate variations of performance within each level.[4,9] Research is in progress to clarify performance specifics.[5]

Lower Cognitive Level Test. In this assessment developed by Allen, the patient is asked to follow the therapist's lead and clap three times in specified rhythms. This tool is designed for use with low functioning individuals. This assessment is described in Allen's *Occupational Therapy for Psychiatric Diseases: Measurement and Management of Cognitive Disabilities.*

Routine Task Inventory. This inventory is described as an observation guide, although it is recommended that either patients or caregivers provide the information covered to avoid the lengthy time that would be needed to observe patient performance. Fourteen task areas are covered, and are said to be taken from an inventory developed by Lawton for assessing the elderly.[16,17] Task areas rated relate to bathing, dressing, grooming, walking, food preparation, housekeeping, finance, medication compliance and travel. The scoring guide provided places patient performance according to Allen's levels 1 through 6. This assessment is described in Allen's *Occupational Therapy for Psychiatric Diseases: Measurement and Management of Cognitive Disabilities.*

Routine Task Inventory (Expanded). The routine task inventory previously described is expanded to include therapeutic exercise, child care skills, a communication scale (written and verbal skill), and a work scale (including skills related to following a schedule, following instruction, and getting along with others).[9]

Work Performance Inventory. As described by Earhart,[8] this assessment was developed to improve communication with sheltered workshops, vocational counselors, and other non-occupational therapists. It describes the patient's work habits, work relationships and emotions as they affect work performance. It assigns a cognitive level from 1 through 6, and makes recommendations regarding the patient's needs in task selection and therapist supervision.

Treatment

Acute Care

The thrust of Allen's discussion is in relation to acute or short term care. She admonishes, "Descriptive studies of long-term cognitive disabilities are scarce and therapists are well-advised to have experience working in acute facilities before attempting this confusing and often demoralizing area of practice."[2] It should be noted that this does not mean that patients with chronic problems are not treated using this framework, but rather, that they are treated during the stage of acute exacerbation in their illness.

Treatment Goals

Treatment goals for acute care have been discussed throughout this chapter and are summarized as follows:

1. To assist with differential diagnosis;
2. To assist with the titration of medication;
3. To assist with discharge planning, including the determination of legal competency if needed;
4. To observe and monitor acute symptoms in the task environment.

Moreover, specific treatment goals are identified relative to each of the six cognitive levels identified by Allen and for many of the *DSMIII* diagnostic categories.

Behavior Management

The management of patient behavior and symptom suppression are identified as key treatment strategies. Because patients are assumed to do the best they can, given their cognitive ability, the way to manage behavior is to give patients tasks at which they can succeed. Meticulous attention is paid to the demands of the task and the task environment so that the patient will not be bombarded with cues or stimuli that he or she cannot handle or asked to perform beyond his or her cognitive capacity.

A task that is beyond the patient's capability will "often elicit more severe symptomatic behavior or a desire to stop working on a project."[2] Although the therapist might choose to observe symptomatic inappropriate behavior as a part of his or her evaluation, the purpose of treatment is to suppress symptoms and the therapist is instructed to "intervene to suppress symptoms as soon as possible."[2] According to Allen, a "catastrophic reaction" can occur "when patients recognize, to some degree, that they are unable to do a simple task and the personal disaster of a mental disorder becomes apparent."[2] By aiming to foster a pleasant experience and minimizing unpleasant experiences, the therapist can help the patient to avoid such emotional reactions as distress, fear, anger, confusion and apathy.[2]

Individual Case Example

The following case example provided by Allen illustrates the manner in which a patient management plan is thought through using this frame of reference.

Case Illustration
Depressive Episode

History

Mabel is a 66 year old woman who was admitted because of severe depression, which has been worsening for the last two years since the death of her husband. One year ago she retired, having worked successfully as a special education teacher for 30 years; nine months ago she was forced to admit her mother to a nursing home, about which she feels guilty. During the last two years she has lost 40 pounds, has had intermittent difficulty with sleeping at night, and has been progressively unable to manage at home. She has been seeing a psychiatrist as an outpatient; the psychiatrist has been treating her with antidepressants and chlorpromazine, but there is some question of her reliability in taking medication.

OT Interview

When seen, Mabel sat huddled in her chair in a wrinkled dress, hair half-combed, with slight perspiration, probably caused by her constant leg and hand movements. Her response to questions was minimal, with no identification of interest or goals. Mabel stated that she wanted out of "jail", but knew the name of the hospital. She made a vague effort to do the ACL but then stopped, listing a number of reasons: "I can't do anything anymore. I never will. You'd better try someone else. My eyes are too bad to see this. They'll never let me out of this place."

Questions

1. List the diagnostic symptoms of depression that are identified in the history and OT interview (DSM III criteria).
2. Cite examples of task behavior that you can anticipate.
3. After two weeks, the therapist notices that Mabel is showing some improvement; she has been smiling, and her personal appearance is better. Mabel completes the steps in level 4 tasks, but shows no initiative in varying her actions or in exploring the relationship between objects. Her task behavior is limited to 30 minutes. The physician must evaluate the effect of medication at this point.
   a. Write your observations of Mabel's performance; include observations and terminology useful to the physician.
   b. Write an interpretation of the observations.
   c. Write your plan.[2] The answers to these questions are also provided by Allen and reproduced with permission.

Case Example XI

1. DSM III criteria for depression in this case are weight loss, sleep disturbance, diminished ability, and loss of interest or pleasure.
2. Anticipate OT observations: loss of energy with slow movements; indecisiveness in making choices; and resistance to, or reluctance to attend OT activities.
3. a. Mabel's functional performance corresponds with the improvement in her personal appearance. She is able to sustain performance for about 30 minutes and shows interest in completing tasks selected by the therapist.
   b. Current level of function is typical of level 4. Level 5 behaviors were not observed. Her functional history indicates that her quality of performance should improve to at least a level 5 and probably a level 6.
   c. Plan. Continue to observe for higher level performance as her medication is titrated.[2]

The preceding is from pages 206 and 207 of Claudia Allen's *Occupational Therapy for Psychiatric Diseases: Measurement and Management of Cognitive Disabilities*, Boston, Little Brown and Company, 1985 and is reprinted with permission.

Therapeutic Group

Similar Cognitive Levels. Allen and her associates support seeing patients at similar cognitive levels in groups specific to cognitive function. As a general rule, patients at levels 1 and 2 will not be seen in the clinic environment, although the therapist may assess their cognitive function on the treatment ward. Allen suggests that patients in occupational therapy activity groups be at a level 3 or higher, and that they be predictable, nonviolent and cooperative.[2] Earhart,[8] however, describes a movement group for patients at level 2. Level 3 and 4 groups typically extend for an hour and use activities that have familiar tools and materials and obvious visual and tactile cues. Such groups may be devoted to basic crafts, activities of daily living, basic woodworking, basic sewing or grooming.

Higher Level Groups. Patients functioning at levels 4 through 6 are offered special interest groups, including a work group (using a limited number of vocational skills), a senior group for patients over age 55, and a medication group.

Patients at the two highest levels, 5 and 6,

are given an opportunity to learn new craft and sewing skills at an advanced level; however, patients at these higher levels are not those to whom this framework is primarily aimed. According to Allen, higher functioning patients are treated by other professionals, presumably psychologists and social workers.

Safety. Because the cognitively disabled are characteristically in need of supervision, the therapist must carefully monitor the treatment environment, including tools and supplies, to ensure patient safety. Allen provides specific recommendations regarding the use and storage of occupational therapy materials.[2] These recommendations are consistent with safety precautions as addressed in other frameworks.

Summary

Knowledge pertaining to the practice of occupational therapy is expanding dramatically. Specialization has been one consequence, and in a sense, the cognitive disabilities frame of reference represents one kind of specialization. The thrust of intervention in this frame of reference is toward the assessment of cognitive level, particularly of cognition that manifests in certain voluntary motor acts.

Activity Focus

Having identified activity as a focus, the therapist must ask the following: "Based on the patient's cognitive ability, at what activity can he or she succeed?" Occupational therapy intervention is not expected to influence the disease process; however, the identification of cognitive level can be used to document changes in patient function, help to promote success experiences for the patient, monitor effects of medical intervention on the disease process, and can assist in the selection of appropriate post-treatment placement.

Challenging Occupational Therapy Assumptions

The cognitive disabilities framework challenges many of the assumptions on which other frames of reference and occupational therapy have rested. Primary among these assumptions is that occupational therapy should serve patients who function at a full-spectrum of cognitive ability. Another assumption that is challenged is the belief that occupational therapy can or should expect to improve patient function. It disputes more specifically behavioral and holistic assumptions about the ability of a cognitively affected person to learn, as well as psychological and cognitive-behavioral theories that place importance on feedback and insight.

Cognitive disabilities as a framework shares with several models an adherence to the traditional medical model. The expectation is that diagnosis of specific psychiatric diseases is integral to the assessment and management of patients.

Chronic Cognitive Disability

The cognitive disabilities frame of reference identifies itself as especially suited for use in response to the problems of chronically cognitively disabled persons in the context of an acute care setting. In fact, occupational therapists without experience are advised to avoid the "confusing and often demoralizing" area of chronic care practice.[2]

Contributions and Limitations of the Cognitive Disability Frame of Reference

Contributions

The thrust of this frame of reference has been to gain quantifiable, objective data about patients' abilities to perform motor behavior in a controlled environment and, by implication, to function in their everyday environment. Cognitive disabilities proponents have embarked on the arduous task of implementing research that can be expected to provide an increasing amount of information about the role of cognitive limitations in behavior performance during task and craft activities.

Because the role of occupational therapy is limited to cognitive assessment of the specific type discussed, the therapist is guided in compiling concise data that he or she can share with colleagues. This approach complements the increased pressure in acute care to assess and place patients. This circumscribed role also helps keep the therapist from trying to be all things to all persons and thereby has a practical advantage. Similarly, data obtained through a relatively simple assessment process have become increasingly accepted as a means to identify appropriate placements and to decide competency issues. As a result, the therapist has something workable and specific to offer among a plethora of treatment services.

By creating an environment in which the patient can be expected to succeed, the therapist provides a humanizing and positive treatment experience that may build patients' confidence and acceptance of their own limitations.

Limitations

Some of the limitations of the cognitive disabilities frame of reference are self-imposed. Its advocates decry the involvement of occupational therapy in trying to treat too broad a range of problems. Increasingly in the literature, this framework is discussed in relation to patients placed on the continuum of sublevels comprising levels 3 and 4. Allen says quite clearly that because the majority of patients seen by occupational therapists aren't going to improve in her view, occupational therapist should get out of the business of trying to improve them. For individual therapists to limit their practice as suggested is, of course, their choice, but when Allen's exhortation is to the profession to limit itself, the issue becomes much more complex. With many patients currently seeking treatment who are not cognitively disabled by Allen's definition, and with other information demonstrating that even the

cognitively disabled can continue to learn, such a limitation of practice could be short-sighted. The issue is complicated, too, because proponents of this framework, using cognitive disability guidelines, have influenced public policy in some states regarding third-party reimbursement.

Allen's assertion that the cognitively disabled cannot be expected to improve as a consequence of occupational or social intervention challenges the position taken by adherents of other models of practice, most directly the organismic, sensory-integrative and behavioral models as discussed in this text. Future research may help to strengthen the arguments made by all of these treatment frameworks.

Although medication can help patients think clearly and can alleviate symptoms, it is not a magic cure, as evidenced in the many patients who continue to require care. The medical literature frequently expresses the view that chronic patients need to improve both their social and work-related skills. Such skill building is judged as important in helping to shorten the length of hospitalization, to avoid future hospitalization, and to build patient confidence.

Allen's assertion that the therapist can keep patients from having negative emotional reactions to task experiences seems presumptuous. Further, to assume that any of us can help but learn about our limitations, or that such information need always be catastrophic seems contradictory to much human experience.

This framework trusts that the response to craft activities can be generalized to home and community environments, but the literature rarely describes this relationship. Given that the person's response to a leather craft provides evaluation data that contribute to major decisions that affect a person's life (e.g., conservatorship), the link between patient responses in hospital and community environments needs to be carefully evaluated.

Even cognitively limited patients may function well and problem-solve at a higher level on occasion or in different environments.

Although Piaget's 2-year-old has never been capable of adult-level understanding, an adult now demonstrating a predominantly lower level of cognitive function may have integrated many adult experiences, memories and behaviors into his or her learning repertoire. No direction is given within this framework to help the therapist make positive use of instances of higher functioning or to respond to the cognitive dissonance that may result when these instances are ignored.

As noted earlier, theoretical postulates continue to evolve within this framework, and the door remains open to address these issues in the future. However, Allen's practice of using theoretical concepts loosely, as with those of Piaget, makes it difficult to identify a theory base and to compare it to other established theories. Although it may be tempting to take advantage of the practical benefits and relative ease with which this framework can be used with patients, the lack of rigor and consistency in the theory base could seriously weaken its position in the future.

References

1. Allen CK: Independence through activity: The practice of occupational therapy (psychiatry). *Am J Occup Ther* 36(11):731–739, 1982.
2. Allen CK: *Occupational Therapy for Psychiatric Diseases: Measurement and Management of Cognitive Disabilities.* Boston, Little, Brown and Company, 1985.
3. Allen CK: Activity: Occupational therapy's treatment method. *Am J Occup Ther* 41(9):563–575, 1987.
4. Allen CK: Cognitive disabilities. In Robertson S (Ed): *Mental Health Focus: Skills for Assessment and Treatment.* Rockville, MD, American Occupational Therapy Association, 1988, pp. 3.18–3.33.
5. Allen CK: New developments in cogntive dysfunction theory. Lecture series. Los Angeles, July 26, 1991.
6. Allen CK, Allen R: Cognitive disabilities: Measuring the social consequences of mental disorders. *J Clin Psychiatry* 48:185–190, 1987.
7. Averbuch S, Katz N: Assessment of perceptual cognitive performance: A comparison of psychiatric and brain injured adult patients. *Occup Ther Mental Health* 8:57–71, 1988.
8. Earhart C: Occupational therapy groups. In Allen CK: *Occupational Therapy for Psychiatric Diseases: Measurement and Management of Cognitive Disabilities.* Boston, Little, Brown and Company, 1985, pp. 235–264.
9. Earhart C, Allen C: *Cognitive Disabilities: Expanded Activity Analysis.* Pasadena, CA, Authors, 1988.
10. Heimann N, Allen CK, Yerxa E: The routine task inventory: A tool for describing the functional behavior of the cognitively disabled. *Occup Ther Pract* 1:67–74, 1989.
11. Heying L: Research with subjects having senile dementia. In Allen C: *Occupational Therapy for Psychiatric Diseases: Measurement and Management of Cognitive Disabilities.* Boston, Little, Brown and Company, 1985, pp. 339–365.
12. Katz N: Research on major depression. In Allen CK: *Occupational Therapy for Psychiatric Diseases: Measurement and Management of Cognitive Disabilities.* Boston, Little, Brown and Company, 1985, pp. 299–313.
13. Katz N, Josman N, Steinmetz N: Relationship between cognitive disability theory and the Model of Human Occupation in the assessment of psychiatric and non-psychiatric adolescents. *Occup Ther Mental Health* 8:31–43, 1988.
14. Kotarbinski A: *Praxiology: An Introduction to the Science of Efficient Action.* New York, Pergammon Press, 1965.
15. Landsmann L, Katz N: Concrete to formal thinking: Comparison of psychiatric outpatients and a normal control group. *Occup Ther Mental Health* 8:73–94, 1988.
16. Lawton MP: Assessment, integration and the environment of older people. *Gerontologist* 10:38–46, 1970.
17. Lawton MP: The functional assessment of elderly people. *J Am Geriatr Soc* 19:465–481, 1971.
18. Leontyev A: *Activity, Consciousness and Personality.* Englewood Cliffs, NJ, Prentice-Hall, 1978.
19. Leontyev A: *Problems in the Development of the Mind.* Moscow, USSR, Progress Publishers, 1981.
20. Mounoud P: Revolutionary periods in early development. In Bever T (Ed): *Regressions in Mental Development: Basic Phenomena and Theories.* Hillsdale, NJ, Lawrence Earlbaum Associates, 1982.
21. Partida A, Price M: Chemical dependency: Objective changes in function and treatment modalities. Paper presented to the American Occupational Therapy Association National Conference, Phoenix, AZ, 1988.
22. Skinner S, Denton P, Levy B: In press. A descriptive study of inpatient schizophrenics functioning in an occupational therapy open clinic and task group. Rockville, MD, American Occupational Therapy Foundation.
23. Vygotsky LS: *Thought and Language.* Cambridge, MA, M.I.T. Press, 1962.
24. Wilson D, Allen CK, McCormack G, Burton G: Cognitive disability and routine task behaviors in a community based population with senile dementia. *Occup Ther Pract* 1:58–66, 1989.

Chapter 11

Holistic Frame of Reference

Focus Questions

1. How does a holistic approach for treatment of organic disorder differ from other cognitive approaches described in this text?
2. What is the difference between organic and functional mental disorders?
3. Describe the holistic relationship of the functional systems of the brain.
4. Describe the holistic approach to cognitive assessment.
5. What are the cognitive elements assessed by the occupational therapist using a holistic framework?
6. Describe an individualized treatment approach for a person with organic brain disorder or cognitive disability.
7. What are the treatment strategies frequently used to improve cognitive performance?
8. Describe therapeutic responses to the affective changes that can occur with organic brain disorder.

Introduction

A group of students was asked to point to that part of their body that they felt most represented them, their essence so to speak. Three, perhaps the romantics in the group, pointed to their hearts. The rest pointed to their heads.

For most of us, our thinking and feeling self seems localized in our brain or head. The prospect of our losing control of the ability to accurately perceive and think about the environment is experienced as an assault on our integrity. By **thinking** we refer to the ability to select, analyze, and intentionally respond to objects and events in a meaningful way. Beyond this, we are able in our thinking to reflect about ourselves; we are able to experience our sense of "I." How frightening and overwhelm-

ing it could be to realize that this thinking function was being compromised, because with it goes the ability to make sense of events in the world.

Organic Mental Disorders

According to *DSM-R* the **organic mental disorders** are those in which thinking is compromised and behavioral abnormalities result from permanent or temporary cerebral dysfunction.[3] Implied is that there exists structural or biochemical changes within the matter of the brain. As summarized in one general psychiatric test, organic disorders are distinguished from **functional disorders** such as schizophrenia and affective illnesses in that "they have known biologic causes and pathophysiologic mechanisms, whereas the functional disorders do not."[10] As such, organic mental disorders are subgrouped according to etiology as **presenile and senile dementias**, **substance-induced disorders** (such as that of cocaine or alcohol abuse), and **physical disorders with etiology unknown** (as in delerium and organically induced hallucinations).

As medical sophistication increases, so does the amount of evidence suggesting that functional disorders are also related to structural abnormalities in the brain. Especially studied has been schizophrenia.[5,15,43,60,66,76]†

The clinical meaning of this information is not clear. Perhaps as King[41] suggests, a day may come when all mental illness will be considered organic in origin and the classifications now used considered obsolete.

Even with increased knowledge of brain chemistry and anatomy, however, dramatic changes in the treatment of either functional or structural illnesses have not occurred, and the complicated relationship of biology to social and psychological systems has been consistently reaffirmed. Put another way, there is continued support for a holistic or mind-body-environment approach to both structural (organic) and functional disorders.[4,16,21,32,42,61,65,73,74]

Treatment in Mental Health Settings

Traditionally in occupational therapy, the personality or psychological system has been emphasized in the treatment of functional disorders, most often in settings designated as a part of the mental health delivery system. Persons with identified brain abnormalities, such as those associated with stroke, Alzheimer's disease, trauma, or birth-related, are more often treated at centers specializing in physical or cognitive training, with relatively less emphasis given to the psychological system by the occupational therapist. The notable excep-

tions to this tradition have been in the application of Allen's cognitive disabilities framework and in the physiological focus of the movement-centered framework.

Individuals with organic mental disorders, either identified or as yet undiagnosed, are at times treated in mental health settings. As commonly used at these settings, the term "organicity" is used to describe a variety of brain related dysfunctions, and one may hear that an individual is "organic." This term is vague and misleading and even dehumanizing to many lay persons. The global use of the term "organic" may serve, for some, to mask their lack of specific information about brain dysfunction and may reflect discomfort in working with persons with brain impairment. Especially in the psychosocial treatment setting, the patient with an organic mental disorder may be an anomaly within the patient group. The staff may feel ill prepared, assuming that problems associated with brain disease are very different from functional disorders. Or, the staff may believe that brain abnormalities suggest a poor prognosis.

When the individual with brain impairment is admitted to a psychosocial setting, he or she may not be recognized initially as having central nervous system (CNS) damage. Because brain insult can result in significant behavior changes, loss of control, anxiety and other so-called psychiatric symptoms, the brain-injured person may be brought into traditional psychosocial treatment because his or her behavior appears primarily social or psychological in origin.

In some instances, persons having some brain impairment but with a good functioning ability (e.g., those with mild retardation, those in early stages of vascular change) or those with residual damage from traumatic head injury may be in treatment with functionally impaired patients learning to deal with behavioral or affective issues. For example, it is common for those with organic syndromes to have a need to control episodic anger or depression, to learn or relearn effective problem-solving strategies, to manage altered feelings

---

†For instance, many, though not all, persons diagnosed with schizophrenia have been found to have one or more of the following: ventricular enlargement, especially of the third and lateral ventricles, cortical atrophy, and cerebellar atrophy.[5,26,37,38,44,59]

about the self, or to improve the ability to interact socially.

Treatment in Physical Rehabilitation Setting

Therapists working in the areas of physical or cognitive rehabilitation with organically challenged persons do not always feel comfortable approaching psychological and social issues with these patients. This apprehension raises concern because an individual's response to organic changes and treatment intervention is expected to be influenced by psychological factors such as personality and favored style of relating, premorbid adjustment, current social and psychological stressors, and the extent of socio-environmental support.[10]

Holistic Approach

Whatever the treatment setting, the organically impaired individual presents multiple challenges. When brain abnormalities result from remediable exogenous factors, treatment staff will be mobilized to eliminate them. When a diagnosis of organic mental disorder has not been established, the occupational therapist may see behavioral signs indiciating that testing for organic etiology is needed. When brain assault is irreversible or progressive, or both, the occupational therapist tries to help the individual cope at the highest functional level, to exert as much control as possible over his or her own life, to maximize appropriate independence, and to maintain self-respect.

This chapter orients the reader to problems and treatment principles for managing brain impairment from an organismic or holistic premise. The assumptions in this framework are in rather direct contrast to the cognitive disabilities frame of reference articulated by Allen and discussed in Chapter 10, although both frameworks speak to treating a cognitively impaired population. Instead the material is in many instances quite compatible with the stance presented by movement-centered therapists (see Chapter 9), and the reader is encouraged to compare and contrast these three chapters carefully. The organismic frame of reference is implied in the writing of those occupational therapists who address the need to treat the whole person, a seminal and enduring theme throughout the history of occupational therapy. Although no single aspect of neurology or rehabilitation can be extensively developed, this overview discusses the framework with regard to neurological syndromes.

Definition

The term holism comes from the Greek root *holos* meaning whole or complete. In health care, holism has also been referred to as **organismic theory**, as used by neuropsychiatrist Kurt Goldstein.[27,28] Holism is closely related to other social and treatment frameworks such as system theory, Gestalt theory, and human ecology.

Holism identifies each person as a unique individual who behaves and must be understood as a unified whole. The mind, body and spirit can not be separated, but rather function together to achieve and maintain a state of constancy, organization and equilibrium. Health and balance are the most natural state of the organism, and there is an underlying belief in the ability for recompensation and the presence of an internal drive toward balance and self-healing.[28,61,73]

Holism stands as a counterpart to reductionistic models such as behaviorism, and many models used in neurobiology.[5] The organismic position articulated by Kurt Goldstein continues to be echoed in the more recent work of scholars, as for example in occupational therapy by Toglia and Abreu. It is interesting to recognize that the physician Adolph Meyers, a pioneer advocate of occupational therapy, is also identified as an early supporter of holism within the medical community.[30] Whereas Goldstein emphasizes the relationship of mind to body, later proponents have stressed the inclusion of the environment in the holistic unit.[53,75]

System theory, as its name implies, is a way to think about how a system works. The simplest system in technology is often depicted conceptually as a feedback loop, in which energy is depicted coming into the system as **input**, being processed as **throughput**, being displayed as **output**, and being integrated into the system as **feedback**. Biologist Ludwig von Bertalanffy[69] proposed a more encompassing system theory that pertained particularly to living systems, which he termed **general system theory**. As discussed by von Bertalanffy, all parts of a living system interact with all the other parts, and the only way to appreciate the richness of the entire system is to look at the whole and the relationship and interdependence of all its parts and subsystems.

Kurt Lewin worked with other men in post World War I Germany in a movement that came to be identified as the origination of **gestalt psychology**. Lewin's contribution, which was known collectively as **field theory,** was an attempt to explain both personality and social behavior. Its chief premise is that behavior is a function of the whole context or "field" that exists when a given behavior occurs. Lewin proposed that the individual and the environment could be depicted mathematically in terms of postive and negative forces (or **vectors**) moving the person toward or away from life events.

Human ecology or ecological theory is identified with Urie Bronfenbrenner,[12] but draws from the work of Kurt Lewin, George Mead, Wofgang Kohler and many other psychologists who preceded him. It was developed and is used in systematic study of the interaction between individuals and their multilevel environment. The levels include the most immediate personal setting of roles and social relationships that constitute the **microsystem**; the **mesosystem**, made up of the multiple environments in which the person interacts (e.g., home, school and work); the **exosystem**, the setting in which events occur that influence the person's life but in which he or she does not directly interact (e.g., government); and the **macrosystem**, the culture or subculture created by one's attitudes, beliefs and ideologies.

Theoretical Development

To understand the person with brain impairment holistically, the therapist is always aware that every part affects the whole organism. The holistic view has three principles that influence the evaluation and conceptualization of deficit and the strategies for compensation, remediation and optimum function. These principles are highlighted as follows:

1. "A part not functioning within the whole tends to be brought into harmonious function within the system."[73]

   In other words, the organism mobilizes to restore equilibrium. This characteristic is reflected in the use of compensation or **functional adaptation** by covert sensory-perceptual, motor and cognitive systems within the brain, as well as in the overt compensations demonstrated by the individual.[47] For example, an 86-year-old home-health patient being treated for a hip fracture also had moderate arteriosclerotic brain disease. When the occupational therapist asked about the patient's deceased husband the patient responded, "Now, what was his name? I was married to him for 50 years; you'd think I could remember his name!" The patient then laughed heartily. The laugh was repeated many times during the interview and appeared genuine. This woman compensated for her memory loss by laughing about it, allowing herself to manage her memory loss without a disruption of emotional equilibrium.

2. "If a portion in the whole is perceived by the organism as unfilled, the organism will tend to fill it."[73]

   On a sensory level, the individual attempts to fill a sensory vacuum. If, for example, there is sensory deprivation, hallucinations (a kind of sensory self-stimulation) may result. If an individual is blind, sensations coming in through the other sensory systems may be perceived as relatively louder or stronger. A frequent behavioral response to a memory deficit is confabulation. In

confabulation, an individual with memory gaps constructs a story to fill in the gaps. A young woman suffering from acute brain hypoxia was an inpatient at the treatment center. When asked what she had for breakfast that day she could not remember. But, after only a brief pause, she answered with animation, "Pancakes . . . and eggs . . . and bacon. My but it was delicious, I ate everything!" The occupational therapist, knowing oatmeal and fruit was breakfast fare, recognized her response as confabulation.

3. The organism has an innate need to give structure or meaning to chaos. For example, unable to find the correct word, a patient with visual agnosia (the inability to name objects viewed) frequently describes the object's purpose, properties or use. Unable to understand why misplaced articles at home are lost, the confused individual often becomes convinced that visitors in the home are stealing the misplaced items.

This chapter explores the previous principles of holism within the following relationships that influence brain dysfunction: 1) the holistic interaction of functional systems within the brain and brain stem, 2) the relationship between physiological change and personality, and 3) the holistic relationship between the person with brain impairment and the environment.

Holistic Relationship of Functional Systems in the Brain

Traditionally, the CNS has been investigated in terms of discrete units and functions. As most students remember, each portion of the human body is represented geographically on the brain's cortex and each functioning system such as vision, hearing, smell, taste, speech, fine movement, gross movement, vestibular-proprioceptive sense and all of the autonomic functions are represented in specialized areas and developed through specified pathways or patterns throughout the nervous system. Many of us have seen film demonstrations in which a portion of the living brain is electrically stimulated and the patient's right toe wiggles, or he exclaims, "I smell smoke!"

Specialized Brain Function

The 1960s and 1970s brought an increased understanding of the specialized function of each hemisphere in the brain.[20,22,23,46-48,56,57,63,64,71] The left hemisphere, usually dominant, is connected to the motor center of the right side of the body and is primarily devoted to analytical or logical thinking, especially in verbal or mathematical functions. The left hemisphere in most right-handed individuals is dominant for the learning of fine skilled motor movements and usually dominant for the development of language. The right hemisphere processes information more simultaneously than the left; it manages information holistically, and has a primary responsibility for spatial orientation.

Students are frequently taught about the split between sensory and motor function. Not only are separate sensory and motor centers identified within the brain, but texts also conceptualize afferent ascending sensory nerve tracts bringing information into the brain, with efferent descending motor pathways leading to the musculature.

Although such a reductionist approach to neurology simplifies and clarifies understanding of a complex system and aids in the differential diagnosis of brain lesions, too often an appreciation for the brain's functional sharing and ultimate plasticity is lost. As suggested by Goldstein, although certain symptoms are more directly related to damage within specific brain sites, the effect of brain disease must be viewed as a "dynamic process which occurs in the entire nervous system, even in the whole organism."[28]

Plasticity

Plasticity within the CNS refers to the ability of other portions of the brain to take over function when one part is damaged, and is especially striking in the cortex. In recent literature, the work of the late Aleksander Luria[46–48] is most consistently cited in support of the concept of CNS plasticity. Josephine Moore,[52] whose investigation of functional anatomy has significantly influenced occupational therapy theory and practice, also supports this concept of plasticity. These two investigators, the seminal work of Goldstein, and the very persuasive exposition of the holistic position by Miller in *Meaning and Purpose in the Intact Brain*[51] are reflected in this chapter.

As demonstrated by Luria[47] and reiterated by Moore,[52] at different stages of development, brain organization changes and the same task can be carried out by different neural constellations. Moore notes that old pathways, perhaps replaced by newer, cortical constellations, retain the latent ability to integrate a task. Fundamental to Luria's observations about brain function is the conceptualization of functional systems. He contends that no one structure within the CNS is responsible for a single function or behavior.[47] Rather, all behavior and thinking is made possible by the extensive interaction between a diversity of structures throughout the brain—structures that work together as a functional unit. Luria assails the premise that vision, hearing, tactile sense, or any other function is mediated by one zone or lobe. He further stresses that what we call higher cortical function or conscious thinking is mediated throughout the brain. When one cortical pathway is derailed, it is possible for another pathway in a nontraumatized area to carry the same information. Luria applies the term **functional adaptation** to this ability. This concept has significant implication for rehabilitation.

Moore explains how specific structures within the brain can assume a diversity of roles. She describes the development of **interneurons**, nerve cells confined within the CNS, pointing out that CNS interneurons are not exclusively sensory or motor; they do not carry pain, touch or motor information, per se. Rather, they carry coded messages that are modified and changed at every synapse.[52] Thus, one can speak of the polysensory capability of neurons, suggesting that when a specific informational tract is damaged, others have the potential to carry the same message.

Bilaterality

Although it is true that each hemisphere of the brain tends toward a unique approach to comprehension and function, a strong tendency exists for bilateral function within the nervous system. This tendency is especially evident when assessing those functions maintained at the subcortical level, such as body tone and balance.[52] Not only is the CNS structured to provide constant feedback and relatedness of both sides of the body to both brain hemispheres and all dimensions of the environment, but when one side of the brain is injured, the other hemisphere also becomes functionally impaired. According to Moore, the impaired hemisphere loses some of its ability to send information to the noninvolved side. The so-called good hemisphere suffers from sensory deprivation.[52] Again, one is reminded that the brain, as a holistic organ, must be affected as a whole to an assault on any part.

Because all brain structures and systems interrelate, a so-called focal problem affects the entire organism's ability to comprehend and adapt. This principle is evident when working with individuals with brain impairment. Even with localized insult, one encounters a group of functionally related symptoms or what Luria calls a **symptom complex**.[47]

To illustrate: A lesion in the left (dominant) parietal lobe produces some combination of the following symptoms: diminished ability to read and write, right-left disorientation, finger agnosia, difficulty with calculation, loss of pain appreciation (pain asymbolia), ideomotor apraxia, and various aphasic disorders.[67]

CNS Reorganization

Because the brain structures are interrelated and because discrete portions of the CNS are capable of carrying out a variety of functions, an assault to one part—whether a single cortical path or a larger portion of brain mass—causes the brain to reorganize in response in a compensatory effort to maintain its integrity. When the brain impairment is gradual and the brain has time to deal with the insult, a great deal of function may be carried out by intact tissue. This ability is repeatedly demonstrated in patients who exhibit minor symptomatology despite extensive neural damage from slow-growing tumors. When the brain assault is sudden, as from a car accident, the brain has not had the opportunity to compensate, and the results of the trauma are immediately evidenced. However, during the posttrauma period the intact portion of the brain can often reorganize to restore much function.

Nowhere is the brain's reorganizational ability more strikingly illustrated than in the follow-up of **hemispherectomy**, the surgical removal of one hemisphere of the brain. Glees[24] cites the longitudinal study of three individuals who underwent hemispherectomy; two had a right hemisphere removed, one had a left. All three had a rather remarkable recovery. They were able to walk, to read, write and maintain a relatively normal social life. Although one individual needed to work within a sheltered workshop setting, another was able to complete his university studies and hold down an administrative position. Glee's discussion highlights dramatically the potential for functional adaptation by the CNS. Although function may be less precise and performed more slowly than before the procedure, the remarkable plasticity of the human brain.

Current Practice in Occupational Therapy

Holistic Relationship of Physiology to Feelings and Behavior

The integral holism between brain and emotion is both obvious, yet not obvious. Clearly, the ability to feel emotion, or to conceptualize what it means when we are about to encounter an unexpected quiz, or when someone says, "Will you marry me?" depends on intergration within the CNS. How this integration happens, and where it occurs is not so clear.

Reticular Activating System

The ability of the **reticular activating system**, located at the core of the brain stem, just above the spinal cord and below the thalamus and hypothalamus, and having direct connection with the limbic system, cerebellum and cerebral cortex, to deflect or stimulate feelings of arousal and excitability has been frequently noted.[25,46–48,50,52,71] The reticular activating system, which consists of activating and inhibiting neural tracts, plays a significant role in screening out irrelevant stimuli, in inhibiting inappropriate response, and also in "charging up" the individual for action.

The Limbic System

The **limbic system**—the central part of limbic activity being in the hypothalamus—is believed to be the substrate for innate drives (e.g., eating, sexual desire, fear); memory; and emotional behavior.[67] As with the reticular activating system, the limbic system has complex interrelationships with other portions of the brain, including the cortex, thereby enabling the learned or volitional expressions of mood, drive and use of memory.

Compromise in any part of the reticular activating or limbic systems, themselves closely interrelated, may result in altered consciousness, altered moods, aggressive behavior, anxiety or lethargy, disorientation, inappropriate sexual response, confabulation and memory disorders.[25,67] It is generally suggested that focal lesions not affecting arousal or limbic centers are less likely, but not necessarily unable, to cause emotional and personality change.

Considering our discussion of functional systems, one might underscore the "not necessarily" since even a so-called focal lesion ultimately affects so much of the brain and has the potential to disrupt vocational and social behavior. Brain impairment often assaults brain tissue in diverse brain areas, and not necessarily in an easily interpretable way. Therefore, it seems useful to broaden the understanding of emotional response in brain disease.

Depression

When recognized by the individual, brain injury represents a significant loss. There is frequently loss of function and loss of control; the individual may look different; he or she may be infantilized by others. There is a disruption of cognitive processing, and with it, a lessening of self-esteem. Finally, there is frequently a loss of vocational and family roles. The reaction of grief, shock, and dismay by the individual is to be expected and may, in fact, need to be facilitated as part of assisting the individual to move toward a gradual acceptance of the loss. When brain assault is progressive, as with the presenile and senile dementias, the grief issue may need to be approached several times as more and more function is lost.[34]

The therapist should encourage the patient to express feelings, and provide accurate information about what can be hoped for in therapy. Therapists can communicate their knowledge about the brain's ability to compensate, but they need to be honest in stating that most frequently the premorbid state of function will not be achieved. Although the brain can compensate, usually efficiency is lost; problem-solving may take longer; motor function, if retrainable, may not be as precise; memory deficits tend to continue to be problematic. Creating false expectations will ultimately decrease trust and increase depression.

Depression is also influenced by other factors. As an individual adjusts to disability and tries to build compensatory patterns, he or she encounters frequent frustration. As one patient said, in disgust, "Things just don't work right!" Attempts at compensation are fatigu-

ing, and the individual may be exhausted after working 20 minutes. Especially when brain impairment is progressive, the patient has many concerns about the foreboding unknown. Patients wonder, "How will I take care of my family?" "Will I be institutionalized?" "Will my family love me, or pity me?" Depression may be reflected as self-deprecating comments, withdrawal from activity or others, passivity, loss of self-esteem and sad affect. Frequently, the loss of peer contact and social relationships is not evident until three to six months after the patient returns to the community.[58] The list of worries can become overwhelming. Suicidal ideation is quite common and is an important concern with patients with brain impairment.

Emotional Lability

Loss of emotional control is a second frequent adjunct to brain assault. When an individual moves quickly from laughter to tears without apparent cause or without control, the term **lability** of affect is often applied. Compromise to the normal regulation of arousal centers can play a significant role in this lability. When cortical control of arousal and limbic centers is damaged through assault in the frontal lobes, there may be an inability to suppress inappropriate response, a lack of goal directedness, apathy or euphoria, irritability and/or a lessening of moral constraints.[58,67,70]

Other influences must be considered, such as any general loss of cognitive function. When this occurs, there is less ability to accurately assess a problem or situation. There is often difficulty with organizing information, ascertaining the relative importance of data, and developing a planned response, which may be due to the lessened ability for abstract thinking, a common sequela in organic brain syndromes. As a result, behavioral responses may appear quite inappropriate.

Second, with a cognitive compromise there is frequently lessened ability to postpone immediate gratification and to be aware of and regard the feelings of others. In Freudian terms, one could say the individual loses some ego and superego function; in developmental terms, one might say he or she seems more child-like or has regressed. The person becomes more concerned with meeting personal desires and less concerned with social politeness. The result may be a more primitive emotionality (e.g., temper tantrums with frustration, raucous laughter or giggling with pleasure).

One must also consider the plethora of problems brought on by brain impairment. The emotionality may be an understandable reaction to the individual feeling overly taxed. The individual coping with brain insult may, by necessity, become very focused on personal struggles and withdraw. A loss of perspective results: victories and setbacks may loom much larger with the shrinking of one's personal sphere.

Motivational Problems

Apathy or lethargy may result from brain impairment. The individual appears to lack motivation or drive. If the arousal centers or medial frontal cortex are insulted, the difficulty may be a physiological problem with self-arousal. That is, once external stimulation is removed, the individual is unable to sustain attention. He or she may be inaccurately assessed as resistive, stubborn or depressed.[70] As with other personality components, apathy may be related to the individual's style of responding to stress before the brain insult. Further, the person may have learned to be helpless as a means to gain attention in treatment centers.[68]

Goldstein[28] cautions against assuming that the individual is just malingering. He proposes that patients sometimes avoid tasks to avoid failure, and thereby maintain emotional equilibrium. Goldstein also observes that the brain-compromised person is more sensitive to failure. He suggests that the variable nature of the patient's performance (successful on a given task on one day, unsuccessful the next)

relates in part to changes in the patient's level of self-confidence.

Just as with the patient with nonorganic impairment, the patient with a brain injury needs to recognize the reason for doing the tasks he or she is being asked to perform in therapy. To give patients endlessly repetitive, boring tasks implies that the patient's need to have variety and social contact is less that in than the so-called normal person.

The therapist's ability to communicate reasonable expectations, provide rest breaks, to break up therapy into manageable units, and to be personally available and supportive may influence the patient's success at using newly devised means to problem-solve. Success then fuels further investment of energy.

Suspiciousness

Depending on the nature and extent of CNS damage, suspiciousness, or its extreme, paranoia, may result from an individual's inaccurate assessment of the environment, disturbance in mood, or may be due to organically induced hallucinations. Diminution in sensory-perceptual processing also frequently results in suspiciousness. In a range of sensory-related dysfunctions termed **agnosias** (e.g.,tactile, visual, and auditory), the individual may have a severely restricted ability to recognize objects or faces, to distinguish or localize sounds, or to comprehend what is said to or about the person. When patients cannot trust their own senses to give accurate and meaningful information about the environment, they are tremendously vulnerable. This vulnerability can only be compounded when, as in expressive aphasias, there is interference with the ability to verbalize one's own needs. In such instances, suspiciousness may be viewed as an understandable exaggeration of the organism's attempt to protect itself. It may act as a mechanism by which the individual slows down a social process in order to gain extra time to understand it.

The therapist can take some simple measures to communicate through those senses that are intact, for instance, approaching the individual from a visual field from which he or she will not be surprised, or assisting the person to identify scrambled sensory data, communicating slowly, and allowing sufficient time for cognitive processing. These measures can help to increase the individual's confidence in his or her own ability to understand and be understood and ultimately to increase trust. In addition, anything the therapist can do to build the patients' sense of power and control over current circumstances may help patients manage their concern about what is going to be done to them and move the focus to what they can learn to do for themselves.

One element of paranoia may have a realistic component. Even when an individual's cognitive processing is slowed and some situations misjudged, there may remain an ability to respond, perhaps on a more primitive or intuitive level, to the feelings of those nearby. For example, individuals with brain injury may be aware that others are uncomfortable, or regard them as strange, as the following example demonstrates.

Marguerite was kept home-bound by her severe emphyzema. The visiting nurse suspected that she had moderate organic impairment, although this had not been formally tested. Nursing notes described her "unduly suspicious," citing Marguerite's comments that, "My neighbors don't like me" and, "They gossip about me." Following an initial visit by the occupational therapist, the OTR was in the hallway, where she was seen by a neighbor who invited her in for coffee. Sensing an opportunity to learn more about Marguerite's social environment, the therapist chatted briefly with the neighbor, who immediately barraged her with comments about Marguerite's unseemly behavior and her "lack of character." Marguerite's suspicion that neighbors didn't like her and took advantage of opportunities to talk about her was, in fact, accurate.

The therapist may have little influence over the reaction of neighbors, but is accountable for his or her own attitudes. Care and respect play as important a role with the person with brain impairment as with anyone, and one could argue, even a more important role. Although some communications depend on higher functioning to be perceived or processed, caring is communicable and receivable at the most basic level.

The Individual in the Personal Environment

The Function of Activity

All of us have an impact on our environment, and all of us are affected by it. Ultimately, the environment will either respond in a helpful or antagonistic way to our well-being.

Brain injury often brings with it a decreased ability to do everyday activities that at one time were easily accomplished. For the person with brain impairment, there may be a diminution in skills related to perceiving, selectively blocking, or processing environmental information. Those concerned with helping the patient to gain access to usable information may place considerble effort in simplifying or clarifying messages.

Activities may be used in concert with adaptations that make visual, tactile, or auditory data bolder. Tasks and the environment may be rearranged or modified to emphasize alternate, intact sensory systems or to make alternative problem-solving strategies viable.

Holistic Context

One factor that makes treating the individual with a compromised brain so challenging is that this person may be able to succeed at some high level task, yet have difficulties with other skills that might be considered simpler. To use activities successfully, the therapist needs to identify the relationship between skills and problem-solving and performance strategies that the individual uses.

Activities are also chosen to be compatible with the expressed needs and desires of the patient and to have the potential to build functional capabilities, independence, and quality of life at home, at work, or in an avocational setting. It is helpful for the patient to know how a therapeutic task relates to his or her function outside of the treatment setting. This information helps to provide a meaningful, holistic context for the activity. Although a brain compromise often changes the way information is used, in a holistic approach learning or relearning can continue to occur, and activities are a vehicle for this learning.

Role of the Occupational Therapist

The therapeutic relationship contributes to the emotional environment, and the quality of caring is of great importance to the healing process. The patient is encouraged to be as autonomous as possible and relate as an equal partner. Attention is given to his or her personal or qualitative report regarding therapy, and behavior is understood as the whole organism's attempt to cope with the disease and the environment and to restore balance.[17,28]

In addition to the occupational therapist's attitudes, the patient rebounds against the attitudes of family, work associates, and friends, all of whom contribute to the emotional environment. With the initial diagnosis of organic brain syndrome, family members often experience as much grief, confusion and even chaos as does the patient. Family members often feel overwhelmed by experiences that seem so removed from anything they have had to cope with previously. For example, they may be frightened by this family member who now behaves so unpredictably, or who seems to get angriest at them, the people who love him or her most. They can be distraught about how to care for the patient at home.

Therapist's Dual Role

The therapist often has a dual role in the relationship with the family. On the one hand, the therapist assesses the nature of family roles and the extent to which the family can be involved in caring for and supporting the patient. On the other hand and along with other health personnel, the therapist recognizes the family's need to control the situation. The therapist helps educate the family about the nature of the disease and its expected progress, provides the family with other information such as that related to symptom management and environmental considerations that support function, and validates the feelings they may be experiencing.

Theoretical Assumptions

In summary, to understand the person with brain impairment from a holistic perspective, the reader is guided by the following principles:

1. The person with brain impairment is best understood as a whole, integrated being, not as a set of discrete systems that function independently. Occupational therapists must understand that purposeful activity (e.g., baking a cake, creating a collage, hammering nails, using a computer, or enjoying a concert or a walk) cannot be localized to any portion of the brain.
2. An assault on any part of the person will result in a reorganization and effort to accommodate to that change, from the microscopic to the macroscopic level, as the person strives to restore equilibrium and achieve meaning.
3. The individual affects and is influenced by the environment. By withdrawing from situations that he or she cannot cope with, the patient tends to shrink his or her environment.
4. Behavior is understood within its context as subjectively experienced and as a part of larger systems.
5. The individual's qualitative (personal and subjective) report is as important as quantitative data.
6. The holistic therapist is concerned with quality of life and not just quantity of skills and experiences.
7. Caring on the part of the therapist influences the healing process.

8. Holistic treatment is concerned with the physical, emotional, and spiritual parts of the person and the person's environment.
9. The patient with brain impairment is considered still capable of learning.

Evaluation

Orienting to the Assessment Process

This text will not describe extensive sensory, motor, or cognitive neurological assessment; nor would such assessment typically be pursued by the occupational therapist in many general psychosocial settings. However, the therapist needs to be knowledgeable about the scope of evaluation that occurs in working with a person with brain injury and must be able to contribute to the continued assessment of functional changes.

In the broadest terms, the therapist may need to gather and interpret data and monitor change in relation to the following:

1. Sensory perception, analysis, and integration;
2. Motor function;
3. Higher cognitive function;
4. Problem-solving, especially as it relates to self-care, activities of daily living, work, and avocational interests;
5. Social facility;
6. Emotional and affective parameters.

The goal of gathering and evaluating information in these areas will be to:

1. Aid in differential diagnosis, when necessary;
2. Identify specific strengths and limitations;
3. Target areas that can best be remediated or where function can be improved;
4. Clarify the conditions under which success is most likely to occur;
5. Establish specific goals;
6. Aid in gauging progress.

Before addressing each area, we underscore that each system functions in relation to

a unified whole. What is especially important in this frame of reference is ascertaining the effectiveness of all systems in contributing to successful problem-solving and meaningful activity. Both the quality and quantity of the person's ability must be addressed; quality of function can be judged within the context of a functional unit.[2] Although the assessment areas are the same as those typically approached by occupational therapists in a diversity of treatment areas, the discussion in this text highlights functional problems especially common to brain injury.

Sensory Perception and Sensory Synthesis

Chapter 7 discusses perception in some detail; here we add to that information. **Perception** is the ability of the CNS to detect or discern sensation; the faculty to discriminate or know what that sensation is and to distinguish it from other sensation; and to retain in memory the impression of that sensation, and hypothesize about it long enough to respond to it purposefully. Once accurately perceived, the organism must then be able to simultaneously relate or integrate sensory data coming from a variety of sources and through a variety of sensory modes through a process frequently called **synthesis** or **integration**. Synthesis occurs at all levels of the brain: cortex, cerebellum, and brain stem. The organism must also be able to screen out or ignore irrelevant sensory information, an ability that is separate from perception and synthesis but complementary to them.

Owing much to the work of Luria, researchers and clinicians have become more aware of the important and integral role played by language in mainstreaming sensory data. By language or speech, one refers to the ability to think in words rather than images. Speech production is itself a motor act, but the comprehension of language and verbal reasoning do not require motorization.

When the individual receives sensory information, upon recognizing it he or she tends to categorize the data by assigning it a name or quality. Thus, an individual doesn't see random lines; he or she sees shapes or identifiable objects or feels textures that are rough or smooth or cool or wet. Because of the functional relationship of speech to all modes of perception, it often follows that when a sensory system is assaulted, speech may be impaired; or, when a speech center is adversely affected, sense perception or sense synthesis is disturbed. Because of the integration of vast amounts of sensory data, at both the conscious cortical level and at subcortical levels, the individual is able to know where he or she is in space, to develop a meaningful body scheme, and to derive meaning from the objects and events encountered in the environment.

Hierarchy of Complexity

The occupational therapy literature conceptualizes a developmental hierarchy of increasing complexity in perception and synthesis, as in the following example:[54,1-2]

Simple Visual Perception Tasks:

1. Focus the eyes on an object;
2. Recognize shapes, colors, objects.

Intermediate Visual Perception Task:

1. Distinguish a shape from within a field of distracting shapes (figure-ground perception);
2. Recognize that foreground objects are closer, and background is farther in a photograph (depth perception).

Complex Visual-Auditory Synthesis:

1. Derive meaning from a television program

With each sense modality, vision, touch, kinesthetic input from joints and muscles, vestibular input, smell, taste, and hearing, the individual learns, as he or she develops, first the simplest, then increasingly complex ability to perceive, analyze, synthesize and make mean-

ingful sensory data. When brain insult occurs, frequently, although not always, the more complex sensory perceptual and sensory synthesis skills demonstrate impairment. For example, stimuli received via one sense at a time may be interpretable, but the ability to understand multidimensional data may be interrupted; or, subtle differences or changes in sensation may not be perceived. However, because of the ability to substitute other intact sensory-perceptive constellations for those that cannot, the individual may not exhibit the dysfunction until his or her skills are pressed. Luria cites the following deficit. When there is a temporal lobe compromise and problem with phonemic hearing patients may be able to hear (sound registers in the CNS) but have difficulty synthesizing sound. They might be able to reproduce a rhythm only if it is slow enough to be counted; or, they may have difficulty comprehending speech when sounds are similar, but not when sounds are distinctly different.[46]

Organic brain syndromes do not equate to a linear developmental regression in skill. Further, not everything is unlearned or lost; rather, pockets of function remain, using higher and lower level skills and cognitive processing.[28]

Agnosia. The inability to comprehend sensory information due to CNS damage is termed **agnosia**. The agnosias most commonly tested and discussed in the literature are visual agnosias, tactile agnosias and auditory agnosias. Actually, all sense perceptions, including taste, smell, and kinesthesia may be disturbed. The agnosias are further categorized to best describe the exact nature of the perceptual problem (Appendix J).

To compensate for milder sensory dysfunction, the individual may do one or more of the following:

1. Restrict the sphere of attention.
2. Respond only to the obvious or unambiguous aspects of a sensory message.
3. Create barriers and isolate oneself to cut

down on the amount of auditory, visual or stimuli coming into the CNS.

4. Avoid touch or being touched.
5. Demonstrate a slowed, more deliberate response.
6. Demonstrate a quickened or more irritable response.

The therapist in the psychosocial setting may or may not perform an extensive sensory evaluation. Regardless, he or she needs to be aware of the presence of sensory-perceptive deficits. It is virtually impossible in the clinic setting to ascertain the existence of sensory-perceptual problems without including some dimension of motor function; that is, the patients must do something to indicate that they understand sensory messages. Therefore, sensory perception and synthesis are typically assessed, formally or informally, within an individual's sensorimotor performance. Tasks typically cited as representative of sensory function are listed in Appendix I, with options for formal assessment described later in the chapter. The performance of so-called sensory or motor tasks cannot be separated from the ability to concentrate, to process intellectually, or any number of other cognitive variables. The therapist needs to be aware of the holism of function.

Body Awareness Synthesis. An important dimension of sensorimotor and cognitive synthesis relates to the ability of the person to interpret sensory data to ascertain the body's position in space. Included is the ability to know where each body part is in relation to the others, to understand concepts of directionality (right-left and up-down) to synthesize information received from all environmental and body planes and in relation to gravity, and to coordinate activity in three dimensions. In this discussion we view spatial relationship and vestibular-kinesthetic synthesis as directly influenced by and influencing each other as well as body awareness.

Spatial Awareness. **Spatial relationship synthesis**, or **spatial awareness**, includes the ability to orient oneself in space, and to visualize what an object looks like from all angles; to know where sounds are coming from; and to know where body parts are in space. It is easily disturbed by visual and tactile agnosias, when the individual has impaired ability to localize and synthesize sensory data. Less obvious to the person unfamiliar with neurological problems is that a disturbance of spatial relationship results in a disturbance in understanding all directional and comparative relationships. For example, patients may be unable to tell time, or to place an object to the right of, or left of another. Or, they may be unable to understand the comparison, "Tom is lighter than Harry, but heavier than Marge." Further, mathematical computations involving multicolumn numbers (e.g., 192 + 468) cannot be conceptualized as representing "one hundred, nine tens and two ones."[47]

Vestibular-Kinesthetic Synthesis. **Vestibular-kinesthetic synthesis** refers to the ability to discriminate and evaluate data received about the pull of gravity and position in space, through the vestibular apparatus within the ears and from the kinesthetic receptors in joints, tendons and muscles. The work of Ayres, Moore, and King has contributed significantly to the knowledge of how vestibular-kinesthetic synthesis is achieved and maintains smooth body movement. Vestibular-kinesthetic synthesis relates directly to the ability to maintain balance, eyes open and closed, and the ability to orient and potentially right oneself in three-dimensional space.

Much vestibular-kinesthetic synthesis occurs in the CNS at the subcortical level, where information is assessed and corresponding muscle tone mediated without the necessity of the individual thinking about coordinated and balanced movement. When brain assault interferes with automatic, subcortical regulation of movement, tone, timing, and balance, the individual may try to compensate by thinking consciously about movement. The result is a loss of stability and fluidity in movement and a diminution of coordination or lessened movement so that the individual might eliminate or lessen the amount of sensory input that needs to be synthesized.

Interference with spatial synthesis and vestibular-kinesthetic pathways at any level of the CNS may result in one or more of the following:

1. Loss of smoothness and fluidity in motor function;
2. Loss of timing;
3. Loss of stability and balance;
4. Unilateral neglect or tendency toward neglect;
5. Lessened movement or rigidity, which ultimately affects gross and fine motor performance.

Motor Synthesis. Purposeful activity requires the ability to perceive and synthesize sensory data, use higher cortical function typically in a language-related process, to analyze the dimensions of a motor problem, plan action, and synthesize movement into a meaningful whole.

Disturbance of voluntary or purposeful movement at the CNS level is termed **apraxia**. Apraxias are further labeled to describe more exactly the specific nature of the deficit (Appendix J). Frequently, as with deficits in sensory perception, simpler or more familiar motor schemes may be intact, whereas more complex or unfamiliar schemes demonstrate the deficit. The deficit may be exhibited as a slowed or jerky response, or there may be a loss of ability to stop one movement pattern and go on to the next.

For example, a person asked to clap might be unable to stop clapping. The inability to interrupt a motor pattern is called **perseveration**. It is frequently seen when patients are asked to copy a visual pattern, and may appear as an obvious continuation of a visual pattern (Figure 11.1) or as scribbling, when an individual gets stuck on one portion of a given scheme (Figure 11.2) Perseveration is also often evidenced in speech, with a compromised individual unable to change topics. In contrast,

there may be an inability to sustain a motor action, termed **motor impersistence**.

When the intention for planned movement is intact, but the ability to mobilize in action is assailed, patients may verbalize their wishes but they are unable to execute them.

Although all portions of the CNS are involved in the smooth execution of intentional activity, the reticular activating system is considered especially significant in the ability to select from a large range of learned behavior patterns the appropriate motor response, while suppressing inappropriate responses.

The attempt to compensate or reorganize in adjustment to assaults on motor performance links lead to a constellation of the following:

1. Avoiding novelty;
2. Staying rigidly with familiar schemes, or in contrast using an unusual or circuitous means to accomplish a task;
3. Slowed response;
4. Tendency to focus on one part of a motor task, with resultant failure to respond to the whole;
5. Fatigue, due to the extra effort needed to synthesize movement.

The tasks typifying motor function are listed in Appendix I.

Speech Synthesis. The ability to think using private speech, to communicate through language, and to comprehend language is a complex function that is depends on the ability to attend to synthesized sensory data, organize thoughts through use of cognitive process, and use speech-motor pathways. Adult language involves five basic processes: 1) understanding spoken language, 2) verbal reasoning, 3) speech production, 4) decoding written language, and 5) writing.[67] An impairment in speech or language is called **aphasia**. Specific categories of aphasia are outlined in Appendix J.

Although damage to the left hemisphere in the right handed person is often found in individuals with aphasia, due to its complex representation throughout the brain, speech is derailed by insult in diverse brain areas. Therefore, even though the therapist is not primarily concerned with the evaluation of

speech, the occupational therapist must be aware of the potential impact of language difficulties on activity. In a response pattern similar to that seen with sensory and motor syn-

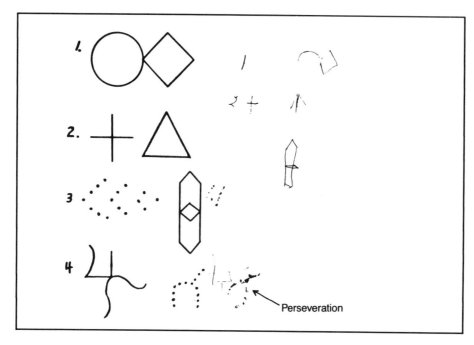

FIGURE 11.1 Perseveration due to organic brain syndrome.

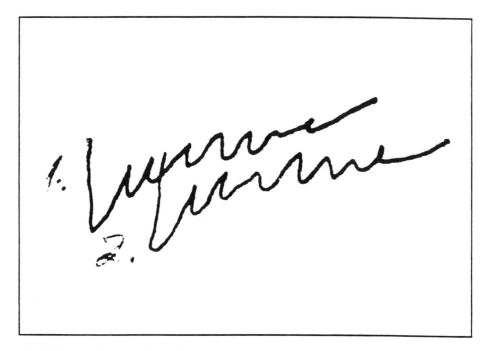

FIGURE 11.2 Perseveration of pattern done by man who twice attempted to write his name.

thesis, interference with language pathways may, in milder deficits, be exhibited as a slowing of language comprehension or language response. For instance, the individual may falter; be unable to find the right word without much deliberation; may need to have the speaker talk more slowly, use shorter phrases, or repeat; and may seem to have a limited vocabulary or may have increased pausing.

Functional Communication. The occupational therapist is concerned with not just speech per se, but the ability for what Kent-Udolf[39] calls **functional communication**. This is the ability to participate in casual everyday conversation and includes the ability to understand implied meaning and to enjoy humor.[39] Limitations in the ability for functional communication will seriously interrupt socialization and may result in social isolation by the patient, isolation typified by the patient's withdrawal, or the withdrawal of others who find social interaction with the patient to be awkward.

When language reception or communication is impaired, the individual may respond to open-ended conversation with irrelevance, confabulation or with very abbreviated replies.[39] It should be recognized that the patient's ability to comprehend speech is not necessarily best evaluated by asking complex or open-ended questions. Such questions require much more than verbal comprehension. It may be more useful, when language comprehension is a concern, to ask patients to follow simple commands or to ask questions that can be answered "yes" or "no" or with a nod.[67]

At its heart, the ability for language is the ability to think in words, not images. When this ability is impaired, the ability to read, write, and mathematically compute is also interrupted. Further, because the ability to use higher cognitive functions (to be addressed later) is generally judged by speech facility, when there is an impairment of language, the individual may be inaccurately perceived as having limited intelligence. The result may be

a further tendency by others to talk around the individual, as if he or she were not there.

When there is a language impairment, the occupational therapist may wish to consult with a speech or language specialist to help ascertain the strategies that could help the patient better communicate. Without effective communication, the individual is in an intolerable position of frustration and isolation. Communication deficits may also present safety barriers. Patients who are unable to call for help can solicit assistance by blowing a whistle or ringing a bell to alert a caretaker of the need for assistance.

In summary, speech and language impairment may result from or lead to deficits in sensory synthesis, motor performance or cognition. It can easily impede social process and the ability for meaningful activity. Attempts to compensate and reorganize may be demonstrated in the individual as follows:

1. Restricted use of language, limited vocabulary;
2. Requests to others to speak more slowly or repeat;
3. Responding to only one part of verbal request;
4. Avoidance of reading, writing, and calculation;
5. Social withdrawal;
6. Slowness to respond to a verbal request.

Cognition

The most complex cortical function is cognition. Cognition includes the ability to assimilate and assess sensory data, retain information over time in memory, and to consciously manipulate it in problem-solving. Higher cognitive function is made possible by the extensive association of multifaceted information at the brain's cortex. Such function is also predicated on vast subcortical activity charged with handling background stimuli, keeping irrelevant detail from awareness, and maintaining a normalized, nonconscious homeostasis that frees conscious, cortical function from a devotion to survival concerns. As discussed in Chapter 7, the higher cognitive processes are frequently perceived as those that enable the individual to proceed past the concrete or tangible aspect of stimuli and problems, to respond symbolically or ideationally, to imagine, to create, and to generate multiple alternative and hypothetical solutions to problems. This is referred to as the ability for **abstraction**.

The following traits are frequently cited in psychiatry as elements basic to cognition and differ in emphasis from the aspects of cognition discussed previously. They are summarized in this general format because many medical assessments are oriented this way. These labels are somewhat arbitrary, however, and always interrelate both theoretically and functionally.

Attention.   **Attention** refers to the ability of the CNS to focus on relevant stimuli or information while screening out or keeping from conscious awareness irrelevant information. Further, the CNS must be able to sustain attention over time. Attention occurs at both the cortical and sucortical levels. At the subcortical level, the CNS must be able to maintain necessary arousal or alertness while dampening any overarousal.

In practice, the ability to attend is often assessed by the individual's motor performance: Does the individual display an ability to focus on the salient features of a task, conversation or problem? Further, is the individual able to maintain attention to these salient features? Attentional difficulties might be described clinically as irritability, distractability, overarousal and hyperactivity or apathy, dullness, or underarousal. The therapist might discern significant differences in the ability of the individual to attend in various environmental settings (e.g., in a dyadic conversation, in a small group interaction, in a familiar setting, or in an unfamiliar setting) as well as differences in the ability to attend to varying kinds or intensities of sensory input and to input coming

from varying positions in the environment (e.g., from the patient's right or left side).

The patient attempting to compensate for his or her attentional difficulties may do the following:

1. Describe noises, lights, and other environmental stimuli as annoying or confusing;
2. Seek social isolation from the stressful environment and try to reduce stimulation;
3. Limit the task to which he or she attends;
4. Use strategies to help maintain attention (e.g., talk aloud, follow along with a finger as he or she reads);
5. Use self-stimulation.

When attentional dysfunction is excessive, patients may feel barraged with meaningless stimuli, and they understandably respond with anxious, confused, or non-goal-directed behavior. They may be so under-aroused that relevant information goes unnoticed. Or, the ability to sustain attention may be sporadic, yielding unpredictable, inconsistent cognitive and motor behavior.

Concentration.   Closely related to attention, **concentration** refers to the individual's ability to maintain attention for longer periods in order to keep thoughts directed toward completing a given task or bringing closure to a given cognitive scheme. Concentration also requires a homeostatic balance of sufficient arousal, while avoiding over-arousal. Individuals unable to concentrate refer to "losing my train of thought." Others may perceive these individuals as daydreaming, switching from one subject to another, rambling, or being unable to finish tasks once started. There may be a strong affective component to the ability for concentration as is demonstrated by our everyday difficulty with keeping our thoughts on a task when we are especially worried about or looking forward to a meaningful encounter. Concentration problems result in a lack of goal-directed behavior.

Orientation.   **Orientation** refers to a specific kind of personal attention, knowledge and memory—the knowledge one has about his or her relationship to the environment. Frequently referred to as orientation to *time, place,* and *person* (sometimes written as orientation x3), it includes the awareness of one's own name, roles, likes, dislikes; the names and roles of significant others; the awareness of one's own physical location; and the awareness of time or day. In an initial assessment, patients are frequently asked to give their name (orientation to person) and the name of the interviewer (orientation to person); to indicate their whereabouts in the treatment setting (orientation to place); and to state the day, time or month and year (orientation to time). Orientation is an ongoing reassessment of one's own relationship within the environment. Loss of orientation is most often evidenced by mild to extreme confusion.

It is quite common, however, for patients who have been hospitalized for any length of time to become somewhat disoriented, especially to date and time. This problem occurs because they no longer have the familiar guidepost of their jobs and home routines to orient them, or because they may not be aware of expected hospital behavior. One patient was asked by a physician whom he had met only once before, "Do you know what my trade, or job is?" The patient later recounted, "I thought he was a doctor, but I told him 'No, I don't know your trade' because I figured if he was a doctor, surely he wouldn't have to ask me what his job was!"

Knowledge. Incoming data become knowledge when it has meaning to the individual. Guidano and Liotti[29] speak of the acquisition of both preverbal (tacit) knowledge and verbal (explicit) knowledge. **Tacit knowledge** includes the incorporation of images, affect and instruction in early childhood and ultimately permits the internal representation of objects, events and persons. **Explicit knowledge** allows for the unconscious manipulation of ideas over time and includes the symbolic-representational knowledge that is language encoded (Chapter 7). Explicit knowledge is most frequently assessed when working with persons with brain impairment. When explicit knowledge becomes less available because of severe impairment, the patient's behavior often appears to reflect a reliance on tacit knowledge. That is, the individual responds nonverbally to familiar tastes, touch and smells, and behavior takes on a primitive quality.

The ability to acquire explicit knowledge may be understood developmentally, as discussed by Piaget and cited by Flavell.[18,19] Essentially, it is the ability to experience objects and events as separate from oneself, name objects and events and recognize their basic properties, categorize objects and events according to similarities and differences, infer cause and effect in the observance of action, seriate events, infer logical relationships in terms of concrete (observable events), read signs and symbols, and infer logical relationships in abstract or hypothetical events.

In clinical practice, knowledge has often been assessed in terms of fund of knowledge. For example, the individual is asked to name the current governor or discuss current events. This is viewed by some therapists as a restricted use of the term knowledge and a more functional understanding, as follows, is suggested.

One cannot separate the evaluation of knowledge and the assessment of memory. Permanent knowledge may be conceived as including three kinds of information: 1) sensory-perceptual, 2) procedural-motoric, and 3) propositional beliefs.[11] **Sensory-perceptual knowledge** includes knowledge of images and internal maps for finding one's way around. **Procedural-motoric knowledge** is knowledge of how to do things, including motor, speech, and intellectual function (e.g., knowing how to ride a bike, solve a math problem, or bake a cake). **Propositional beliefs** include beliefs about self and others, knowledge and concept of word meanings, knowledge of objects and events over time, and knowledge about values.[11]

The therapist assessing knowledge may find it useful to have patients demonstrate knowledge representative of learning in each of the preceding areas (see Appendix I). Persons with knowledge deficits may appear immature or unskilled if their behavior does not appear grounded in prior experience. They may be described as impulsive when their actions do not appear to anticipate probable outcomes. They may be described as intellectually deficient when their fund of common information appears limited or their command of language is compromised. Mild deficits in knowledge synthesis are often difficult to separate from misperception and memory deficits. Generally, knowledge insufficiency may be exhibited by the individual through the following:

1. Ineffective or inappropriate task and social behavior;
2. Withdrawal from former work-related tasks;
3. Avoidance of new tasks;
4. Rigidity in problem-solving;
5. Expressions of frustration over one's own inability to think or function;
6. Denial or confabulation or both to cover deficits;
7. Obvious inaccurate recitation or manipulation of data (including verbal, written, mathematical).

Memory. Memory is a complex, as yet only partially understood, function. It involves the ability of the CNS to take in information (**input**); code, categorize and store information (**maintenance**), as well as the ability of the individual to willfully retrieve or remember that information (**retrieval**). As discussed by Guidano and Liotti[29] and Flavell[18,19] memory is an exquisitely personalized process by which the individual actively selects data and interprets it or gives it meaning in the context of personal experience. **Memory** is not static maintenance but a process in which old information may be constantly reevaluated and remembered differently as new experiences are integrated. Think, for example, of the way you remember your first bicycle, or first date. First, you may have remembered the bicycle as huge. Later the bicycle may have been remembered as smaller and less significant. Your first date may also be remembered quite differently now than it was remembered 10 years ago.

Memory includes both the explicit holding of information as verbal knowledge, as well as the more primitive preverbal (tacit) experiencing of the infant.† Tacit or unconscious memory may be viewed as providing a contextual background without which explicit information cannot be sought and maintained in memory.

Mental health clinicians have frequently referred to and assessed three temporal divisions of memory: immediate recall, short-term memory and longterm memory. These divisions apply to the ability to recall newly given information, frequently as given by the practitioner in assessment:

- **Immediate recall**: The ability to recall information within one minute of its being received.
- **Short-term memory**: The ability to recall information within one minute to one hour after it is received.
- **Long-term memory**: The ability to recall information after one hour (including over weeks, months, years).

Short-term Memory and Long-term Memory. The recent cognitive literature speaks more often to two major divisions: the separation of short-term memory from long-term memory, conceptualizing the two as being stored differently.[7] **Long-term memory** is the repository of permanent knowledge and skills (sensory-perceptual, procedural motoric and propositional). **Short-term memory**, or working memory, is of limited capacity, as it constantly provides a context for current activity and manages new information.[11]

Think for a moment about what has happened in your experience over the last hour. Although events may be easily recalled at this moment, a year from now very little, perhaps none, of the information in this short time

---

†Jung's hypotheses regarding the integration of a collective unconscious have been postulated as the acquisition of tacit knowledge by the celluar matter of the individual before his or her birth.

span will be a part of long-term memory. Short-term memory is prone to deception by attentional difficulties or distraction. Consider, for example, of how quickly you forget to turn off the stove if something distracts you, or how quickly you forget the name of a newly introduced acquaintance if you are not really paying attention.

The ability for information to transfer from short-term to long-term memory appears related to its repetition or rehearsal during the short span and is also facilitated by the ability of the individual to make meaningful or personal associations between the new information and knowledge already contained in long-term memory.[11,47] Bower and Hilgard[11] refer the interested reader to Craik and Lockhart[14] for a more extensive discussion of the role of association in memory.

Theorists are starting to believe that the ability to draw on or retrieve memory is like opening a locked treasure chest, requiring just the right key or retrieval cue.[11] **Cues** are words, images, sounds, or perceptions that are associated with and elicit the memory. For example, the smell of baking bread may act as a cue for remembering days spent at Grandma's house; or the word "wrinkled" may be the cue to the memory of ironing.

The therapist assessing memory both formally and informally would assess effective memory as related to the following:

1. Short-term memory/long-term memory;
2. Meaningful (personal) memory/nonmeaningful (impersonal) memory;
3. Sensory-perceptual/procedural-motoric/propositional memory.

The therapist would also assess the role played by cueing, including the patient's own cueing as well as cues provided by the therapist, as well as noting the role played by attentional function or dysfunction in short-term memory.

It is quite common in persons with organic syndromes to see daily fluctuations in memory: In other words, the patient who appears quite clear one day or one hour may have less functional memory at another time. Memory is also influenced by affective components. For exmple, we all are often less able to remember when we are very anxious or depressed.

Individuals experiencing mild memory problems may describe themselves as forgetful (e.g., unable to remember appointments, anniversaries, or the names of acquaintances). They may find themselves in the midst of an errand, and forget what they had gone for; or in the midst of a conversation and lose tract of their thoughts. They may misplace household items put away for safekeeping.

Efforts to compensate for mild memory loss include:

1. Making lists;
2. Writing notes to oneself;
3. Asking others to remind oneself;
4. Confabulation;
5. Rambling or talking around an event not remembered;
6. Perseveration;
7. Avoiding tasks requiring good memory.

Severe memory loss is frightening, disorienting and immoblizing. The individual loses a sense of continuity over time and with events. He or she becomes incapable of deriving meaning from everyday events and from negotiating the tasks of daily living.

Insight and Judgment. Sometimes addressed separately, judgment and insight are here discussed as closely related. **Insight** refers to the ability to see into a situation and imagine what would happen if, or what has happened because. In applying **judgment**, the individual anticipates the likely consequences of one's actions, including the likely social acceptance, and plans behavior accordingly.

The person with insight is freed from the necessity of trying out a series of actions to ascertain their appropriateness or likely outcome. Rather, the person can hypothesize based on past learning. Further, when an event has occurred and the person looks at it in retrospect, he or she generates a reasonable hypothesis about why it happened. For example, individuals with insight can state why they are in the treatment setting; hypothesize why another patient is angry about missing the bus; or describe what will happen if they don't pay a parking ticket.

In the psychosocial setting, much of the ability to engage in meaningful process-oriented group interaction depends on the patient's ability to understand insightfully the actions and interactions of others.

Frequently, with mildly lessened insight the patient's behavior is described as indicative of **poor judgment**. This would be exemplified by mismanagement of finances, loss of social polish, failure to observe safety precautions (e.g., while driving, or when using tools), or lack of apparent concern regarding dress, hygiene or eating.

Judgment and insight can be assessed by asking questions about why events occur or what behavior would be considered appropriate in given situations (Appendix I). Judgment and insight, however, are most accurately assessed through the observation, over time, of an individual's task and social behavior.

Abstraction. **Abstract thinking** is the ability to derive meaning from an event or experience beyond the tangible aspects of the event itself. It involves being able to perceive the symbolic or conceptual nature of an object and event and to extrapolate the similar and unique features of objects and events beyond the concrete. For example, when one reads *Moby Dick*, he or she can understand that in addition to being a story about a man hunting a whale, it is a depiction of the struggle between good and evil. Abstraction includes the ability to decenter and imagine the feelings of others. It includes the ability for Piaget's formal operational thinking and complex, hypothetical problem-solving.[18]

Some individuals seem naturally more or less comfortable with and able to respond effectively in the abstract domain. The individual with limited ability for abstraction has spe-

cial difficulty imagining "what would happen if" in a hypothetical problem. The ability for insight becomes in a practical sense closely related to the ability for abstraction.

Mild Impairment. With milder impairment, the patient frequently may be able to describe one appropriate (and, most likely, familiar) strategy for solving a problem, but remains stimulus bound and cannot generate any alternative approach. The patient cannot discern the moral of the story when others speak and cannot, therefore, derive the most significant meaning in social events. The classic test in psychiatry for the ability to abstract has been in the interpretation of proverbs (e.g., What is meant by "people in glass houses shouldn't throw stones"?)

A reduction in the ability for abstract thinking frequently leads to behavior that is described by others as rigid, egocentric, opinionated, or missing the point. Because of its relatedness to insight and judgment, limited ability for abstraction is frequently associated with behavior described as inappropriate, narrow, thoughtless, or careless. Goldstein[28] asserts that many of the so-called personality changes associated with organic brain syndromes are due to the diminution of the ability for abstract thinking. To assess the ability to abstract, the therapist, using a functional assessment approach, observes the patient's ability to function in a diversity of problem solving tasks, and to appreciate subtlety, humor, hypothesis and implied meaning in social interactions.

Summary of Cognition. In summary, cognition is a complex, internally mediated process by which the individual attends to internal and external information, analyzes the meaning of objects and events, and retains and manipulates data toward the ultimate end of successful engagement with the environment. A breakdown in any step in cognitive function is detrimental to the entire thinking process. Compromise in cognitive function is a frequent result of brain assault and is often the most distressing residual dysfunction for individuals and their families. Although treatment strategies can assist in the regaining of cognitive ability or in building compensatory behaviors, most often the premorbid level of cognitive function will not be restored.

Problem-Solving and Functional Performance

As discussed in Chapter 7, the traditional approach in problem-solving has been for the therapist to identify the existence and efficacy of the following seven general steps: 1) identify that a problem exists, 2) analyze the problem and identify its salient features, 3) identify alternative solutions for solving the problem, 4) select one of the alternatives, 5) make a plan of action, 6) implement the plan, and 7) evaluate the outcome.

In assessing problem-solving, the therapist attempts to determine how all the threads of function come together in handling both the practical and more esoteric events of living. Keeping the sequence in mind, Bara's broad categories are useful in pinpointing specific kinds of problems that a patient can or cannot manage effectively. Bara[8] identified six classification of problems: 1) formal, 2) mundane, 3) physical, 4) interactive, 5) personal and 6) self-problems (Chapter 7). These categories should not be conceived as located in a specific area in the brain.

One cannot separate the assessment of problem-solving from the assessment of knowledge (e.g., the existence of knowledge needed to solve the problem), memory, sensation, motor ability, and other components of function. Indeed, for a person with limited function any daily task can present a difficult problem. Typically, however, in assessing problem-solving occupational therapists have selected problems that allow opportunity for the use of such higher cognitive processes as those involved in insight and hypothesis. The therapist is also interested in ascertaining the patient's ability for conjecture or the ability to act on more than one solution to a problem. Therefore, he or she frequently selects problems in assessment that have two or more reasonable means of resolution and then asks the patient to identify these alternative means. The

Analysis of Activity Complexity in Appendix I may be helpful in judging the relative complexity of a range of problem-solving tasks.

Assessing Affective States

As discussed previously, brain dysfunction frequently results in significant personality or emotional changes. These changes may be a result of brain trauma to specific arousal or control centers or a result of increased physiological and psychological stress.

With mild brain dysfunction, the personality may be described as similar to the premorbid personality, but personality traits or affective reactions may be more exaggerated. It is generally held that those defense mechanisms used before the organic breakdown will continue to be used, often to a more extreme but less functionally effective degree.[10] In some instances, the individual is described by others as having a marked personality change. With diminished sensorimotor function and lessened or slowed cognitive synthesis, a frequent constellation of two or more of the following affective reactions develops:

1. Increased frustration or lessened ability to deal with frustration;
2. Poor impulse control;
3. Dimunition or alteration in body image;
4. Affective change related to under-arousal or over-arousal;
5. Loss of self-esteem;
6. Anxiety or irritability;
7. Worry about the future;
8. Feelings of hopelessness;
9. Feelings of helplessness;
10. Feelings of depersonalization;
11. Depression or euphoria;
12. Suspiciousness and distrust.

The assessment will attempt to establish the relationship between premorbid personality variables with current affective states, as well as to note affective changes as influenced by task demands and the social and environmental setting.

Social Parameters

Impairment of brain function frequently jeopardizes the individual's ability to function successfully in a social context. This inability may be due to lessened social astuteness, loss of judgment, lessened affective and behavioral control, diminished ability to perceive and respond to verbal and nonverbal messages, and attentional or arousal difficulties. Additionally, there may be withdrawal by the individual who has a diminished self-esteem or social isolation by others who find his or her behavior discomforting.

The therapist will assess the individual's ability for appropriate social discourse in the dyadic relationship. Additionally, if possible, the patient should be observed in one or more group settings. The therapist may make observations about the following:

1. What skills facilitate the patient's interaction with others?
2. What behaviors interfere with successful interaction?
3. Does he or she approach others? In what manner?
4. Do others approach the patient? Isolate the patient?
5. Does he or she comprehend direct statements, questions or feedback?
6. Can the patient comprehend the group's theme? Concrete meaning? Implied or subtle meaning theme?
7. Does he or she seem to comprehend when others are speaking but not directing their conversation to him or her?
8. Does he or she maintain appropriate eye contact?
9. Is he or she able to share materials? Share space?
10. Is he or she able to cooperate in a task?
11. Does the patient's behavior suggest that he or she values self within the setting?
12. Does the patient's behavior suggest that he values others in the setting?
13. What role does the patient take in the setting? Is he or she able to appropriately assume more than one role?
14. In what kind of environment and social setting does the patient appear most successful?

Given these observations, the occupational therapist can use knowledge of group structure and group dynamics and select social, therapeutic experiences in which the patient can experience success or regain social skill and confidence.

Assessment Process

The occupational therapist working in the psychosocial setting may not have a formalized assessment battery for use with patients with organic brain syndromes because persons with organically induced deficits are not the primary population in many of these settings. Therapists need to be able to adapt the assessment with which they are familiar, whether they are standardized or idiosyncratic to the setting, or, they may wish to select from one or more of the testing procedures highlighted in this chapter.

Addressing Primary Concerns. When considering which approach to take in evaluation, the therapist should consider the ability of a given assessment or procedure to give the kind of information which is of most concern. For example, if primarily concerned about an individual's ability to functon independently at home, the therapist selects an assessment that provides information about the patient's ability to do practical tasks of daily living and to approach problems in an organized fashion. If the patient's referral describes a presenting problem with socialization, the therapist may use an evaluation that primarily addresses social skills and skill components. If more extensive sensory-perceptual, sensorimotor, or cognitive testing is needed, the therapist selects an assessment tool that provides baseline data to which later comparisons can be made.

Assessing Skills and Strategies. As discussed by Abreu and Toglia,[2] occupational therapists have traditionally used a skills-specific approach in assessing cognitive-perceptual processes, establishing a quantifiable score that may be useful in identifying the presence and extent of a given dysfunction, but not necessarily saying much about the ability to function. Their suggestions, proposed to facilitate the assessment of quality of function, include the following: 1) tests should not be terminated when the patient fails to accomplish tasks with standardized instruction, but rather adapted instruction, environmental changes or cues should be tried to determine what might facilitate or hinder performance; and 2) strategies or styles used by the patient should be evaluated to determine whether and when they are effective or ineffective.[2] These suggestions are consistent with Goldstein's earlier observation that patients with organic brain syndromes often succeed in a roundabout way, and that important information is learned when the assessor can analyze these indirect approaches. A broadly based assessment, designed to gain information about a patient's ability to function in a variety of task, social, and environmental situations would be consistent with a holistic framework.

Before beginning an assessment, the occupational therapist considers two factors: a person with brain impairment frequently has difficulty with maintaining attention for any extended time, and performance tends to be irregular, that is, good on a given task on one day, and poorer on another, without predictability. With these two factors in mind, the therapist usually gains more reliable information by extending the evaluation process over two or more brief evaluation sessions.

Preassessment Preparation. The therapist typically reviews available medical history, including any input from other professionals who have worked with the patient. This approach assists the therapist in selecting the evaluation procedures that are most likely to accommodate the patient's limitation and skills. Finally, it is consistent with Goldstein's suggestion that the therapist conduct an initial interview followed by less formal interaction.

Such an interview, in addition to helping to establish rapport, helps the therapist gain insight into the patient's style of communication, strengths and limitations, and ability to sustain attention. Fatigue and loss of attention are suggested by an increase in perseverative behaviors, signs of irritability, and signs of drowsiness. During the initial interview, the therapist may use some of the questions or topics of exploration suggested in Appendix I to elicit information specific to patient's cognitive abilities, including orientation, memory, general awareness of events, and ability for abstract as well as concrete thinking. From this interview, the therapist can also learn more about the patient's moods, attitude toward treatment, and concerns and expectations for self and others. With this information, therapists adapt the assessment to specific patient needs.

In general, no single evaluation battery can be expected to accommodate all patients, nor all types of difficulty. If the therapist does this preliminary preassessment groundwork, he or she may be able to avoid a plethora of initial testing, testing that can overwhelm a patient. If, in the course of treatment more specific information is needed, additional test batteries may be administered.

While a variety of assessment material is available in occupational therapy, no standardized occupational therapy assessment batteries specific to organic brain syndromes are currently available. If the therapist is concerned primarily with gaining baseline information about an individual's ability to function on given tasks, this may not present a problem; however, if the therapist is unclear about what is normal adult function, what is subnormal, and what is directly indicative of brain dysfunction, he or she may need to select a battery outside the usual occupational therapy domain.

Assessment Instruments

The following assessments are representative of those used in the preliminary evaluation of persons with brain impairment.

Bay Area Functional Performance Evaluation (BaFPE) (Revised). This evaluation is identified with behavioral and occupational behavioral treatment. Although it is not designed for the assessment of organic brain dysfunction, it does provide the opportunity to assess a broad range of functional performance, language, social and cognitive skills including the observation of the patient in five specific situations. The therapist must have knowledge about brain dysfunction to use the text diagnostically. The test manual and materials are available from Consulting Psychologists Press, Palo Alto, Calif.[72]

Magazine Method of Testing. This method is a nonthreatening, nontestlike task, which can be easily performed in a clinic or home setting. A magazine is opened to a two page advertisement with pictures. The individual is asked to read the text aloud, name the objects, and describe the purpose or message in the advertisement. The therapist can note the patient's ability to read (large and small print), to name objects, to attend to a full visual field, to visually scan, and to discern abstract as well as concrete meaning. It is not a standardized test and the therapist must be an astute observer.[33]

The Person Drawing. The person drawing may be conceived of as an assessment tool in itself, or, as a part of a larger assessment battery. The request for a person drawing is, for example, a part of the Schroeder-Block-Campbell, BaFPE and other evaluations described in this text.

King[40] supports the use of a person drawing as one means to detect dysfunction in the CNS, noting that the ability to depict a person in a visual symbol depends on the ability to abstract, successfully integrate body awareness and spatial orientation, and to integrate visual and motor planning. Loss of integration or loss of wholeness in the person drawing is a frequent adjunct to brain dysfunction and is different from simplification seen in normal children's drawings.[31] The interested reader is referred to Cohn's *The Person Symbol in Clinical Medicine*[13] for a thorough discussion of how brain impairment may manifest in figure drawings.

Flower-House-Self. The patient draws a person and copies a house and flower. Designed for use with an adult stroke population, this test looks for unilateral neglect, body visualization, and space concepts.[62]

Bender-Gestalt Test. This standardized assessment is based on the work of Lauretta Bender. The individual is shown and asked to duplicate nine geometric figures, given one at a time in the order of maturational difficulty. After completing the test, the person is asked to duplicate from memory those figures he or she can recall. This test has been used by occupational therapists as a screening tool for perceptual and motor function and by psychologists as a projective test. The assessment is also discussed in the literature as a screening tool for organic impairment.[35,36] It is available from the American Orthopsychiatric Association, New York, NY.

Schroeder-Block-Campbell Sensory-Integration Evaluation (SBC). The SBC is an evaluation designed to assess sensory integrative function in the adult psychiatric population and not specifically designed for assessment of brain dysfunction. However, it provides many opportunities for the therapist to test perceptual synthesis and body awareness synthesis (Chapter 9).

Benton Neuropsychological Assessment. This test is designed by Benton,[9] a neuropsychologist, includes a series of 12 separate neuropsychological tests designed specifically for screening for and specifying the nature of CNS deficit. The manual gives a description of each test and provides sample forms, administration and scoring procedures, and normative data for normal as well as dysfunctional adults. Of the 12 tests, some can be replicated from reading in the manual, whereas others require special materials available from the author. The 12 tests described are for the assessment of the following:

1. Temporal orientation;
2. Right-left orientation;
3. Serial-digit learning;
4. Facial recognition;
5. Judgment of line orientation;
6. Visual form discrimination;
7. Pantomime recognition;
8. Tactile form perception;
9. Finger localization;
10. Phoneme discrimination;
11. Three-dimensional block construction;
12. Motor impersistence.[9]

Although the primary author is a neuro-psychologist, the tests are very similar to those long used by occupational therapists. This assessment is recommended because of its clarity and because normative data are given for many groups, including normal children, older adults, normal adults and persons with brain injury. A similar type of test referenced by occupational therapists is the Luria-Nebraska Neuropsychological Battery, available from Western Psychological Services, Los Angeles, Calif.

Key Performance Variables

Regardless of the assessment chosen, the occupational therapist needs to assess the following important variables:

1. The ability to maintain attention and persist on a task;
2. The ability to maintain attention to the environment;
3. The method of responding to frustration;
4. The ability to manage distracting stimuli;
5. The ability to recognize error;
6. The ability to correct error;
7. The ability to recognize alternate means of problem-solving;
8. The predominant sensory, motor or cognitive approach taken during task performance;
9. The relative effectiveness of strategies used;
10. The influence of the environment in improving or diminishing patient performance;
11. The consistency of performance over time;
12. Changes in affect and emotional tone;
13. Comments made about self and one's performance;
14. The ability to ask for clarification or assistance as needed.

Assessment of the Environment

As part of the evaluation process, the therapist often gathers information about the patient's academic or work history, including the current educational and employment status, premorbid and current interests, the nature of family roles and interactions, and the nature and demands of the environment in which the patient will function. The patient may be able to give this information, or the therapist may need to gather some information from medical records, family members or other professionals.

Patient Dialogue. It is advantageous to gather this information from dialogue with the patient. It is not just the history, per se, but the patient's current attitudes and interests in activities and roles that is especially important. Through discussion the therapist and patient can often begin to understand the complex interplay of function and dysfunction in all areas of the individual's everyday world.

Activities of Daily Living. The therapist tries to ascertain the degree to which social activities have been maintained or curtailed. Frequently, persons with brain impairment, even when highly functional, regard themselves as different or handicapped and will tend to be isolated within the community. In some communities, the therapist may be aware of support groups created especially to meet the needs of persons with brain injury.

The therapist looks at activities of daily living in the broadest sense. Even when dressing, eating, and hygiene are easily accomplished, the individual may be restricted in other activities of special significance. For example, he or she may be restricted from strenuous physical activities and no longer able to participate in the sports previously enjoyed. Or, the person may not be allowed to drive an automobile or use other machinery. These restrictions may dramatically alter his or her life-style, academic and vocational plans, and sense of purpose.

In many instances, the therapist's assessment at the conclusion of treatment is used to aid in determining whether the individual can return home or will need partial or full care. The scope and focus of the assessment may need to be individualized to accommodate this issue.

Final Comments Regarding Assessment

Although the preceding discussion may suggest a high demand in the area of assessment, the occupational therapist need not let the assessment get in the way of knowing the patient. Learning about a patient is an ongoing, unfolding process, and as conceived within a holistic frame of reference, a process that goes beyond the formal assessment. As discussed by Goldstein, a wealth of information emerges when the therapist comes out from behind his or her tests to learn about the patient and the world as the patient experiences it over a period of time.[28]

Treatment

Establishing Treatment Goals

Having identified specific areas of function and dysfunction, treatment goals will be established with the individual. Lynch[49] suggests making a problem list, from which priorities can be established regarding the urgency of the problem for the patient and the feasibility of solving the problem within the treatment setting. This step is especially important because the list of problems may be long, and the duration of treatment short.

Abreu and Toglia[2] recommend an emphasis not on individual tasks but on the strategies that underlie task performance. For example, such strategies as planning ahead and check-

ing work can be emphasized in a variety of situations. In most treatment programs, there will be a mix of specific tasks and strategy building goals. When possible, the treatment goals will be established in the areas in which the individual desires to improve and toward the goals identified. Treatment success is measured in relation to changes in the individual's own function, not in relation to his or her ability to meet the norm.

Some patients may be able to make only global statements about treatment hopes (e.g., they may state they wish to "remember better" or "get around town more" or "learn some games to help pass time"). It is the therapist's responsibility to break down global goals or problems into manageable, accomplishable smaller units that will lead to goal attainment.

When working with persons with brain impairment, the therapist looks carefully at the complexity of sensory and motor skills involved, the manner in which information is organized and processed, and the influence of the environment on performance. When activities are to be accomplished stepwise, the individual needs to know how each step leads to the attainment of desired goals. When there is an impairment of cognitive function, this relationship of steps to the final outcome may not be obvious to the patient, and the therapist needs to make sure that the relationship is understood. Once goals are established, they will be communicated to family and other involved staff.

In addition to the pursuit of formalized treatment goals, the therapist often has the opportunity for more casual encounters that can help to increase the individual's awareness of everyday events and social expectations, and to increase his or her ease in social encounters. These are discussed further as reality orientation.

Individualization

No single technique or strategy or combination is best for all patients; a variety of treatment tasks may be individualized to meet an individual's specific strengths and limitations.

The literature describes strategies that are primarily reality-oriented, behavioral, cognitive, cognitive-behavioral, or sensory integrative. Using a classification proposed by Neistadt,[55] these treatment strategies could be grouped into two major categories: those that promote compensation and adaptation to the environment and those that are remedial and seek recovery or reorganization of the impaired CNS.

Though emerging from diverse treatment frameworks, strategies may overlap. Be aware, however, some principles basic to sensory integration are in contradiction to those primarily cognitive strategies. The reader will find also that many strategies involve the direct manipulation of the environment and activity; others speak to the therapist-patient interaction.

Treatment Strategies

Making Treatment Meaningful. As previously stated, the activity(s) selected for treatment need to have personal relevance for the patient so that he or she will sustain interest in the therapy process. An activity or task has meaning on a sensory level when sensory data are received and understood by the nervous system. The therapist must be certain that the sensory stimuli integral to an activity are clear enough, slow enough, and given through sensory avenues that the individual can integrate.

Relating Task Experience to Goal. On a task level, the individual must perceive how a given task is designed to lead to the goal of treatment. For example, if the patient wants to build skills that will enhance the ability to return to work, the therapist may begin with simple, repetitive tasks designed to increase sustained attention, or to rebuild familiar motor schemes. These initial tasks may be in the form of a game or as part of a craft. Or, the therapist may analyze the patient's job and break it into component parts, which can be relearned or practiced.

In the psychosocial setting, persons with brain impairment may perceive themselves and their problems as far different from those of other patients. This belief can lead them to perceive ward meetings and group activities as irrelevant. The therapist can assist by highlighting for the patient the parallel or common problems shared by many of the patients in the treatment environment. The therapist can also highlight for patients the manner in which hospital or clinic situations parallel the social or work or activities of daily living demands that will be encountered at home or in the community. When possible, it is useful to provide opportunities for the patient to return to the community and respond to real life situations rather than the simulated experiences of the clinic.

Simplification. In simplification, the requirements of a task, be it work, play, activities of daily living, or social, are reduced to a level at which the patient can succeed. Gradually, the complexity of the task is increased as each step or task is successfully accomplished. **Simplification** may be conceived of in two ways: Some activities are inherently more simple than others. For example, the therapist may select a simplified method for attaining a desired outcome (e.g., weaving on a hand-held or cardboard loom is simpler than weaving on a floor loom). Or, a therapist may be able to simplify a complex task, making it ultimately attainable, by breaking it into its component parts and reteaching one part at a time. To illustrate, a patient may indicate a desire to be able to play a card game. The occupational therapist might begin by seeing if the patient can recognize and sort the playing cards according to color. After sorting in this way, the patient can try to sort the cards according to suit. Or, the therapist may give a demonstration and request that the patient imitate and practice until sorting by suit is easily accomplished. During subsequent treatment sessions, activities are broken into integral parts and the patient practices each new skill until it is overlearned or performed without hesitation, even automatically.

As discussed previously, however, sometimes high level skills are retained, with lower level skills compromised. The success of the patient in actual task performance will depend in part on the patient's use of remaining, automatic, and newly developed performance strategies.

Retraining Through Repetition. This principle is taken from physical rehabilitation. The approach is relearning through practice. The therapist determines the patient's specific skill level and then sets small goals to keep just ahead of the patient. As described in reference to learning a card game, each step is practiced until it comes easily, before a new skill is attempted. The therapist should strive to add only one new behavior or skill at a time. For example, a patient learning to dress may practice putting his or her arms into the sleeves of a shirt until this maneuver was easily accomplished. Then, he or she would practice getting buttons properly aligned, and finally, approach the task of buttoning the shirt.

The principle behind such repetition is the recognition of the brain's ability to establish alternate pathways for function. Further, it has been demonstrated that repetition enhances the likelihood that short-term memory will be translated into long-term memory. Integral to the development of these new pathways is consistent feedback to the CNS regarding its own success. For example, the therapist will draw the patient's attention to the success of each attempt.

Although repetition and practice are essential in relearning, an important caveat must be given. When an activity becomes too repetitive, it begins to lose its meaning.[11,52] On a sensory level, the individual may begin to ignore sensory stimuli. This development is termed CNS **habituation**. On an attentional level, the individual may decrease attention. Consider your own reaction to repetitive music; you may habituate to it and stop hearing it. Or, consider your reaction to piano or typing drills; they become boring. The therapist may be able to assist by providing simple variation through interacting with the patient. Enthusiastic comments and a slight touch to the hand

can bring back the patient's attention. Drills, per se, are less consistent with a holistic approach.

Feedback. Patients attempting to relearn a skill need frequent and immediate reinforcement of success. When sensory-perception or synthesis or cognitive processing is impaired, patients may not be aware that they have succeeded without this reinforcement. For example, if an individual is sorting cards in preparation for a game of cards, very clear statements such as, "Good, you put the *red heart* (verbal emphasis) with the *red hearts,*" gives specific information regarding success and reaffirms to the reintegrating nervous system the accuracy of what it has perceived. Feedback also includes correction of error: "Oops! You put a *black heart* with the *red hearts.*"

Feedback is important both in validating patients' successes and in helping them to eventually monitor and correct their own errors. Because perseveration is common in patients with organic brain syndromes, a patient aware of his or her errors may still continue with an incorrect response. In this case, the therapist may interrupt the perseverative behavior or bring the patient's attention to alternative approaches. (See Brainstorming and Guided Search.)

Feedback is equally important in the social setting. An individual may have difficulty perceiving the theme or meaning of a group interaction. Therefore, the therapist may place the patient in a smaller, less demanding group setting, and pays close attention and encourages the individual's appropriate response in the group. This strategy may involve responding to the person's affect and not just his or her verbalization (e.g., "I see the smile on your face, Tom, and I can tell you enjoyed Mr. Barr's story as much as I did").

The therapist is engaged in a constant process of giving the patient feedback. She or he does this through verbal and nonverbal responses: praise, smiles, frowns, and by the enthusiasm communicated. The communication of genuine caring is important for all patients.

Amplification. Amplification is also called **highlighting**.[39] The therapist using this strategy helps an individual compensate for sensory losses, attentional, arousal or cognitive problems by making stimuli louder or bolder, and making the salient features of a problem more obvious. For example, a patient experiencing visual perception problems might be better able to attend to data with larger, thicker, lettering or outlining. The therapist can assist a patient with attentional difficulties by talking louder or by using more voice intonation. A patient with tactile perception problems may dress more easily by using larger buttons or zippers.

The individual may become more aware of the important aspects of a living or social problem if the therapist highlights its significant features. For example, an individual may not understand why another patient has responded abruptly or angrily, or why the neighbors regard his or her dress as odd. The therapist can assist by drawing attention to the key qualities of the person's behavior and the key features of appropriate behavior.

One additional way that a given message is made more obvious is by the elimination or dampening of distracting messages. It is often appropriate for a therapist to select an environment or create a place in the environment that is especially quiet or visually nonstimulating and that is without the usual traffic of patient and staff. This environment permits the individual to perceive the essential sensory messages in an activity.

Substitution. In **substitution,** one intact perceptual or motor system, or one intact behavior is substituted for another that is impaired. For example, an individual with visual agnosia may be able to enjoy the talking books available at libraries and on cassettes. An individual who can no longer wash and iron clothes may be taught to use the local cleaners. The successful use of substitution requires the therapist to be knowledgeable about the exact nature of a patient's deficient and intact processing systems. Substitution is also at the heart of many memory strategies wherein visual or auditory messages take the place of memory.

Modeling and Physical Guidance. Especially in reteaching functional motor skills, the therapist may use modeling and physical guidance. If teaching a patient to tie a simple macrame knot, for example, the therapist would give directions, model, and if necessary, physically guide the patient's hands through the scheme. Initially, patients may need hands-on guidance. Gradually, the therapist provides less and less guidance until the patient can complete the procedure independently.

As another illustration, an individual having difficulty with pathfinding around the treatment center might be guided by the therapist through a specific path many times, until it was familiar. No new or alternate paths would be shown until the first one was clearly established. The path might be made more obvious or highlighted by adding visual cues (e.g., red tape along corridors). Once established, the cues might be removed.

Brainstorming and Guided Search. Malec[50] suggests brainstorming and guided search as a means to generate more potential solutions in problem-solving. Frequently, patients with impaired brain function are stimulus-bound in problem-solving. That is, they cannot get beyond the obvious features of a problem, or they cannot generate more than one possible solution to a problem. One patient, for example, verbalized concern about what she would do if Meals on Wheels would forget to bring her meal. The only solution she could come up with was, "I'd call my daughter," but she then perseverated on the fact that her daughter is "never home."

Through brainstorming and with some prompting from the occupational therapist, she was able to develop two other possibilities: notify Meals on Wheels or ask a neighbor for assistance. These solutions were not as obvious to the patient as they might be to the reader and by being able to essentially draw from her own information and come up with these alternatives, she was able to re-establish a significant cognitive link.

Brainstorming involves three basic steps:

1. The individual is asked to generate as many solutions to a problem as possible. Any ideas, even the most ridiculous "off the top of the head" are encouraged. The therapist may have to pick up on words or gestures to bring the idea to fruition.
2. The therapist lists the ideas and reviews them with the patient. The most appropriate are either discussed or attempted.
3. A decision is made to select the most effective one or two solutions. These may then be practiced.[50]

A **guided search** may be used as a part of the brainstorming procedure. Through guided search, the patient is cued to help identify relevant information needed for problem-solving.[50] For example, a patient unsure of who to call to ask for help might be asked "Who are your friends?" or "Who lives next door?" An individual uncertain of the day of the week may be asked: "What activity did you do this morning? Bowling? Then it must be Monday because Monday is the day on which the group goes bowling."

Generalization. Whether trying to build work-related, leisure, activities of daily living, or social skills, it is essential that any skill learned in therapy be able to be applied into a wide variety of settings and contexts. The therapist conducting home care is in the best position to assure that this carry over occurs. However, he or she must be aware that his or her approval may be serving as a significant reward for behavior, and that once treatment is discontinued, other naturally occurring or intrinsic rewards must sustain the behavior.

The therapist working in a hospital or clinic setting would frequently profit from a home visit to become familiar with the key features of the home environment so that they may be approximated more closely in the therapy setting. This concern regarding generalization is especially important because with cognitive loss, the individual's ability to see the similarities in given situations frequently is impaired. One way that generalization can be facilitated is to practice a new skill in a variety of similar settings.

For example, a patient who has relearned to use a telephone may be initially taught on the clinic phone and then may practice with a pay phone or a touchtone phone. A patient regaining social confidence might begin with one primary social group, then be encouraged to try out his skills in different kinds of groups. Role playing and rehearsal in a therapeutic setting may also be used. The therapist could assist by pointing out the similar features and expectations across groups.

Reality Orientation. **Reality orientation** is a term applied to an ongoing process, used especially with confused patients. Although most often discussed in relation to nursing home care, it may be effective for use with any individual experiencing cognitive dysfunction. Confused individuals are continuously reminded of names, places, events and temporal relationships.[33] Upon greeting the individual the therapist says, "Hello, Mr. Barnes. I'm Mary and it's 10 o'clock, time for occupational therapy." During the therapy session, the patient might be reminded, "Let's look out the window . . . It's snowing very hard today. What a cold Tuesday we're having, Mr. Barnes." The occupational therapist speaks slowly and clearly and supplements speech with nonambiguous, nonverbal messages. To assist in establishing orientation, calenders and clocks will be conspicuous in the clinic. Where at all possible, the schedule and routine will be rigidly followed.

To facilitate appropriate responses, the therapist frequently encourages conversation around specific tasks or events. For example, rather then asking "What's new?" the therapsit might say, "I saw your daughter and you visiting in the day room today. Did you enjoy your visit?'' To help the patient succeed, prompting can assist a patient to give a correct answer. For example, if another patient asks, ''Did you watch that musical special on T.V. last night?'' the patient might be prompted by the therapist who says, ''Yes Mr. Barnes, wasn't that Perry . . .'' (allowing the patient time to complete his response).

An important part of reality orientation is the interruption of confabulation and confused talk through appropriate feedback. To readdress a previous example, if a patient states incorrectly, ''I had pancakes, eggs and bacon for breakfast,'' the therapist might gently disagree, without diminishing the individual's self-esteem. He or she might say, ''Well, I believe I saw oatmeal and fruit, but I can understand how one day might seem like the next.''

Another way of interrupting confabulation and perseverative talk is to interrupt the discourse, direct the patient to a specific subject in the here and now, and require a response: ''Oh, Mr. Barnes, I see you have a haircut. Did you go to the barbershop today?'' In some cases, the therapist may be able to ascertain an underlying feeling or concern that is in part generating the individual's discourse. The therapist might then be able to respond to the affect displayed.

The reader wishing to know more about the use of reality orientation with individuals and in a group context is referred to Holden and Woods, *Reality Orientation: Psychological Approaches to the Confused Elderly.*[33]

Compensatory Memory Strategies. When the function of the brain is compromised, the person frequently does not automatically use the memory strategies described in the previous chapters. Therefore, the therapist may teach the patient to use compensatory memory strategies. These memory strategies are designed to 1) increase the likelihood that a given message is perceived, 2) help in storing information in an easily retrievable form, 3) provide cues for retrieval and 4) rebuild long-term memory through repetition and associa-

tion. The environment needs to be arranged to decrease distraction while maintaining necessary arousal. In some instances, memory of stimuli or of an event will be enhanced by the attempt to incorporate all or many senses. Accordingly, a patient will be instructed not only to see an object, but also to touch and even smell it. Further, he or she may be asked to incorporate speech pathways, being directed to describe verbally aloud what is seen and what is occurring. This multisensory approach can provide extra sensory cues and extra associations for memory.

Repeating a task many times during a short span, as in practicing a tennis swing, may increase the likelihood of storage as long-term memory. Events being remembered are more likely to be retained when the individual can make meaningful association. Thus, the therapist may attempt to draw out these associations, for example, assisting the patient to state aloud the memories or images that a task is triggering.

Patients may be taught to use substitutions for memory. They may be taught to make lists, put visual or written reminders in conspicuous places (or others may be asked to do this for them), and they may be taught to tape record or log important information for easier retrieval.[39]

Memory losses in persons with brain impairment are not usually recoverable. It is most often helpful to assist the individual in reestablishing associative links for functional information. For instance, the patient may be reintroduced to familiar objects with a multisensory approach in an effort to trigger intact memory pathways or rebuild memory associations. Further, the individual may be taught compensatory memory strategies, such as those involving substitution to support his or her function in everyday life. It is unlikely, however, that the patient will again have what one calls a good memory. This inability must be considered as the person looks ahead to employment objectives.

Adapting the Environment. Many of the

treatment strategies discussed incorporate adaptations within the environment. For example, the dampening or amplification of stimuli in the treatment setting is an obvious adaptation.

In many cases, it will be necessary to make changes in the environment to ensure patient safety. A patient who cannot remember to turn off hot stoves or irons will need to have family or community support in his or her selfcare. An individual who remains confused about medications may not only need to be assisted with these substances, but may need to have all potentially hazardous materials removed from his or her home.

Support groups in the community may help patients become aware of available community resources including special public transportation and social groups.

Responding to Affective Changes.   In working with the patient, the therapist needs to be aware of affective changes as influenced by the activity, environmental setting, and social process that provide parameters in which the individual functions. The therapist must be especially attuned to the need to provide an emotionally and physically safe, consistent, and trustworthy interactive and environmental framework for treatment. Essential in establishing this trust is the therapist's verbal and nonverbal congruence, genuineness, and regard for the individual. One must remember that simply stating "I want to help you," or "I care about you," may be quite insufficient when cognitive impairment has interceded.

Consistent, caring behavior must be communicated through all means. While indepth psychotherapy may be inappropriate, the person with brain impairment is always viewed as a person whose feelings and emotions are as important as those of anyone else. At times patients may wish to talk about their own emotional concerns. The therapist may be able to assist them by the following measures:

1. Help the patient clarify current feelings.
2. Validate feelings and emotions as having worth.

3. Be perceptive about and responsive to nonverbal as well as verbal messages.
4. Provide alternative means of communication when verbalization is ineffective.
5. Be patient in allowing the individual to gather and concretize current thoughts.

Many times the less medical, more functional qualities of the occupational therapy setting provide a naturally facilitating atmosphere in which, given the opportunity and encouragement, the individual will draw on experiences, develop associations, and eventually integrate important feelings.

The individual who is suspicious, angry, and uncooperative in treatment presents special difficulties. It is sometimes helpful for the therapist to:

1. Help the patient with reality orientation when perceptual distortions are at play.
2. Understand that some of this affect may be due to fright, as the individual tries to retain a sense of dignity.
3. Avoid touching the patient unless he or she indicates comfort with touch.
4. Approach the patient from a position and in a manner that will not be a surprise.
5. Speak slowly and clearly and be certain communication is understood.
6. Support the individual's efforts to realistically and reasonably exert influence over the treatment program.
7. Assure and be sure that the patient will not be allowed to be in a position to harm others.
8. Give maximal information to the patient about what you, the therapist, are doing and why.
9. Provide the patient with opportunities for time-out from interaction and therapy.

The individual who is experiencing feelings of depression, loss, and grief is encouraged to communicate these feelings while being informed of the progress he or she has made or can reasonably expect to make. The therapist may consider the following:

1. Avoid the over-solicitous, "Everything will be all right."
2. Provide realistic information about function, dysfunction, treatment, and goals.
3. Provide the individual an opportunity for expression of sadness. This opportunity may need to occur many times, in ways and in duration the patient can tolerate.
4. Validate the individual's right to sadness.
5. Assist the individual to put words or thoughts to affective states and to actions when affect seems random.
6. Help the patient realistically assess losses so that they may be grieved and assessing personal strengths so that they may be maximized.
7. Assist the individual in making memory associations with persons, objects and events to facilitate the expression of grief.
8. Assist in values clarification when values need to be reassessed.
9. Provide avenues for closure, for example, saying goodbye to a relationship, role, or skill as needed.
10. Listen carefully for suicide indicators.

When lability of affect, under emotionality or over emotionality is a problem, the therapist might be able to assist the individual by the following:

1. Moderate the environment and increase or decrease stimuli, as needed.
2. Assess the possible calming effects of soft music, rocking in a chair, and other sensory-integrative approaches.
3. Help the patient become sensitive to his or her own body's cues.
4. Encourage the patient to take time out from activity or interaction as needed and provide a place where this process can occur.
5. Break the activity into smaller, time-limited units.

Whatever the affective state of patients, it may be helpful for them to understand how the physical assault to their nervous system, as well as the psychological assault to their sense of self, has helped lead to the feelings they now experience. This knowledge may free them from the burden of believing that their emotional states indicate that they are bad, selfish, or crazy. When patients have some context in which to understand their emotions, they gain some ability to more successfully manage these feelings and incorporate them in a meaningful way. Without such a context, patients may feel at the mercy of feelings that seem outside of themselves; they may experience depersonalization as they view thoughts, actions, and feelings as without apparent cause, aim, or connection.

Therapeutic Activity Group

A holistically oriented activity group pays special attention to the physical as well as emotional environment, the level and nature of task demands, and the nature of social and communication components. A group activity is especially well suited for building social skills, as it allows participants to receive and respond to feedback about their interactive performance.

The following group description is a summary of information taken from Lundgren and Persechino.[45] Although this group is described as a cognitive group for head-injured adults, it has strong holistic threads, and would seem appropriate for use with a more broadly mixed adult psychiatric population in which organic syndromes are represented.

The group is designed for approximately six patients who will meet five times per week in 30-minute sessions. The life of the group is from 2 to 24 weeks, depending on the specific needs of individual patients and the group as a whole. The group meets in a quiet, distraction-free setting. Depending on the skills of participants, the leader may structure the group so that social interaction is minimized, as for example, when each patient works on their own project. Or, the leader may structure the group to facilitate cooperation and call for verbal sharing.

A sample group might function as follows:

Begin with a review of each group member's activity over the preceding weekend to promote the use of memory. Move to the activity of the day, which on this day asks participants to role play various telephoning situations (e.g., ordering a pizza; using directory assistance). Group discussion and feedback then follows. In closing, a word is assigned to each member who will at the beginning of the next meeting be asked to recall and repeat his or her memory word. The memory words relate to the group's activity and could include, for example, the words "dial," "operator," or "touch-tone."[45]

Summary

The Founding Father of Psychiatry, Sigmund Freud, never gave up his belief that the secrets of the human psyche would someday be uncovered in the matter of the brain itself. To some extent, he may have been proved correct. The stacks of any medical library attest to the vast amount of information that has been gathered about the brain and its function. Even with the information now available, however, a great deal yet remains a mystery. The holistic framework provides a basis for understanding brain function and responses to dysfunction and not only is capable of integrating what is known about the brain, but also is flexible enough to accommodate what is unknown. At its heart, holism proposes that the sum is more than the total of the parts. In terms of the brain, this means that what we call consciousness, purposeful behavior, and personality are not fully understood by dissecting the brain. Rather, they can best be appreciated as changing or fluid in their representation throughout a nervous system that is constant itself only in its vigilance toward the aim of making human experience meaningful.

Contributions and Limitations of the Holistic Frame of Reference

A holistic orientation to treatment is endogenous to occupational therapy, although it is not without its detractors. It must be remembered that one of the first persons to articulate holism in psychology, Kurt Goldstein, based the tenets of holism on his work with patients with brain injury, whom he saw for over 10 years. Thus this theory cannot be criticized in a way that many other theories have been—namely that information is based on normal or healthy populations and is then used to treat less than healthy populations.

Contributions

It is hard to argue against seeing the individual as a bio-psycho-social whole; as an attitude, holism is broadly accepted. With persons with brain injury, the identification of functional units that cut across anatomical boundaries makes viable the study of the whole person in the context of his or her everyday world.

The holistic framework, however, is more than a mandate to consider the total person in an environmental context. It calls for qualitative as well as quantitative report in assessment and proposes that the longitudinal, single-case study of the person provides a more compelling indication of patient change than do studies of isolated pieces of behavior as exhibited by many patients. This approach challenges the behavioral model now typically used in medical research, but is a research strategy that has been suggested for use within occupational therapy by many proponents of research.

Holism allows the therapist to respond to the most pressing needs as experienced by the patient, needs that could be associated with any of the subsystems—social, cognitive, physical, emotional or spiritual—within the scope set by the use of therapeutic activity. By viewing the organism as one that by nature strives to achieve balance, the therapist has a rationale for considering how seemingly resistive or unhealthy behavior may, in fact, have a healthy component. Taking this a step further, Abreu and Toglia echo the position taken by Goldstein when they assert, "Because it is not the role of occupational therapists to diagnose the disabling condition but evaluate function and dysfunction . . . a portion of the occupational therapy evaluation should emphasize quality more than quantity and function more than dysfunction . . . It is not enough to know that a client cannot perform a task."[2]

Limitations

The strongest opposition to a holistic framework in working with organically impaired patients in occupational therapy comes from Claudia Allen, as discussed previously. Her criticism is especially pertinent, as she, too, presents a frame of reference designed for treating organically caused dysfunction, although she defines organic impairment differently than does the DSM-III-R and chooses not to differentiate between organic and functional disorders. She articulates the most obvious problem inherent in a holistic framework, that is, its failure to define the boundaries in treatment. In practical terms, even a holistic therapist has to set limits on the scope of treatment, and there is no agreement on how these limits should be set, beyond the guide within occupational therapy to use a functional activity focus. Thus, the holistic framework is in large part an attitude about one's concern for the total person more than a dictum that defines particular problems to address. This orientation contradicts Allen's assertion that with this population only cognition as defined by voluntary motor behavior should be the domain of occupational therapy.

The therapist using a holistic model, therefore, must use judgment in determining which assessment(s) will be used, how they will be used if adaptation is called for, what goals will be set for individual patients, and how to best judge their attainment. One could expect disparity when comparing holistically oriented treatment programs.

A lack of agreement persists about the place of subjective or qualitative assessment. Although most persons in health care would seem to agree that how the patient feels about his or her experiences is important, primary respect continues to be given to hard or quantitative data.

For some, the premise of brain plasticity may suggest reaching for goals that are not practically attainable. Although the potential for the brain and the total organism to adjust to brain assault is well documented in particular cases, in many other cases, compensation has been minimal. The concept of plasticity could be viewed as creating such high expectation that when great success is not achieved, blame may be placed on the treatment design, the lack of patient compliance, or lack of adequate time to achieve treatment goals.

References

1. Abreu BC, Toglia JP: *Cognitive Rehabilitation Manual.* New York, authors, 1984.
2. Abreu BC, Toglia JP: Cognitive rehabilitation: A model for occupational therapy. *Am J Occup Ther* 41:439–448, 1987.
3. American Psychiatric Association: *Diagnostic and Statistical Manual of Mental Disorders (DSM III).* Ed 3. Washington, DC, American Psychiatric Association, 1980.
4. Anderson CM, Reiss D, Hogarty G: *Schizophrenia and the Family.* New York, Guilford Press, 1986.
5. Andreason NC: Brain-imaging: Applications in psychiatry. *Science* 239:1381–1388, 1988.
6. Andreason NC, Nasrallah H, Dunn V, et al: Structural abnormalities in the frontal system of schizophrenia. *Arch Gen Psychiatry* 17:136–144, 1986.
7. Atkinson R, Shiffrin R: Human memory: A proposed system and its control processes. In Spence K, Spence J (Eds): *The Psychology of Learning and Motivation.* Vol. 2. New York, Academic Press, 1968.
8. Bara B: Modifications of knowledge by memory processes. In Reda M, Mahoney M: *Cognitive Psychotherapies.* Cambridge, MA, Ballinger Publishing Company, 1984.
9. Benton A, Hamsher K, Varney N, et al: *Contributions to Neuropsychological Assessment: A Clinical Manual.* New York Oxford University Press, 1983.
10. Binder RL: Organic mental disorders. In Goldman HH (Ed): *Review of General Psychiatry.* Norwalk, CT, Appleton and Lange, 1988.
11. Bower G, Hilgard E: *Theories of Learning.* Ed 5. Englewood Cliffs, NJ, Prentice-Hall, Inc., 1981, pp. 422, 423, 427, 446, 447, 492.
12. Bronfenbrenner U: *The Ecology of Human Development:*

Experiments by Nature and Design. Cambridge, MA, Harvard University Press, 1979.

13. Cohn R: *The Person Symbol in Clinical Medicine.* Springfield, Ill, Charles C Thomas, 1960.

14. Craik R, Lockhart R: Levels of processing: A framework for memory research. *J Verb Learn Verb Behav* 11:671–684, 1972.

15. Crow TJ: Positive and negative schizophrenic symptoms and the role of dopamine. *Br J Psychiatry* 139:251–264, 1981.

16. Edelstein B, Couture E (Eds): *Behavioral Assessment and Rehabilitation of the Traumatically Brain Damaged.* New York, Plenum Press, 1984.

17. Ferguson M: *The Aquarian Conspiracy: Personal and Social Transformations in the 1980's.* Los Angeles, Tarcher, 1980, pp. 246–248.

18. Flavell J: *Cognitive Development.* Ed 2. Englewood Cliffs, NJ, Prentice-Hall, Inc., 1977.

19. Flavell J: *Cognitive Development.* Englewood Cliffs, NJ, Prentice-Hall, Inc., 1985.

20. Franco L, Sperry R: Hemispheric lateralization for cognitive processing of geometry. *Neuropsychologia* 15:107, 1977.

21. Frey W: Functional assessment in the 80's. In Halpern A, Fuhrer M (Eds): *Functional Assessment in Rehabilitation.* Baltimore, Brookes Publishing Co, 1984.

22. Gazzangia M: The split brain in man. *Sci Am* 209:24–29, 1967.

23. Gazzangia M: *The Bisected Brain.* New York, AppletonCentury-Crofts, 1970.

24. Glees P: Functional cerebral reorganization following hemispherectomy in men and after small experimental lesions in primates. In Bach-y-Rita P (Ed): *Recovery of Function: Theoretical Considerations for Brain Injury Rehabilitation.* Bern, Hans Huber, Publishers, 1980, pp. 106–126.

25. Golden C: Rehabilitation and Luria-Nebraska Neuropsychologial Battery. In Edelstein B, Couture E (Eds): *Behavioral Assessment and Rehabilitation of the Traumatically Brain Damaged.* New York, Plenum Press, 1984, pp. 83–120.

26. Golden C, Moses J, Trizelazowski R, et al: Cerebral ventricular size and neuropsychological impairment in young chronic schizophrenics. *Arch Gen Psychiatry* 37:619–623, 1980.

27. Goldstein K: *The Organism.* New York, American Book Co., 1939.

28. Goldstein K: *After-effects of Brain Injuries in War.* New York, Grune and Stratton, 1942, pp. 6, 69–73, 84, 94.

29. Guidano V, Liotti G: *Cognitive Processes and Emotional Disorders.* New York, The Guilford Press, 1983.

30. Hall C, Lindzey G: *Theories of Personality.* Ed 2. New York, John Wiley and Sons, 1970, p. 298.

31. Harris D: *Children's Drawings as a Measure of Mental Maturity.* New York, Harcourt Brace Jovanovich, 1963.

32. Henderson A: Occupational therapy knowledge: From theory to practice. *Am J Occup Ther* 42:567–576, 1988.

33. Holden U, Woods R: *Reality Orientation: Psychological Approaches to the Confused Elderly.* Edinburgh, Churchill-Livingstone, 1982, pp. 124, 156.

34. Horenstein S: Effects of cerebrovascular disease on personality and emotionality. In Benton A (Ed): *Behavior Change in Cerebrovascular Disease.* New York, Harper and Row, 1970.

35. Hutt ML: *The Hutt Adaptation of the Bender-Gestalt Test.* Ed 2. New York, Grune and Stratton, 1969.

36. Hutt ML, Briskin G: *The Clinical Use of the Revised Bender Gestalt Test.* New York, Grune and Stratton, 1961.

37. Jeste D, Kleinman J, Potkin S, et al: Ex uno multi: Subtyping the schizophrenia syndromes. *Biol Psychiatry* 17:199–222, 1982.

38. Kelip J, Sweeney J, Jacobsen P, et al: Cognitive impairments in schizophrenia: Specific relations to ventricular size and negative symptomatology. *Biol Psychiatry* 24:47–55, 1988.

39. Kent-Udolf L: Functional appraisal and therapy for communication disorders of traumatically brain injured persons. In Edelstein B, Couture E (Eds): *Behavioral Assessment and Rehabilitation of the Traumatically Brain Damaged.* New York, Plenum Press, 1984, pp. 23, 32, 56.

40. King LJ: The person symbol as an assessment tool. In Hemphill B (Ed): *The Evaluation Process in Psychiatric Occupational Therapy.* Thorofare, NJ, Slack, Inc., 1982.

41. King LJ: Occupational therapy and neuropsychiatry. In Robertson S (Ed): *Mental Health Focus: Skills for Assessment and Treatment.* Rockville, MD, American Occupational Therapy Association, 1988.

42. Kleinman A: *The Illness Narrative: Suffering, Healing and the Human Condition.* New York, Basic Books, Inc., 1988.

43. Lehmann H: Current perspectives on the biology of schizophrenia. In Menuck M, Seeman M (Eds): *New Perspectives in Schizophrenia.* New York, Macmillan, 1985.

44. Losonczy M, Song I, Mohs R, et al: Correlates of lateral ventricle size in chronic schizophrenia. *Am J Psychiatry* 143:976–981, 1986.

45. Lundgren C, Persechino E: Cognitive group: A treatment program for head injured adults. *Am J Occup Ther* 40:397–401, 1986.

46. Luria A: *Restoration of Function After Brain Injury.* New York, Macmillan Publishing Company, 1963, pp. 28, 36.

47. Luria A: *Higher Cortical Function in Man.* New York, Basic Books, Inc. (Consultants Bureau), 1966, pp. 73, 150–160.

48. Luria A: *The Working Brain.* New York, Basic Books, 1973.

49. Lynch W: A rehabilitation program for brain-injured adults. In Edelstein B, Couture E (Eds): *Behavior Assessment and Reahabilitation of the Traumatically Brain Damaged.* New York, Plenum Press, 1984, pp. 273–312.

50. Malec J: Training the brain injured client. In Edelstein B, Couture E (Eds): *Behavioral Assessment and Rehabilitation of the Traumatically Brain Damaged.* New York, Plenum Press, 1984, pp. 121–150.

51. Miller R: *Meaning and Purpose in the Intact Brain.* Oxford, Clarendon Press, 1981.

52. Moore J: Neuroanatomical consideration relating to recovery of function following brain lesions. In Bachy-Rita P (Ed): *Recovery of Function: Theoretical Considerations for Brain Injury Rehabilitation.* Bern, Hans Huber Publishers, 1980, pp. 27, 29, 36, 74.

53. Mosey AC: *Occupational Therapy: A Configuration of a Profession.* New York, Raven Press, 1981.

54. Najenson R, Rahmani L, Elazer B, et al: An elementary cognitive assessment and treatment of the craniocerebrally injured patient. In Edelstein B, Couture E (Eds): *Behavioral Assessment and Rehabilitation of the Traumatically Brain Damaged.* New York, Plenum Press, 1984, pp. 313–338.

55. Neistadt M: A critical analysis of occupational therapy approaches for perceptual deficits in adults with brain injury. *Am J Occup Ther* 44:299–304, 1990.

56. Ornstein R: *The Psychology of Consciousness.* Ed 2. (revised). New York, Harcourt Brace Jovanovich, 1977.

57. Ornstein R: *The Psychology of Consciousness.* New York, W.H. Freeman and Company, 1972.

58. Rosenthal M: Strategies for intervention with families of brain injured patients. In Edelstein B, Couture E (Eds): *Behavioral Assessment and Rehabilitation of Traumatically Brain Damaged.* New York, Plenum Press, 1984, pp. 23–81.

59. Rosse R, Griese A, Deutsch S, et al: *Laboratory Diagnostic Testing in Psychiatry.* Washington, American Psychiatric Press, 1989.

60. Seeman P: Brain dopamine receptors in schizophrenia. In Menuck M, Seeman M (Eds): *New Perspectives in Schizophrenia.* New York, Macmillan and Company, 1985.

61. Short-DeGraff M: *Human Development for Occupational and Physical Therapists.* Baltimore, Williams & Wilkins, 1988.

62. Siev E, Fershat B: *Perceptual Dysfunction in the Adult Stroke Patient.* Thorofare, NJ, Slack, Inc., 1976.

63. Sperry R: The great cerebral commissure. *Sci Am* 206: 142–152, 1964.

64. Sperry RW: Lateral specialization of cerebral function in the surgically separated hemispheres. In McGuigan F, Schoonover R (Eds): *The Psychophysiology of Thinking.* New York, Academic Press, 1973, pp. 209–229.

65. Stein F, Nikolic S: Teaching stress management techniques to a schizophrenic patient. *Am J Occup Ther* 43:162–169, 1989.

66. Stevens FR, Casanova MF: Is there a neuropathology of schizophrenia? *Biol Psychiatry* 24:123–128, 1988.

67. Strub R, Black F: *Organic Brain Syndromes: An Introduction to Neurobehavioral Disorders.* Philadelphia, F.A. Davis Company, 1981, pp. 10–27, 30, 53, 240, 242–244.

68. Sufrin E: Physical rehabilitation of brain damaged elderly. In Edelstein B, Couture E (Eds): *Behavioral Assessment and Rehabilitation of the Traumatically Brain Damaged.* New York, Plenum Press, 1984, pp. 191–226.

69. von Bertalanffy L: *General System Theory: Foundations, Development, Application.* Rev ed. New York, George Braziller, 1968.

70. Walsh K: Neuropsychological aspects of rehabilitation following brain injury. In Garret J (Ed): *Australian Approaches to Rehabilitation in Neurotrauma and Spinal Cord Injury.* New York, International Exchange of Information in Rehabilitation, World Rehabilitation Fund, Incorporated, 1982 (monograph #19), p. 36.

71. Williams M: *Brain Damage, Behavior and the Mind.* New York, John Wiley and Sons, 1979.

72. Williams SL, Bloomer J: *Bay Area Functional Performance Evaluation.* Palo Alto, CA, Consulting Psychologists Press, 1987.

73. Wolanin M, Phillips L: *Confusion: Prevention and Care.* St. Louis, Mosby-Year Book, 1981, p. 14.

74. Yerxa E: Seeking a relevant, ethical and realistic way of knowing for occupational therapy. *Am J Occup Ther* 45(3):199–204, 1991.

75. Yerxa E: As quoted in Fox S: What is this thing called occupation? *Adv Occup Ther* October 30(12):5, 1989.

76. Zubin J, Spring G: Vulnerability: A new view of schizophrenia. *J Abnorm Psychol* 86:103–126, 1977.

Chapter 12

CONCLUSION

Focus Questions

1. How would you define occupational therapy?
2. State and describe the key elements (components) of occupational therapy.
3. Describe the dynamic interaction that occurs among the elements of occupational therapy.
4. Describe the purposes and value of activity as therapy.
5. How does individual difference influence the choice of a frame of reference for occupational therapy practice?
6. What are the advantages or disadvantages of multiple frames of reference for occupational therapy practice?
7. How does occupational therapy contribute to contemporary mental health care?

Introduction

As we come to the end of our journey through occupational therapy, research and practice we are aware of the wealth of information that exists, the alternative frames of reference that are applied in practice, and the concerns and questions posed by educators, clinicians and students as they look toward their future practice in psychosocial occupational therapy.

When a person completes a journey and reflects on recent travels, he or she may highlight what has been seen and learned. When reflecting on meaningful sites, events and personal encounters, an individual often becomes aware of how he or she has changed since the journey began. This chapter highlights the key elements of occupational therapy and responds to some of the criticisms leveled at multiframework approaches to education and

practice. To suggest what is gained from a broadly based development of knowledge, the psychosocial occupational therapy process that exists regardless of the framework applied is summarized. Finally, the potential value of activity as therapy, as well as the limitations of occupational therapy as a profession contributing to contemporary mental health care, is discussed.

Multiframeworks for Education and Practice

Occupational therapy resides in the realm of applied science, and each of the frames of reference included in this text have had a dual task. First, each must select and organize information and provide logical and internally related assumptions judged to be essential to understanding how an individual engages with persons, objects and events to achieve meaning, identity and purpose in life. Second, each frame of reference must state how this understanding of the person-activity relationship can be applied in the context of therapy to promote an individual's well-being. These frames of reference often (but not always) include statements about the following:

1. Criteria for selecting information into the framework;
2. The nature of man, including the relative relationship of biological, psychological, and social-cultural forces;
3. The person's relationship to the environment;
4. The nature, purpose and organization of activity as it enables persons to achieve meaning;
5. The nature of motivation, including the relative importance of internal and external determinants;
6. What constitutes optimum function;
7. What constitutes dysfunction;
8. The conditions (internal and/or external) believed to promote and sustain optimum function;
9. The means, tools, and criteria for assessing function/dysfunction;
10. What constitutes therapy, including areas identified for remediation, goals and expectations for therapist and patient;
11. Therapeutic principles for implementing treatment;
12. The suitability of the framework to designated patients or clients;
13. Recommendations and parameters for research.

Each frame of reference described in this text places a different emphasis in addressing these issues, and not all issues are treated by each with the same clarity nor conceived as having equal importance. That each of the frameworks is far from complete is evidenced by the relatively vague development and lack of empirical support for many of the theoret-ical assumptions on which the individual frameworks lie and on the very limited research regarding the efficacy of treatment.

Each frame of reference, however, does serve an important function, as it acts as a "pair of glasses," providing a unique perspective on person, activity and therapy. Recognizing that no therapist, indeed no individual, can at any given time attend equally to every aspect of the human condition, the frame of reference helps the therapist determine what is *most* important as he or she she plans, implements and evaluates treatment. Toward this end, each of the frameworks in this text can act as a basis for further and much needed exploration and study; and each adds to the knowledge that occupational therapy offers about how an individual achieves purpose through investment in activity and how activity can best be used as therapy.

If all of the frameworks in this text are useful, the question must be asked: "Useful to whom?" Our supposition throughout this text has been that adult psychosocial occupational therapy is concerned with serving a broad spectrum of adults. This supposition is challenged, by Allen, in her elucidation of cognitive therapy, and by some proponents of the occupational behavior frame of reference. Although these theorists come to some very different conclusions, they share three common general beliefs:

1. Occupational therapy has too much knowledge and/or irrelevant knowledge. Knowledge needs to be confined to a more manageable amount.
2. Theoretical development in and the practice of occupational therapy should be restricted to one frame of reference or just a selected few.
3. Occupational therapists treat primarily the "chronically" disabled and should be most concerned as a profession with meeting the needs of the "chronic" patient.

We respond briefly to these three assumptions and hope that we stimulate critical thinking.

1. In response to the contention that occupational therapy has too much knowledge, we reiterate that the role of a frame of reference is to select and organize information to keep it from being unwieldy. No one person is expected to be expert in all frameworks, nor to have a depth of information in all frames. If one looks at the relative lack of research, the only limited availability of program descriptions and case studies in the literature and the as yet vague development of many theoretical and practice-oriented premises, one could argue that occupational therapy has many areas of knowledge deficit.

2. Should occupational therapy limit itself to development and practice within the confines of a single frame of reference? We believe that no one frame of reference has proved more legitimate for understanding the person-activity relationship, or more helpful when applied within the context of patient care. Not only is the lack of rigorous and broad empirical evidence a concern, but also the denial of individual difference and the limitation of individual preference and option.

In looking about in everyday practice, individual patients seek and profit from different emphases in practice, as a result of their unique needs and preferences. Some patients are concerned strictly with tangible results and find stringently applied behavioral programs a helpful vehicle for monitoring their own success. Others desire to "know themselves better." These patients engage the therapist in "how" and "why" questions, endeavor to clarify their own motives, or find self-expression in media to be a legitimate and helpful endeavor. The individual who needs to learn more self-control may be contrasted with the individual whose over-control renders the person ineffective and anxious.

Some individuals can learn from activity without any need to verbalize about it; others learn more readily when they can talk about the activities in which they have participated. Some individuals lack physical ease and move about in a manner that appears stiff and over-protective; others display physical ease, but disregard social mores. Not surprisingly, therapists also bring to therapy their own strengths, limitations, interests, values, and needs. As a result, they are often much more at home within one frame of reference than another.

Thus far, no one frame of reference has been able to attend to all treatment challenges with comparable effectiveness, and it seems unlikely that any will in the foreseeable future.

If, as some suggest, we put all our professional "eggs in one basket" and attempt to develop one framework to the extent that it addresses "all" the needs of all our patients, will we unwittingly move away from our commitment to the individualization of care? Is individualization of treatment a priority? If, in fact, one frame of reference could be developed to the status of paradigm, is it evident which would best serve this function?

We have indicated both contributions and limitations of all the frameworks discussed. Beyond this, we have tried to present the frameworks in a positive light. It does not appear to us that occupational therapy is so well grounded in psychosocial practice to suggest that now is the time to close our doors on avenues of learning. Where theoretical frameworks are presented with an emphasis only on what they fail to do, then they are unlikely to generate interest or development. Further, the notion is often promulgated that a person can learn only from those things that fit nicely with one's own biases; often, critical thinking suffers.

We believe that any student of occupational therapy, as well as the seasoned professional, profits from being cognizant of the key premises of all the frames of reference in psychosocial practice. This information gives the individual a means to compare and critique theoretical assumptions and a basis to choose the framework in which he or she will go beyond the general and seek expertise.

3. Finally, we address the proposal that occupational therapy should be primarily concerned with meeting the needs of the "chronic" patient. What constitutes criteria for

chronicity, and, perhaps more important, why and in what way the preparation to meet the needs of the "chronic" patient should be different than the preparation needed to meet the needs of the more general population is not clear. If we prepare our new therapists to work only with a select population, however, then obviously, their skills will only be in this area of treatment, and our statistics will show that these are the patients that occupational therapy serves. Given the uncertain and ever-changing nature of public health needs, is this the appropriate preparedness to meet the health needs of the 1990s and beyond? If indeed the profession determines that it will henceforth specialize in the treatment of a select patient population, then we must all recognize that at that point occupational therapy has defined itself in a new way.

Although we propose that all frameworks offer a legitimate girder for therapy, we all are well aware of the need for occupational therapists in psychosocial practice to better clarify and document their contribution in patient care. This need parallels the need within the broader mental health community to better determine what it can and cannot offer the general population.

For all the theories and alternatives in mental health practice, many patients make no demonstrable progress, in neither our nor their estimation. The treatment of psychosocial problems is by no means the exact science anyone might hope it to be. Even where we can predict likelihood or trends in macrostructures of behavior, we cannot make any one patient profit from participation in therapy. However, we have seen in the work of our colleagues, in clinics and research endeavors, and in the literature all of the frameworks discussed in this text, and professionals who are committed to further development of theoretical and practice principles within their area of expertise. Although we wish to encourage therapists to look creatively at what may prove to be new, as yet unconceived ways for conceptualizing therapeutic activity, we must continue to sup-

port and encourage those individuals who continue to learn within their chosen domain.

Psychosocial Occupational Therapy

Whatever the frame of reference, the occupational therapy process in psychosocial practice has consistent boundaries that identify and define psychosocial occupational therapy: 1) purposeful activities; 2) an occupational therapist who is knowledgeable of psychosocial theories, activity analysis, and occupational therapy theory; effectively uses his or her interpersonal skills to work with patients and colleagues, and implements occupational therapy services within the guides of an ethical code; 3) a patient who seeks to change personal knowledge, behavior, increase satisfaction, participate and increase control of his or her environment and to improve the quality of life that he or she experiences; and 4) an environment that has available given (but not unlimited) resources that support the patient in the quest for change and an environment that sanctions certain behaviors. Using these boundaries psychosocial occupational therapy may be defined as follows.

Definition

Psychosocial occupational therapy is a major rehabilitation service, based in theoretical principles that emphasize the role of activity in the development of personhood and the achievement and maintenance of optimum well-being. Psychosocial occupational therapy principles are compatible with many theories within psychology, sociology, education and rehabilitation. Within the theoretical framework, the occupational therapist and patient work together to assess the patient's level of function (physical and psychosocial) within the environment and to target areas needing change and to implement intervention that will use the patient's abilities and promote competent function in the environment.

Competent function indicates that the patient has adequate knowledge, skills and attitudes to function in the environment to communicate effectively, to meet daily needs, to contribute to the community, to participate in recreation and be renewed for work and maintained health, and to use time meaningfully, efficiently and effectively. Change in function is brought about through the dynamic interaction between the therapeutic activity, the patient, and the therapist within the environment.

We can look further at the components of this definition as we summarize what has been posited by the frameworks for therapy discussed in this text.

Activity as Therapy

The choice of activity and the manner in which activities are used by the occupational therapist to promote growth and to facilitate change in function are determined by the frame of reference. Regardless of the theoretical framework, the effectiveness of an activity is determined by the **context** in which it occurs. That is, activity becomes meaningful because of the interaction between patient, therapist, activity and the environment.

This text identifies therapeutic activities as being capable of serving one or more of the following functions:

1. A bridge to the community;
2. A catalyst for social, vocational, recreational and/or task-related interaction;
3. A means for expression;
4. Enabling the creation of an end product by the patient;
5. A desired behavioral outcome;
6. A reinforcer of behavior;
7. A tangible indicator of progress;
8. A means to master developmental tasks;
9. A means to assess the individual's knowledge, skills, beliefs and values;
10. A way to achieve meaning or purpose;
11. A vehicle for trying out or practicing roles or different facets of self-hood;
12. A means to increase competent function

and help the individual achieve a realistic sense of control within the environment;
13. The tools and outcome of the education process;
14. Occupation;
15. Corrective learning experiences;
16. A focus for dialogue;
17. A means to engage the "whole" person in a way that is satisfying, optimizes physical and emotional well-being, and helps to prevent dis-ease and disability.

Roles of the Occupational Therapist

The role of the occupational therapist also depends on the frame of reference within which he or she operates, the work environment, the focus of the treatment/health setting, the needs of the patient, the purpose (function) of the activity, and the desired treatment outcome.

The occupational therapist has multiple role choices: educator-facilitator, motivator, teacher, trainer, role model, participant-observer, observer, resource, and supporting agent. Regardless of the role assumed, the therapist establishes and maintains a therapeutic relationship based on understanding, open communication, and a valuing of change. In this relationship, the therapist facilitates an interactive process between the patient, the activity and the environment, and assures the patient that he or she offers a safe, caring environment, which will assist the patient to "risk" change.

The Patient in Occupational Therapy

The frame of reference chosen influences the therapist's view of the patient's level of function and determines what will be conceived as the optimum or desired level of function for each patient. In this text, the view of the person and his or her behavior is described within the context of particular theories, and guides are provided to determine function or dysfunction.

The patient in occupational therapy need

not be labeled or categorized by a diagnosis in order to determine that occupational therapy services are needed. The patient's knowledge, skills and attitudes and the way in which they influence functioning in the environment are the focus of occupational therapy evaluation and treatment. The therapist asks: Do the patients have the knowledge and skills they need to function competently in the environment? Do they use their knowledge and skills toward an effective outcome? Can they make use of available resources when their level of skill or information base is inadequate? What are their beliefs about themselves and others? Do they feel in control and competent?

Dynamic Interaction in Occupational Therapy

The term **dynamic interaction** connotes *change* in the relationship between patient, therapist, activity and the environment, as each of these four elements constantly influences the other.

This interaction influences the assessment and treatment services that the occupational therapist provides. The interaction in assessment promotes "purposeful inquiry" to gather data that identifies the patient's physical and/or psychosocial level of function in the environment. These data are used to determine short-term and long-term goals, to identify expected functional outcomes, and to evaluate the efficacy of treatment. The data may be used to compare the patient's performance to a norm or may identify and measure the individual's function according to particular performance criteria. Aware of this dynamism, the therapist frequently reassesses treatment goals and is open to making treatment changes that are responsive to the patient's changing needs.

During treatment, the interaction between patient activity and therapist can occur in individual or group situations, and it provides experiences through which the patient can 1) gain knowledge and skills, 2) practice skills and problem-solving, 3) develop coping patterns, 4) learn more about personal abilities

and limitations, 5) better learn the rules for social interaction and role performance, and 6) become more independent.

Theoretical Principles

In this text, the frames of reference provide the guidelines for understanding patients and determining how to use activities to assess function and produce the desired treatment outcome. Thus, the theoretical principles or assumptions of each frame of reference are capable of guiding or influencing the dynamic interaction in the occupational therapy process.

The theoretical assumptions listed with each frame of reference in this text are compatible with and/or within the guidelines of the broader principles that underlie psychosocial occupational therapy. The following assumptions are emphasized in this text:

1. The patients are individuals who need and are capable of change.
2. The therapist's primary and guiding concern is the well-being of patients and the needs they experience within the milieu.
3. Occupational therapy practice is based within identified theoretical and practice frameworks.
4. Occupational therapy is a dynamic process in which therapist, patient and activity interact within and with the environment, and none can adequately be understood in isolation.
5. Occupational therapy uses a combination of tasks and dialogue to facilitate change.
6. Occupational therapy experiences are designed to promote the maintenance or improvement of function.
7. The occupational therapist is concerned not only with remediation of function, but also the maintenance of health and the prevention of further (or future) disability.
8. The individual is understood as an integrated bio-psychosocial "whole" whose health care needs must be addressed accordingly.
9. In practice, occupational therapy activities

are graded to adapt to the developmental and functional needs of the patient and the resources and demands of the environment.

10. Participation in activity provides a means by which individuals can improve skills, broaden their knowledge base, perceive themselves more positively, and become better prepared to meet the expectations of their tomorrow.

The Promise: The Reality

This book has described the potential of therapeutic activity to bring about positive change for the individuals we serve. This potential may be thought of as the "promise" of occupational therapy. In actual practice, the promise has not always come to fruition, and occupational therapy, as well as the mental health care of which it is a part, must be accountable. The following concerns and problems confront occupational therapy in psychosocial practice:

1. The concept of "activity as therapy" is tremendously broad and inclusive. Therapists engaged in practice, education and research must grapple with determining which human "activities" are the legitimate vehicles for occupational therapy intervention and which are the primary concern of other helping disciplines.

2. Occupational therapy is conceived as both an "art" and a science. The profession as a whole and the individual in practice, education and/or reseach must find a way to respect and integrate both aspects of the therapy process.

3. The theory and practice of occupational therapy are poorly understood by the health community, by the public and by third-party payers. Ask even enthusiastic occupational therapy students to describe their chosen field, and the lack of clarity becomes quickly evident. One result is that occupational therapy has varying and often limited support within the mental health care community, and third-party payers are reluctant to reimburse occupational therapy services. Contributing to this dilemma is the limited research in support of the practice of occupational therapy.

4. Although multiple assessment instruments have been developed, few of them have reliability and validity standards. Thus it is difficult for professionals to clarify and document what occupational therapy can reasonably be expected to accomplish.

5. The desire to clarify and better manage the parameters of therapy have led some educators, clinicians and students to limit the theoretical assumptions and practices subsumed within occupational therapy. Without a sound research base, it is difficult to assess which theoretical assumptions and practices should be excluded.

In its desire to be responsive to changes in the health care system, occupational therapy has tended to move quickly from one "bandwagon" to another. It is important to strike a balance between the need to be responsive and also proactive in our service to the public, with the need to be diligent and patient in developing and testing the assumptions we purport. We must educate ourselves before we can educate others in what is not only the promise but the benefit of occupational therapy.

Appendices

OCCUPATIONAL THERAPY CODE OF ETHICS

The American Occupational Therapy Association and its component members are committed to furthering people's ability to function fully within their total environment. To this end the occupational therapist renders service to clients in all stages of health and illness, to institutions, to other professionals and colleagues, to students, and to the general public.

In furthering this commitment, the American Occupational Therapy Association has established the Occupational Therapy Code of Ethics. This code is intended to be used as a guide to promoting and maintaining the highest standards of ethical behavior.

This Code of Ethics shall apply to all occupational therapy personnel. The term *occupational therapy personnel* shall include individuals who are registered occupational therapists, certified occupational therapy assistants, and occupational therapy students. The roles of practitioner, educator, manager, researcher, and consultant are assumed.

Principle 1 (Beneficence/Autonomy)

Occupational therapy personnel shall demonstrate a concern for the welfare and dignity of the recipient of their services.

A. The individual is responsible for providing services without regard to race, creed, national origin, sex, age, handicap, disease entity, social status, financial status, or religious affiliation.

B. The individual shall inform those people served on the nature and potential outcomes of treatment and shall respect the right of potential recipients of service to refuse treatment.

C. The individual shall inform subjects involved in education or research activities of the potential outcome of those activities.

D. The individual shall include those people served in the treatment planning process.

E. The individual shall maintain goal-directed and objective relationships with all people served.

F. The individual shall protect the confidential nature of information gained from educational, practice, and investigational activities unless sharing such information could be deemed necessary to protect the well-being of a third party.

G. The individual shall take all reasonable precautions to avoid harm to the recipient of services or detriment to the recipient's property.

H. The individual shall establish fees, based on cost analysis, that are commensurate with services rendered.

Principle 2 (Competence)

Occupational therapy personnel shall actively maintain high standards of professional competence.

A. The individual shall hold the appropriate credential for providing service.

B. The individual shall recognize the need for competence and shall participate in continuing professional development.

C. The individual shall function within the parameters of his or her competence and the standards of the profession.

D. The individual shall refer clients to other service providers or consult with other service providers when additional knowledge and expertise is required.

Principle 3 (Compliance with Laws and Regulations)

Occupational therapy personnel shall comply with laws and Association policies guiding the profession of occupational therapy.

A. The individual shall be acquainted with applicable local, state, federal, and institutional rules and Association policies and shall function accordingly.

B. The individual shall inform employers, employees, and colleagues about those laws and policies that apply to the profession of occupational therapy.

C. The individual shall require those whom they supervise to adhere to the Code of Ethics.

D. The individual shall accurately record and report information.

Principle 4 (Public Information)

Occupational therapy personnel shall provide accurate information concerning occupational therapy services.

A. The individual shall accurately represent this or her competence and training.

B. The individual shall not use or participate in the use of any form of communication that contains a false, fraudulent, deceptive, or unfair statement or claim.

Principle 5 (Professional Relationships)

Occupational therapy personnel shall function with discretion and integrity in relations with colleagues and other professionals, and shall be concerned with the quality of their services.

A. The individual shall report illegal, incompetent, and/or unethical practice to the appropriate authority.

B. The individual shall not disclose privileged information when participating in reviews of peers, programs, or systems.

C. The individual who employs or supervises colleagues shall provide appropriate supervision, as defined in AOTA guidelines or state laws, regulations, and institutional policies.

D. The individual shall recognize the contributions of colleagues when disseminating professional information.

Principle 6 (Professional Conduct)

Occupational therapy personnel shall not engage in any form of conduct that constitutes a conflict of interest or that adversely reflects on the profession.

This document was approved by the Representative Assembly in April 1988; it replaces the (1977/1979) ''Principles of Occupational Therapy Ethics.''

Reprinted from American Journal of Occupational Therapy, 42(12), 795–796, The American Occupational Therapy Association, Inc., 1988. Reprinted with permission.

STANDARDS OF PRACTICE FOR OCCUPATIONAL THERAPY

Preface

These standards are intended as recommended guidelines to assist occupational therapy practitioners in the provision of occupational therapy services. These standards serve as a minimum standard for occupational therapy practice and are applicable to all individual populations and the programs in which these individuals are served.

These standards apply to those registered occupational therapists and certified occupational therapy assistants who are in compliance with regulation where it exists. The term *occupational therapy practitioner* refers to the registered occupational therapist and to the certified occupational therapy assistant, both of whom are in compliance with regulation where it exists.

The minimum educational requirements for the registered occupational therapist are described in the current *Essentials and Guidelines of an Accredited Educational Program for the Occupational Therapist* (American Occupational Therapy Association [AOTA], 1991a). The minimum educational requirements for the certified occupational therapy assistant are described in the current *Essentials and Guidelines of an Accredited Educational Program for the Occupational Therapy Assistant* (AOTA, 1991b).

Standard I: Professional Standing

1. An occupational therapy practitioner shall maintain a current license, registration, or certification as required by law.
2. An occupational therapy practitioner shall practice and manage occupational therapy programs in accordance with applicable federal and state laws and regulations.
3. An occupational therapy practitioner shall be familiar with and abide by AOTA's (1988) *Occupational Therapy Code of Ethics*.
4. An occupational therapy practitioner shall maintain and update professional knowledge, skills, and abilities through appropriate continuing education or inservice training or higher education. The nature and minimum amount of continuing education must be consistent with state law and regulation.
5. A certified occupational therapy assistant must receive supervision from a registered occupational therapist as defined by the current *Supervision Guidelines for Certified Occupational Therapy Assistants* (AOTA, 1990) and by official AOTA documents. The nature and amount of supervision must be provided in accordance with state law and regulation.
6. An occupational therapy practitioner shall provide direct and indirect services in accordance with AOTA's standards and policies. The nature and scope of occupational therapy services provided must be in accordance with state law and regulation.
7. An occupational therapy practitioner shall maintain current knowledge of the legislative, political, social, and cultural issues that affect the profession.

Standard II: Referral

1. A registered occupational therapist shall accept referrals in accordance with AOTA's

Statement of Occupational Therapy Referral (AOTA, 1989) and in compliance with appropriate laws.

2. A registered occupational therapist may accept referrals for assessment or assessment with intervention in occupational performance areas or occupational performance components when individuals have or appear to have dysfunctions or potential for dysfunctions.

3. A registered occupational therapist, responding to requests for service, may accept cases within the parameters of the law.

4. A registered occupational therapist shall assume responsibility for determining the appropriateness of the scope, frequency, and duration of services within the parameters of the law.

5. A registered occupational therapist shall refer individuals to other appropriate resources when the therapist determines that the knowledge and expertise of other professionals is indicated.

6. An occupational therapy practitioner shall educate current and potential referral sources about the process of initiating occupational therapy referrals.

Standard III: Screening

1. A registered occupational therapist, in accordance with state and federal guidelines, shall conduct screening to determine whether intervention or further assessment is necessary and to identify dysfunctions in occupational performance areas.

2. A registered occupational therapist shall screen independently or as a member of an interdisciplinary team. A certified occupational therapy assistant may contribute to the screening process under the supervision of a registered occupational therapist.

3. A registered occupational therapist shall select screening methods that are appropriate to the individual's age and developmental level; gender; education; cultural background; and socioeconomic, medical and

functional status. Screening methods may include, but are not limited to, interviews, structured observations, informal testing, and record reviews.

4. A registered occupational therapist shall communicate screening results and recommendations to appropriate individuals.

Standard IV: Assessment

1. A registered occupational therapist shall assess an individual's occupational performance components and occupational performance areas. A registered occupational therapist conducts assessments individually or as part of a team of professionals, as appropriate to the practice settings and the purposes of the assessments. A certified occupational therapy assistant may contribute to the assessment process under the supervision of a registered occupational therapist.

2. An occupational therapy practitioner shall educate the individual, or the individual's family or legal guardian, as appropriate, about the purposes and procedures of the occupational therapy assessment.

3. A registered occupational therapist shall select assessments to determine the individual's functional abilities and problems as related to occupational performance areas; occupational performance components; physical, social, and cultural environments; performance safety; and prevention of dysfunction.

4. Occupational therapy assessment methods shall be appropriate to the individual's age and developmental level; gender, education, socioeconomic, cultural and ethnic background; medical status; and functional abilities. The assessment methods may include some combination of skilled observation, interview, record review, or the use of standardized or criterion-referenced tests. A certified occupational therapy assistant may contribute to the assess-

ment process under the supervision of a registered occupational therapist.

5. An occupational therapy practitioner shall follow accepted protocols when standardized tests are used. Standardized tests are tests whose scores are based on accompanying normative data that may reflect age ranges, gender, ethnic groups, geographic regions, and socioeconomic status. If standardized tests are not available or appropriate, the results shall be expressed in descriptive reports, and standardized scales shall not be used.

6. A registered occupational therapist shall analyze and summarize all collected evaluation data to indicate the individual's current functional status.

7. A registered occupational therapist shall document assessment results in the individual's records, noting the specific evaluation methods and tools used.

8. A registered occupational therapist shall complete and document results of occupational therapy assessments within the time frames established by practice settings, government agencies, accreditation programs, and third-party payers.

9. An occupational therapy practitioner shall communicate assessment results, within the boundaries of client confidentiality, to the appropriate persons.

10. A registered occupational therapist shall refer the individual to the appropriate services or request additional consultations if the results of the assessments indicate areas that require intervention by other professionals.

Standard V: Intervention Plan

1. A registered occupational therapist shall develop and document an intervention plan based on analysis of the occupational therapy assessment data and the individual's expected outcome after the intervention. A certified occupational therapy assistant may contribute to the intervention plan under

the supervision of a registered occupational therapist.

2. The occupational therapy intervention plan shall be stated in goals that are clear, measurable, behavioral, functional, and appropriate to the individual's needs, personal goals, and expected outcome after intervention.

3. The occupational therapy intervention plan shall reflect the philosophical base of occupational therapy (AOTA, 1979) and be consistent with its established principles and concepts of theory and practice. The intervention planning processes shall include:
   a. Formulating a list of strengths and weaknesses;
   b. Estimating rehabilitation potential;
   c. Identifying measurable short-term and long-term goals;
   d. Collaborating with the individual, family members, other caregivers, professionals, and community resources;
   e. Selecting the media, methods, environment, and personnel needed to accomplish the intervention goals;
   f. Determining the frequency and duration of occupational therapy services;
   g. Identifying a plan for reevaluation;
   h. Discharge planning.

4. A registered occupational therapist shall prepare and document the intervention plan within the time frames and according to the standards established by the employing practice settings, government agencies, accreditation programs, and third-party payers. The certified occupational therapy assistant may contribute to the formation of the intervention plan under the supervision of the registered occupational therapist.

Standard VI: Intervention

1. An occupational therapy practitioner shall implement a program according to the developed intervention plan. The plan shall be appropriate to the individual's age and developmental level, gender, education, cul-

tural and ethnic background, health status, functional ability, interests and personal goals, and service provision setting. The certified occupational therapy assistant shall implement the intervention under the supervision of a registered occupational therapist.

2. An occupational therapy practitioner shall implement the intervention plan through the use of specified purposeful activities or therapeutic methods to enhance occupational performance and achieve stated goals.

3. An occupational therapy practitioner shall be knowledgeable about relevant research in the practitioner's areas of practice. A registered occupational therapist shall interpret research findings as appropriate for application to the intervention process.

4. An occupational therapy practitioner shall educate the individual, the individual's family or legal guardian, noncertified occupational therapy personnel, and nonoccupational therapy staff, as appropriate, in activities that support the established intervention plan. An occupational therapy practitioner shall communicate the risk and benefit of the intervention.

5. An occupational therapy practitioner shall maintain current information on community resources relevant to the practice area of the practitioner.

6. A registered occupational therapist shall periodically reassess and document the individual's levels of functioning and changes in levels of functioning in the occupational performance areas and occupational performance components. A certified occupational therapy assistant may contribute to the reassessment process under the supervision of a registered occupational therapist.

7. A registered occupational therapist shall formulate and implement program modifications consistent with changes in the individual's response to the intervention. A certified occupational therapy assistant may contribute to program modifications under

the supervision of a registered occupational therapist.

8. An occupational therapy practitioner shall document the occupational therapy services provided, including the frequency and duration of the services within the time frames and according to the standards established by the employing facility, government agencies, accreditation programs, and third-party payers.

Standard VII: Discontinuation

1. A registered occupational therapist shall discontinue service when the individual has achieved predetermined goals or has achieved maximum benefit from occupational therapy services.

2. A registered occupational therapist, with input from a certified occupational therapy assistant where applicable, shall prepare and implement a discharge plan that is consistent with occupational therapy goals, individual goals, interdisciplinary team goals, family goals, and expected outcomes. The discharge plan shall address appropriate community resources for referral for psychosocial, cultural, and socioeconomic barriers and limitations that may need modification.

3. A registered occupational therapist shall document the changes between the intial and current states of functional ability and deficit in occupational performance areas and occupational performance components. A certified occupational therapy assistant may contribute to the process under the supervision of a registered occupational therapist.

4. An occupational therapy practitioner shall allow sufficient time for the coordination and effective implementation of the discharge plan.

5. A registered occupational therapist shall document recommendations for follow-up or reevaluation when applicable.

Standard VIII: Continuous Quality Improvement

1. An occupational therapy practitioner shall monitor and document the continuous quality improvement of practice, which may include outcomes of services, using predetermined practice criteria reflecting professional consensus, recent developments in research, and specific employing facility standards.
2. An occupational therapy practitioner shall monitor all aspects of individual occupational therapy services for effectiveness and timeliness. If actual care does not meet the prescribed standard, it must be justified by peer review or other appropriate means within the practice setting. Occupational therapy services shall be discontinued when no longer necessary.
3. A registered occupational therapist shall systematically assess the review process of patient care to determine the success or appropriateness of interventions. Certified occupational therapy assistants may contribute to this process in collaboration with the registered occupational therapist.

Standard IX: Management

1. A registered occupational therapist shall provide the management necessary for efficient organization and provision of occupational therapy services.
2. A certified occupational therapy assistant, under the supervision of a registered occupational therapist, may perform the following management functions:
   a. Education of members of other related professions and physicians about occupational therapy.
   b. Participation in (1) orientation, supervision, training, and evaluation of the performance of volunteers and other noncertified occupational therapy personnel, and (2) developing plans to remediate areas of skill deficit in the performance of job duties by volunteers and other noncertified occupational therapy personnel.
   c. Design and periodic review of all aspects of the occupational therapy program to determine its effectiveness, efficiency, and future directions.
   d. Systematic review of the quality of service provided, using criteria established by professional consensus and current research, as well as established standards for state regulation; accreditation; American Occupational Therapy Certification Board (AOTCB) certification; and related laws, policies, guidelines and regulations.
   e. Incorporation of a fair and equitable system of admission, discharge, and charges for occupational therapy services.
   f. Participation in cross-disciplinary activities to ensure that the total needs of the individual are met.
   g. Provision of support (i.e., space, time, money as feasible) for clinical research or collaborative research when such projects have the approval of the appropriate governing bodies (e.g., institutional review board) and the results of which are deemed potentially beneficial to individuals of occupational therapy services now or in the future.

References

American Occupational Therapy Association. (1979). The philosophical base of occupational therapy. *American Journal of Occupational Therapy, 33,* 785.

American Occupational Therapy Association. (1988). Occupational therapy code of ethics. *American Journal of Occupational Therapy, 42,* 795–796.

American Occupational Therapy Association. (1989). Statement of occupational therapy referral. In *Reference manual of the official documents of the American Occupational Therapy Association, Inc.* (AOTA) (p. VIII.1). Rockville, MD: Author (Original work published 1969, revised 1980).

American Occupational Therapy Association. (1990). Supervision guidelines for certified occupational therapy assistants. *American Journal of Occupational Therapy, 44,* 1089–1090.

American Occupational Therapy Association. (1991a). *Essentials and guidelines of an accredited educational program for the occupational therapist.* Rockville, MD: Author.

American Occupational Therapy Association. (1991b). *Essentials and guidelines of an accredited educational program for the occupational therapy assistant.* Rockville, MD: Author.

Prepared by the Commission on Practice (Jim Hinojosa, PhD, OTR, FAOTA, Chair).

Approved by the Representative Assembly March 1992.

This document replaces the 1983 Standards of Practice for Occupational Therapy (*American Journal of Occupational Therapy, 37,* 802–804), which was rescinded by the 1992 Representative Assembly.

Standards of Practice reprinted from American Journal of Occupational Therapy, 46, pp. 1082–1085, American Occupational Therapy Association, 1992. Reprinted with permission.

DEVELOPMENTAL GROUPS

Parallel Group

A group composed of patients who have the ability to trust others enough to tolerate being with more than one person at a time. They can acknowledge the presence of other group members through eye contact or casual conversation. The occupational therapist is the leader of the group, and thus provides the group boundaries, explains the purpose of the group, the expectations for behavior in the group, and is responsible for giving feedback to the patients regarding their performance during the group. She provides an occupational therapy environment which is a safe place to work and where the patient can feel accepted and valued. The goal of the group is to have each patient work on his own chosen task while sharing space with other patients. For example, a craft group may be started in which each patient is working on a craft project of his choice.

Project Group

A group experience in which the patients are expected to come together to interact with each other in casual conversation and in order to complete a short term task (about one half hour work period). Patients are expected to work together cooperatively, share space, materials and tools, and be able to cope with limited competition. The occupational therapist is a leader who plans and presents the short term task to the patients and is available during the work period to support, assist, and guide patients as needed. The goal of the group is to provide the patients with an opportunity for trial and error learning, for group interaction around a task, and for a balance of cooperative and competitive experiences. These experiences may be, for example, team sports and games, making holiday decorations, or planning and preparing a patient party.

Egocentric-Cooperative Group

A group in which the patients come together to work on a task that is completed in one or two work sessions (one hour per session). During the task, the patients learn to express their needs, acknowledge the needs of other patients, ask for feedback, and give feedback to the other patients. The occupational therapist is a democratic leader that makes suggestions and allows the patients to choose and carry out the task and group plan. She is a resource for facilitating task completion and a support that promotes an atmosphere of acceptance and safety. The goal of the group is to have a task experience in which the patients will learn to (1) identify group norms and goals, (2) use their own knowledge and skills to respond in the group, (3) experiment with different group roles, (4) identify themselves as a group member with rights, (5) respect the rights of other group members, (6) respond empathetically to group members' needs, and (7) gain satisfaction from participating in the group experience. Examples may include structured learning experiences such as assertiveness, communications skills, or stress management.

Cooperative Group

A cohesive group in which patients come together to express and share their needs, thoughts, and feelings, and in which they listen to each other. The task of this group is used to promote sharing and listening, and does not seek to produce an end product. The occupational therapist serves as an advisor rather than as a leader. She helps form the group and initiate the task experience, and then becomes a participant who freely shares her thoughts and feelings. The goal of the group is to provide an experience for the patients that helps them to share their thoughts, feelings, values, and common interests, and to gain pleasure and satisfaction from this shared experience. Behavior change is not the focus of the group. Examples are art, music, poetry, or other creative experiences which facilitate the discussion of thoughts and feelings; another example is a values clarification group.

Mature Group

A group experience in which patients independently select, plan, and complete a group task which is time limited and produces a specific end product. The occupational therapist is a group member, and not the identified leader. During the task, the function of the group and group needs have priority over the needs of the individual. The task experience is processed in order to help the patients learn the social-emotional and task roles of the group. The goal of the group is to provide an activity that will allow the individual patient to put aside his needs for the betterment of the group, and to help the group accomplish its goal. During the task, from the group "process" discussion each patient will identify the social-emotional and task roles that they assume. Examples of this are a community transition group or group in the community.

Note: Material used for these descriptions is adapted from Mosey A: *Three Frames of Reference for Mental Health*, Thorofare, NJ: SLACK Inc, 1970 (pp. 201–206), and from Mosey A: *Activities Therapy*, New York: Raven Press, Publishers, 1973 (pp. 120–136).

ACTIVITY GROUPS

Evaluation Group

During an evaluation group, the occupational therapist uses a short term activity to observe the patient's interpersonal skills and response to the activity. The specific areas of function which are evaluated are determined by the frame of reference that is applied. Intervention strategies are not planned during this evaluation experience.

Task Oriented Group

A task group is a group which has a tangible outcome (end product or service). During the group, the patient learns from his interactions with others and the activity. He increases his awareness and understanding of himself and other patients. He learns interpersonal skills, practices new behaviors, and explores the interaction of thoughts, feelings, and behaviors that occur. The occupational therapist helps the patient process the activity experience and actively seeks to change the patient's behavior through the group interaction that occurs.

Developmental Groups

This is a group in which the patient learns group interaction skills through sequential, stage specific activities. The therapist uses activities, which are graded from simple to com-plex and short term to long term, in order to provide progressive challenges which require collaborative effort, the ability to compete, and increased independence in problem-solving and task completion.

Thematic Groups

A thematic group is one in which the therapist uses purposeful activities to help the patients gain knowledge, skills, and attitudes necessary for function in a protective environment. The patient learns activities of daily living, work, and leisure skills through didactic, directive, and supportive experiences.

Topical Groups

Topical groups are ones in which the patient learns to independently use in the community the knowledge, skills, and attitudes gained in a protective environment. The two types of topical groups are (1) anticipatory groups in which patients focus on the future and the performance expectations needed in their future environment; and (2) concurrent groups in which patients focus on the knowledge, skills, and attitudes needed to function in the present roles that the patient has in his community. During these groups, the occupational therapist may prescribe activities and facilitate discussion of role expectations, identify the knowledge and skills needed to identify problems, and promote brainstorming and skill practice for solving problems.

Instrumental Groups

An instrumental group is one in which the occupational therapist uses activities to maintain the patient's present level of function and to promote an optimum level of health.

Note: Material for these descriptions is adapted from Mosey A: *Occupational Therapy—Configuration of a Profession*, New York, Raven Press, 1981, pp. 110–112.

DEFENSE MECHANISMS

Defense mechanisms are unconscious intra-psychic processes by which anxiety-producing information or wishes are kept out of conscious awareness. These processes are used by everyone to some degree, but over-reliance on them ties up libido, tends to distort reality, and reduces the opportunity to see a full range of personal option. These processes keep the individual from knowing himself, from being congruent, and from changing. The most common defense mechanisms are:

Denial

This is the process by which an individual protects himself against painful information by refusing to accept its validity. An example of this is when a person who on first hearing that a loved one has died, refuses to believe it.

Displacement

This is a process by which the individual puts his feelings about one person onto another person or object. An example of this is when a student has had disagreements with a teacher, and then comes home and shouts at his roommate.

Projection

This is a process by which a person attributes to another person the feelings he is really having himself. An example of this is: I am unconsciously angry with you, but I believe that you are angry with me.

Regression

This is a process by which an individual reverts back to a more infantile way of meeting his needs. An example of this is when an individual, feeling overwhelmed by a job and personal setbacks, refuses to go to work, stays in bed, snuggles up under the covers, and seeks to be taken care of.

Rationalization

This is a process by which the individual makes excuses for himself, or justifies his own or someone else's behavior—behavior that would otherwise be considered unacceptable or hurt his self-esteem. An example of this may result when a person is late for a job interview, thereby losing his bid for a job. He may rationalize by telling himself that he did not really want the job. Another example is when a person on a diet may overeat, and then rationalize by telling himself that it was a bad day.

Sublimation

This is a rechanneling of unacceptable impulses into personally and socially acceptable channels. It is considered to be a healthy process. For example, aggressive impulses might be channeled into a game of handball. Freud felt that all artistic endeavor, work, and hobbies were a function of sublimation. In poor mental adjustment there is little capacity for sublimation.

Identification

This is the process by which an individual takes on the qualities or attributes of a person he admires. For example, a little boy wears a Superman cape to emulate his hero or a young lady smokes cigarettes to model after her favorite teacher.

Repression

Repression is a process by which the ego pushes painful or anxiety-producing stimuli out of consciousness. Some repression is necessary to deal with unacceptable wishes. Repression is at the core of many of the other defense mechanisms.

Fixation

This is the process by which the individual gets "stuck" at a stage of psychosocial development because there is anxiety associated with moving to the next stage. An example of this is a young lady who can only carry on a flirtation, superficial relationship with men because of her fear of mature heterosexuality.

Reaction-Formation

This is a process by which the conscious thought and feelings that develop in the ego are just the opposite of unfelt, unconscious thoughts and wishes. For example, a person who is highly pious and overly moral might be responding to unconscious wishes to engage in immoral behavior.

Conversion (or Conversion Reaction)

This is a process by which unconscious wishes or thoughts are repressed, then channeled, and make their appearance via a variety of physical or somatic symptoms. An example of this is when an individual who has an unconscious wish to "walk out on" his spouse develops a hysterical paralysis of the lower limbs.

PERSON DRAWINGS

The pictures in this appendix are presented to exemplify the patient's expression of his or her image and concerns as they are presented in figure drawings. These drawings were used as tools for interaction and were not interpreted by the occupational therapist. They facilitated a shared discussion of self-image, roles, interests, likes and dislikes, and patient concerns.

The Patient and His Environment

Patients may depict their environment or objects within the environment that represent a conflict, concern, or problem that they are experiencing.

Figure F1. The patient (a 15–year-old girl) depicts her dilemma as being between continuing her life style as a runaway and staying at home following the rules of her parents. She drew the "welcome" mat, and stated that she wished there was such a mat at her home.

Figure F2. The patient (a 15–year-old girl) reflects her attitude about her "hold and treat" status (hospital commitment). Her primary concern was her loss of "freedom," rather than the reasons for her hospitalization—drug and alcohol abuse, promiscuity, being overweight, and her parents' refusal to have her return home to live.

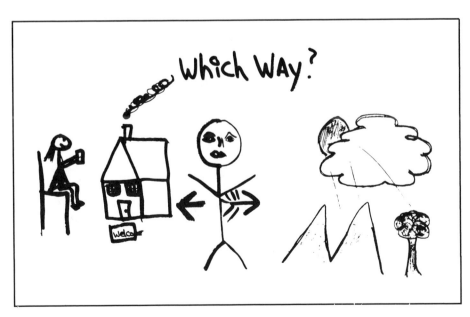

FIGURE F-1.   Dilemma.

Figure F3. The patient (a 20–year-old male) identified himself as a "biker." (A biker is a person who owns a motorcycle and may belong to a particular motorcycle gang or identify with a special group of people. He may choose a transient life style, have an antisocial attitude, and seek power.) This patient was in the hospital for an inability to control his aggression.

Figure F4. The patient (a 30–year-old female) is hospitalized for depression. She states that the chair in her drawing is her only sup-

port and that she needs something to lean on. She expressed feelings of being overwhelmed by the demands of her husband, the responsibilities of her job, and that she had multiple financial concerns.

The Patient and Physical Function

The patient's physical well-being may be seen in patient drawings.

Figure F5. The patient, a 69-year-old male

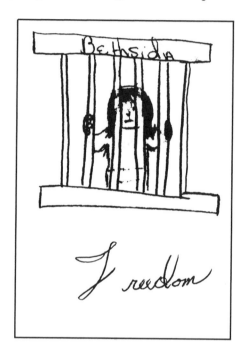

FIGURE F-2.   Hold and treat.

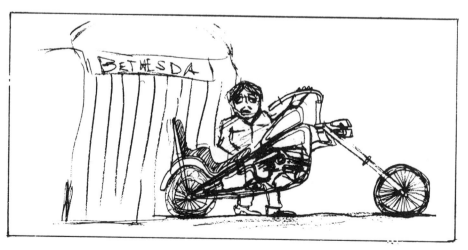

FIGURE F-3.   Biker.

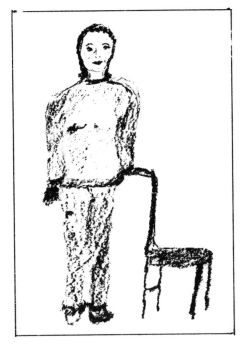

FIGURE F-4.   Chair.

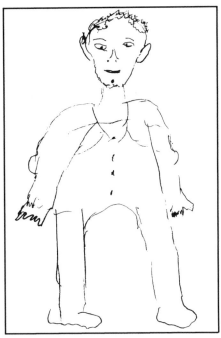

FIGURE F-5.   Organic brain syndrome.

with organic brain syndrome, was hospitalized because of agitation and paranoia. His drawing is typical of one drawn by a patient with organic problems.

Figure F6. The patient (an 18–year-old female) was hospitalized for depression and a suicide attempt. She is hemiplegic due to surgery for removal of a benign tumor. After completing the drawing, she shared her feelings regarding her disability and the hopelessness she felt. Physically, she was more capable than her drawing suggests and than her discussion indicated.

Figure F7. The patient (a 19–year-old female) was hospitalized for anorexia. Her weight at the time of this drawing was 85 pounds. During the discussion which followed this drawing, she verbalized many angry feelings.

The Patient and Symbolic Drawings

The drawings presented in this section are symbolic. Patients who may or may not be reality oriented may choose to express their feelings, concerns, or problems symbolically. Patients who are diagnosed as "psychotic" may have lucid periods. Thus, the patient may be asked to do a self-portrait during the evaluation process, or the drawing may be requested after the patient is stabilized on medications. The occupational therapist may limit the discussion of symbolism if the discussion increases the patient's confusion, promotes agitation, or is otherwise to the detriment of the patient.

Figure F8. The patient (a 30–year-old male) was diagnosed as "psychotic," or not reality oriented. He drew himself as a tree, and ex-

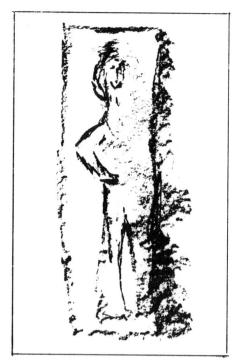

FIGURE F-6.   Hemiplegia.

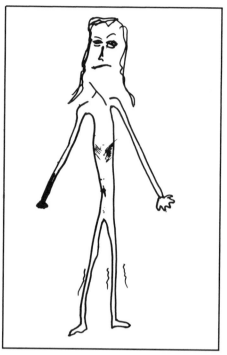

FIGURE F-7.   Anorexia.

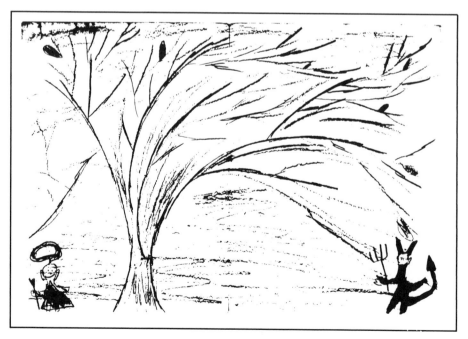

FIGURE F-8.   Tree.

pressed the dichotomy of his conflict in the angel-devil drawings. His discussion focused on issues of right and wrong, good and evil, and God and the devil. The therapist chose to limit the discussion of religious issues and helped him to verbalize his conflicts regarding "right" or "wrong" choices that were affecting his job performance and daily function at home.

Figure F9. The patient (a 19–year-old male) was hospitalized for depression and psychotic episodes due to drug abuse. Through his symbolic self-portrait, he expressed his feelings and identity through his concerns which related to political and social movements.

Figure F10A and F10B. The patients (ages 20 and 30 years old, respectively) were psychotic at the time of the drawings. Each drew herself symbolically and wished to discuss, at length, the symbolism. When this occurs, the therapist must determine the benefits of the discussion to the patient and its usefulness to treatment planning. The therapist may limit the discussion.

Figure F11. The patient (an 18–year-old male) depicted his concerns through symbols that he added to his person drawing. He drew a light bulb and shared his concern with "thoughts that go on in my head"; he described himself as "always getting into trouble," as expressed through "horns" and the "halo" in the drawing.

The Patient and Drawing Emphases

Patients also express concerns and problems through emphases in drawings which may be represented by accentuating body parts, colors used, and pressure of the lines drawn.

Figure F12. The patient (an 18–year-old male) drew body parts to express his concern regarding his male identity and to express "if I'm alive I have a heart."

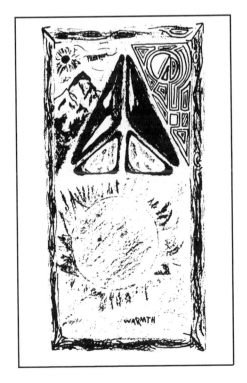

FIGURE F-9. Symbolic rectangle.

Figure F13. The patient (a 28–year-old male) drew his heart and expressed his fear that "something was wrong with his heart." Anxiety was his chief complaint.

Figure F14. The patient (a 16–year-old male) was hospitalized for bipolar depression, manic phase, and verbalized his multiple concerns regarding homosexuality. Note the spontaneous elaboration of the drawing to the right of the main figure.

The Patient and Similarity of Drawings

Figures F15A and F15B. These two drawings were made by two women of triplets (both 19 years old). The women were not in treatment at the same time, but were both hospitalized within the same one and a half year time period. Both were experiencing the adjustment problems of young adulthood.

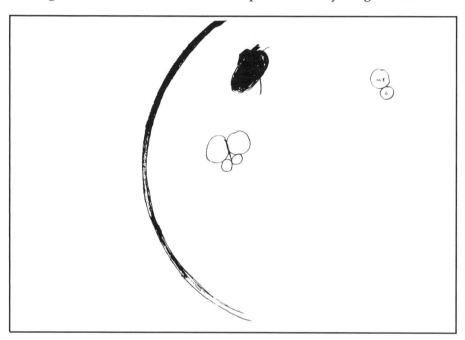

FIGURE F-10A.   Symbolism.

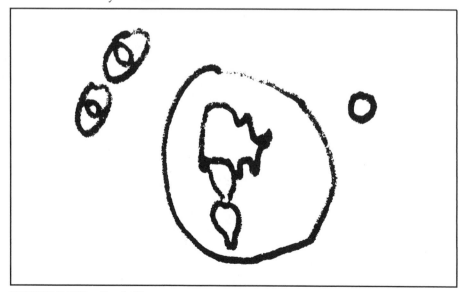

FIGURE F-10B.   Symbolism.

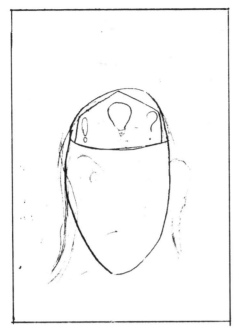

FIGURE F-11.   Light bulb.

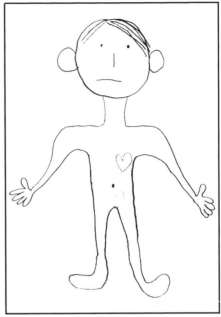

FIGURE F-12.   Heart and male organ.

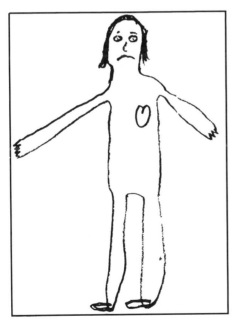

FIGURE F-13.   Heart—anxiety.

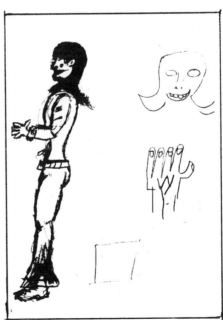

FIGURE F-14.   Homosexuality.

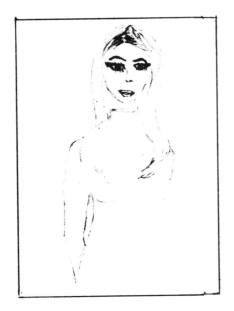

FIGURE F-15A.   Triplets.

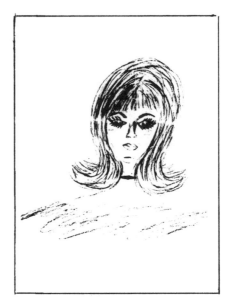

FIGURE F-15B.   Triplets.

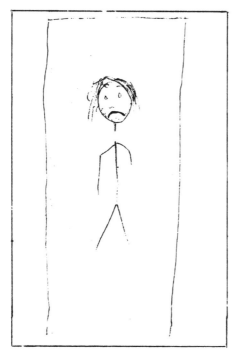

FIGURE F-16.   Depression.

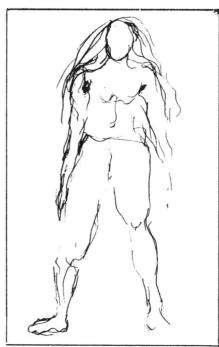

FIGURE F-17.   Suicide.

The Patient and Drawing Ability

The patient need not have artistic ability in order to represent oneself and information that promotes understanding of the patient and his or her problems. Sometimes the patients have creativity that produces a drawing, but they may be unable or unwilling to share views of themselves.

Figure F16. The patient (a 21–year-old man) was hospitalized for depression. He drew a stick figure and verbalized his concerns about "no job and no plans for the future."

Figure F17. The patient (a young woman) was hospitalized for depression, and has artistic ability as depicted in her sketch of a girl. She later committed suicide.

Figures F18A and F18B. The patient (a 15–year-old female) was hospitalized for drug abuse, psychotic episodes, running away from home, and school truancy. She has artistic ability, which is demonstrated in both of her drawings. The symbolic picture was completed shortly after admission to the hospital, and the picture of the young girl was done after six months of treatment. Through symbolism, she discussed wanting to be "like the virgin to crush out all evil . . . like Robin Hood to be able to give to the poor . . . give freedom to men and women."

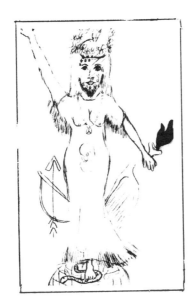

FIGURE F-18A.   Girl at admission.

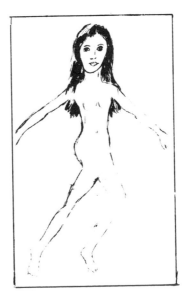

FIGURE F-18B.   Girl after six months.

SAMPLE OF
PSYCHOEDUCATIONAL COURSE MODEL
IN OCCUPATIONAL THERAPY —
INDEPENDENT LIVING IN THE COMMUNITY

Course Modules

General Budget Principles
Community Residence
Preparing for the Move
Community Resources
Money Management
Meal Planning and Preparation
Friends and Community Network
Recreation

Sample Module—Preparing for the Move

Goals include establishing knowledge, developing and practicing skills, and identifying and clarifying values and attitudes.

Knowledge:
1. The patient will identify the furniture, equipment, and supplies needed for his community residence.
2. The patient will identify the public services needed for his residence, and the advance arrangements needed for telephone, gas, electric services, and newspaper.
3. The patient will identify the community resources near his residence, and the nearest physician, dentist, medical emergency serv-

ices, supermarket, shopping center, discount stores, library, and recreation facility.

Skill:
4. The patient will make an itemized list of moving costs.

Attitude:
5. The patient will identify the value of planning and budgeting to reduce stress and ease his move into the community.

Learning Activities

1. Conduct a brainstorming session in which patients in the group make a list of the possible furniture, equipment, and supplies needed for an apartment.
2. Using the general list compiled during brainstorming, each patient will make an individual list for his residence, identifying bathroom, kitchen, bedroom, and living room needs.
3. Using newspapers, the *Sears Catalog, Montgomery Ward Catalog,* or other consumer information, each patient will list the cost of each item on the supply-equipment list and determine the total cost of his apartment needs.
4. Each patient will then evaluate independently, or with the assistance of the thera-

pist or his peers, the compatibility of the furniture, supply, and equipment costs with his monthly budget. (The budget would have been established during a previous module, "Budgeting Principles.")

5. Conduct a brainstorming session in which patients in the group make a list of the necessary community facilities, advanced arrangements, and costs for these facilities, i.e., telephone, gas, lights, and television.

6. Using the telephone directory, city maps, and newspapers, the patients will learn to use the physician and dentist referral resource, and identify where supermarkets, secondhand furniture stores, shopping centers, discount stores, church, and library are located.

7. Assign as homework that two or more patients visit some of the community resources previously listed in learning activity six.

Learning Resources:

(Examples of materials that may be used by the therapist during class experiences.)

1. Handout—Budget format for itemized lists and costs;

2. Newspapers, magazines, catalogues, and telephone directory;

3. Sample utility bills to explain facility costs; and

4. Mover's pamphlet from local moving company.

Knowledge Gained:

Budget principles;

Community resources; and

Basic principles of home management.

Skills Practiced or Learned:

1. Group and individual decision making;

2. Task oriented problem solving;

3. Budget analysis and implementation; and

4. Communication skills.

Note: The patient's needs and abilities, the group composition, and the treatment setting will determine learning goals, course modules, the learning activities, and the learning resources that the occupational therapist may use. These are not all inclusive, but are a representative sample.

This sample educational model is based upon information shared with the authors by Ms. Judith Talbot, OTR, West Haven Veterans Administration Hospital, New Haven, Connecticut.

SEVEN ADAPTIVE SKILLS

Perceptual-Motor Skill

The ability to receive, integrate, and organize sensory stimuli in a manner which allows for the planning of purposeful movement.

1. The ability to integrate primitive postural reflexes, to react appropriately to vestibular stimuli, to maintain a balance between the tactile subsystems, to perceive form, and to be aware of auditory stimuli.
2. The ability to control extraocular musculature, to integrate the two sides of the body, and to focus on auditory stimuli.
3. The ability to perceive visual and auditory figure-ground, to be aware of body parts and their relationships, and to plan gross motor movements.
4. The ability to perceive space, to plan fine motor movements, and to discriminate among auditory stimuli.
5. The ability to discriminate between right and left, and to remember auditory stimuli.
6. The ability to use abstract concepts, to scan, integrate, and synthesize auditory stimuli, and to give auditory feedback.

Cognitive Skill

The ability to perceive, represent, and organize objects, events, and their relationships in a manner which is considered appropriate by one's cultural group.

1. The ability to use inherent behavioral patterns for environmental interaction.
2. The ability to interrelate visual, manual, auditory, and oral responses.
3. The ability to attend to the environmental consequence of actions with interest, to represent objects in an exoceptual manner, to experience objects, to act on the bases of egocentric causality, and to seriate events in which the self is involved.
4. The ability to establish a goal and intentionally carry out means, to recognize the independent existence of objects, to interpret signs, to imitate new behavior, to apprehend the influence of space, and to perceive other objects as partially causal.
5. The ability to use trial and error problem solving, to use tools, to perceive variability in spatial positions, to seriate events in which the self is not involved, and to perceive the causality of other objects.
6. The ability to represent objects in an image manner, to make believe, to infer a cause given its effect, to act on the bases of combined spatial relations, to attribute omnipotence to others, and to perceive objects as permanent in time and place.
7. The ability to represent objects in an endoceptual manner, to differentiate between thought and action, and to recognize the need for causal sources.
8. The ability to represent objects in a denotative manner, to perceive the viewpoint of others, and to decenter.
9. The ability to represent objects in a conno-

tative manner, to use formal logic, and to work in the realm of the hypothetical.

Drive-Object Skill

The ability to control drives and select objects in such a manner as to ensure adequate need satisfaction.

1. The ability to form a discontinuous, libidinal object relationship.
2. The ability to form a continuous, part-libidinal object relationship.
3. The ability to invest aggressive drive in an external object.
4. The ability to transfer libidinal drive to objects other than the primary object.
5. The ability to invest libidinal energy in appropriate abstract objects and to control aggressive drive.
6. The ability to engage in total and diffuse libidinal object relationships.

Dyadic Interaction Skill

The ability to participate in a variety of dyadic relationships.

1. The ability to enter into association relationships.
2. The ability to interact in an authority relationship.
3. The ability to interact in a chum relationship.
4. The ability to enter into a peer, authority relationship.
5. The ability to enter into an intimate relationship.
6. The ability to engage in a nurturing relationship.

Group Interaction Skill

The ability to be a productive member of a variety of primary groups.

1. The ability to participate in a parallel group.
2. The ability to participate in a project group.
3. The ability to participate in an egocentric-cooperative group.
4. The ability to participate in a cooperative group.
5. The ability to participate in a mature group.

Self-Identity Skill

The ability to perceive the self as an autonomous, holistic, and acceptable object which has permanence and continuity over time.

1. The ability to perceive the self as a worthy object.
2. The ability to perceive the assets and limitations of the self.
3. The ability to perceive the self as self-directed.
4. The ability to perceive the self as a productive, contributing member of a social system.
5. The ability to perceive the self.
6. The ability to perceive the aging process of the self in a rational manner.

Sexual Identity Skill

The ability to perceive one's sexual nature as good, and to participate in a heterosexual relationship which is oriented to the mutual satisfaction of sexual needs.

1. The ability to accept and act upon the bases of one's pregenital sexual nature.
2. The ability to accept sexual maturation as a positive growth experience.
3. The ability to give and receive sexual gratification.
4. The ability to enter into a sustained heterosexual relationship.
5. The ability to accept physiological and psychological changes that occur at the time of the climacteric.

Reproduced with permission. Mosey A: *Three Frames of Reference for Mental Health.* Thorofare, New Jersey: SLACK Inc., 1970, pp. 134–136.

Note: In Mosey A: *Psychosocial Components of Occupational Therapy*, New York, Raven Press, 1986 there are six adaptive skills: sensory integration skill, cognitive skill, dyadic interaction skill, group interaction skill, self-identity skill, and sexuality identity skill.

COMMONLY ASSESSED SENSORY, MOTOR, AND COGNITIVE TASKS

Visual Perception:
Focus on a single stimulus
Scan a visual field
Identify shapes and colors
Identify common objects, shown individually
Identify object (from photograph or in actual presentation) from a variety of perspectives
Identify objects or shapes depicted in distracting visual field
Describe the purpose of objects viewed
Remember visual data

Visual-Motor Synthesis:
Write familiar schemes (i.e., name)
Copy simple shapes
Duplicate with blocks a two-dimensional or three-dimensional pattern
Draw a designated object without the aid of a pattern to copy

Auditory Perception:
Comprehend familiar schemes, i.e., "Hello, what is your name?"
Localize where sounds are coming from
Attend to one auditory stimulus and screen out irrelevant ones
Comprehend complex or new auditory scheme
Recall auditory information

Auditory Motor Synthesis:
Follow simple, familiar commands (i.e., wave goodbye or shake hands)
Duplicate a rhythm with finger (or pencil); change rhythm as therapist changes it
Follow commands, less familiar schemes, i.e., touch your right elbow with your left hand

Spatial Relationship Synthesis:
Follow direction to go left, right, up or down
Mimic hand directions of interviewer
Deal with spatial ideas (i.e., tell time, draw hands on a clock)
Place objects above, below or to the right of
Understand arithmetic computations

Body-Awareness Synthesis:
Cross body midline in reaching, and in tasks
Name body parts
Indicate where body parts are in space (eyes closed)

| | Imitate postures of interviewer sitting across from or next to the individual assessed |
| | Draw an integrated person-symbol |

Vestibular-Kinesthetic Synthesis:

Maintain balance (one leg and two legs, eyes open)
Maintain balance (one and two legs, eyes closed)
Maintain trunk balance when interviewer applies pressure (individual seated and standing)
Walk straight line (forward and backward)

Tactile Perception:

Recognize tactile qualities (cold, warm, pressure, or pain)
Locate tactile stimuli applied to body
Indicate specified fingers
Recognize textures (rough, smooth, or bumpy)
Discriminate objects by shape and feel

Motor Synthesis:

Initiate and stop movement of large muscle bodies
Use both sides of the body in purposeful movement
Cross body midline
Accomplish gross-motor purposeful movement (i.e., jump, hop, skip, clap, and catch a large ball)
Use smaller muscle groups in purposeful movement (i.e., write name or open lock with key)
Persist in motor task (i.e., keep hand in air until therapist says to put it down)

Cognition/Attention:

Maintain eye contact
Attend to visual stimulus
Attend to interviewer's verbal directions
Attend to conversation in a group structure
Sustain involvement in a task (1 minute, 10 minutes, 1/2 hour)

Cognition/Concentration:

Sustain involvement in a task (1 minute, 10 minutes, 1/2 hour)
Able to subtract from 100 by 7's or from 30 by 3's

Cognition/Orientation:
  (To person)

Answers: What is your name? Your occupation? How old are you? Do you remember who I am? What I do? Who is that person? (Point to significant other)

  (To place)

Answers: Where are you now? What is the name of this hospital (if not at home)?

  (To time)

Answers: What day (of the week) is it today?
What is the calendar date?
What is the season of the year?

Cognition/Knowledge:
  (See also "memory" and "problem solving" tasks)

Seriates numbers
Sorts objects according to same and different
Discusses simple current events
Does simple math
Reads (therapist begins with single words, and then reads phrases and sentences)
Writes

	Demonstrates knowledge of motor process(es), procedures, and social expectations in daily encounters
Cognition/Insight and Judgment:	States why in treatment
	Describes strengths, limitations, and needs
	Discusses family's feelings about treatment
	Describes the view others have of him or her
	Interprets proverb
	Demonstrates judgment in tasks of daily living, i.e., dresses and grooms appropriately; clothing is clean; asks for assistance from the OTR or nurse as needed; eats adequate meals
	Uses tools appropriately (observes safety precautions)
	Follows norms of social politeness

Cognition/Memory:
  (Some common examples,
  illustrative only)

Personal (and long term):
Gives accurate personal history
Able to describe events of last 24 hours prior to treatment (when an appropriate question)
Can answer: what did you do last Christmas, who were you with, and where were you? (Therapist can use any significant day)
What was for breakfast this morning?
What did we do in therapy yesterday?

Impersonal (and short term):
Remembers three unrelated items: five minutes to 1/2 hour
Remembers content of paragraph he reads: 2 to 15 minutes

Procedural-motoric (long term):
Demonstrates how to dial a phone or find a phone number
Demonstrates how to play checkers, play badminton, or pot a plant (if this was a skill formerly in his or her learning repertoire)

Sensory-perceptual (short or long term):
Demonstrates way to hospital room (or other familiar site)
Can find bathroom, dining room, or other landmark in the hospital or his or her home
Accurately recalls what is heard or seen in the environment

Cognition/Problem-Solving Tasks:
  (Combines knowledge,
  memory, and insight in
  higher cognitive function)

Generates one (or more) solutions to:
obtain an unknown phone number, trace a route on a city map, read a bus schedule, and describe how to get from one place to another
Balances a simple checkbook ledger
Makes change
States what he or she would do in a medical emergency
Constructs a 3–D box, given a piece of paper, tape, and scissors

Analysis of Activity Complexity

Parameters	Less Complex	More Complex
Sensory	Requires attention to primarily one sensory mode	Requires multisensory integration
	Requires little attention to detail	Requires attention to detail or subtle change
	Sensory input given slowly and boldly	Sensory input given quickly and less boldly
	Errors easily perceptible	Errors difficult to discern
Temporal	Can be completed in short time	Task extends over time
	New information given slowly	New information given quickly
	Task can be done slowly	Task to be done quickly
	Allows opportunity for pause or rest	Little opportunity for rest
Motor	Requires gross motor skill	Requires fine motor skill
	High unilateral demand	High bilateral demand
	Makes no use or simple use of tools; use of familiar tools	Complex use of tools; unfamiliar tools
	Highly repetitive	Requires many changes in motor response
	Done slowly	Done quickly
Cognitive	Involves only familiar schemes	Introduces new schemes (novel schemes)
	High degree of predictability	Little predictability
	Can be learned through imitation	Requires creativity and spontaneity
	Uses knowledge already acquired	Requires assimilation of new information
	Depends on ability to perceive concrete relationships	Depends on ability for abstraction
	Cause-effect is obvious	Cause-effect is not obvious
	Requires little memory	Requires sustained memory
	Demands little attention and concentration	Requires attention and concentration
External vs. Internal Control	Obvious benchmarks for passage of time	No obvious benchmarks for time passage
	Has obvious rules	Rules not obvious
	Has written or verbal instructions	Instruction retained in one's memory
	Others signal when activity is started and stopped	Person must signal self to stop or start
	Errors pointed out by others	Self perceives errors
Social	Social group limited to two to four members	Social discourse in large group
	Group has familiar others	Group of unfamiliar others
	Task-oriented	Process oriented
	Low expectation for self-disclosure	High expectation for self-disclosure
	Low expectation for cooperation and sharing	High expectation for cooperation and sharing
	Social group has one permanent leader	Changing leadership
	Group homogeneous	Group heterogeneous
	Minimal change in membership	Social membership changes frequently
	Social "rules" obvious	Social rules subtle

THE APRAXIAS, AGNOSIAS AND APHASIAS

Apraxia

Apraxia is the impairment of voluntary or purposeful movement not attributable to muscle deficit, or lack of comprehension.

1. *Ideomotor apraxia*—The person understands what the therapist asks the patient to do, but cannot organize the sequence of behavior necessary to accomplish the task, i.e., he or she may be able to "automatically" put on glasses when picking up a magazine, but cannot follow the therapist's request that he or she (intentionally) put on glasses.
2. *Ideational apraxia*—The person cannot create the idea of what motor behavior is desired, i.e., when asked to "button your sweater," he or she cannot create the idea of what is meant by this. However, well established automatic responses may be retained.
3. *Constructional apraxia*—The person can demonstrate isolated purposeful movement, but cannot put them together; he or she cannot apply skills to a new situation, i.e., the individual is unable to construct a "star" from matches, or draw a clock to show a depicted time, or to assemble Lego© blocks according to a desired pattern.
4. *Dressing apraxia*—The person has an inability or difficulty with dressing; he or she does not know which limb goes in which part of his or her clothing, and has a problem with sequencing the events in dressing.

Agnosia

Agnosia is an impairment in object recognition not due to a deficit in the sensory systems or ignorance.

1. *Visual agnosia*—The person cannot name objects by sight alone (he or she may be able to describe their attributes). (Object recognition will typically be better for "real" objects than for "pictures" of objects.)
2. *Tactile agnosia*—The person cannot recognize an object by touch alone.
3. *Prosopagnosia*—The person is unable to recognize familiar faces (may be able to identify familiar others when he or she hears the voice).
4. *Finger agnosia*—The person is unable to name his or her own fingers or those of the therapist.
5. *Spatial agnosia*—The person experiences spatial disorientation, he or she is unable to find the way around familiar surroundings, and the person loses understanding of directionality. This may include inability to locate one's own body parts.
6. *Unilateral neglect*—Related to body agnosia, the person ignores one side of the body, or fails to use it upon command, i.e., when asked to comb his or her hair, the person combs only one side, or to put on his shoes, he or she puts on only one shoe. The neglected body side may be used appropriately in spontaneous, coordinated acts.

Aphasia

Aphasia is a speech or language disorder, evidenced in problems with word choice, grammar, or comprehension, and is not due to motor disturbance or ignorance.

1. *Wernicke's aphasia* (also known as receptive aphasia). In this case, the person does not understand what is being said to him. His or her speech may be fluid and well articulated, but is out of context and is senseless, and he or she has associated difficulty with naming objects, reading, and writing. This condition leads to unusual and even bizarre behavior.
2. *Broca's aphasia*—In this case, the person has limited ability for verbal expression. This can range from a complete "loss of words" to mild problems with word finding. The written and spoken word are well comprehended. Residual speech is more likely to contain nouns and verbs. Automatic phrases like "good morning" may be retained. Reading, writing, and calculation are impaired.
3. *Global aphasia*—The most severe aphasia. There is a major deficit in word comprehension and a lack of meaningful speech.
4. *Conduction aphasia*—The person can produce meaningful spontaneous speech, but cannot repeat back what is told him.
5. *Transcortical aphasia*—The person can repeat back what he or she hears, but has difficulty with spontaneous speech production.

The information in this table is compiled from the following:

Strub R, Black FW: *Organic Brain Syndromes: An Introduction to Neurobehavioral Disorders.* Philadelphia: F.A. Davis Company, 1981, pp. 217–236.

Holden U, Woods R: *Reality Orientation: Psychological Approaches to the Confused Elderly.* Edinburgh: Churchill Livingstone, Incorporated, 1982, pp. 114–121.

Luria A: *Higher Cortical Functions in Man.* New York: Basic Books, Incorporated, 1966.

Williams M: *Brain Damage, Behavior, and the Mind.* New York: John Wiley & Sons, Incorporated, 1979, pp. 64–109.

Appendix K

TASK CHECKLIST

Directions: Circle number in appropriate column and add for total.	Rarely / Sometimes / Often			Circle rater/student familiarity − 1 2 3 4 5 +	Rarely / Sometimes / Often			Name _____ Rater _____ Date _____	Rarely / Sometimes / Often		
I. ENTRY LEVEL				**IV. RELATIONSHIP LEVEL**				**VII. ACHIEVEMENT LEVEL**			
States desire to attend	0	1	2	Seeks approval	0	1	2	Assumes self-responsibility	0	1	2
Stays through classes	0	1	2	Accepts feedback	0	1	2	Completes tasks	0	1	2
Hallucinates/delusional	2	1	0	Is outgoing and friendly	0	1	2	Manages stress	0	1	2
Is easily distracted	2	1	0	Interacts with peers	0	1	2	Is able to abstract	0	1	2
Stays on topic/coherent	0	1	2	Seeks reinforcement	0	1	2	Is self-motivated	0	1	2
Is disruptive/combative	2	1	0	Works productively 1-1	0	1	2	Generalizes	0	1	2
Speaks & acts at normal pace	0	1	2	Gives compliments	0	1	2	Competent in ADL skills	0	1	2
Observes limits	0	1	2	Receives compliments	0	1	2	Makes discharge plans	0	1	2
Affect is appropriate	0	1	2	Uses staff appropriately	0	1	2	Seeks independence	0	1	2
Threatens suicide	2	1	0	Shares feelings with others	0	1	2	Generates + self-statements	0	1	2
TOTAL		2	0	TOTAL		1	9	TOTAL		1	0
II. ACCEPTANCE LEVEL				**V. EXPLORATORY LEVEL**							
Attentive	0	1	2	Asks questions	0	1	2				
Suspicious, guarded	2	1	0	Seeks new situations	0	1	2				
Answers questions	0	1	2	Makes suggestions	0	1	2				
Engages others	0	1	2	Tries new behaviors	0	1	2				
Is rude or indifferent	2	1	0	Requests feedback	0	1	2				
Keeps appointments	0	1	2	Initiates activities	0	1	2				
Withdraws/lacks trust	2	1	0	Reveals feelings	0	1	2				
Refuses feedback	2	1	0	Considers goals	0	1	2				
Denies problems	2	1	0	Role plays	0	1	2				
Accepts contacts with staff	2	1	0	Expresses concern for others	0	1	2				
TOTAL		2	0	TOTAL		1	8				
III. ORDER LEVEL				**VI. MASTERY LEVEL**							
Appears neat and orderly	0	1	2	Makes decisions	0	1	2				
Follows rules	0	1	2	Problem solves	0	1	2				
Adheres to schedule	0	1	2	Exercises good judgment	0	1	2				
Acts impulsively	2	1	0	Sets treatment goals	0	1	2				
Organizes tasks	0	1	2	Self-reinforces	0	1	2				
Is rigid or compulsive	2	1	0	Generates alternatives	0	1	2				
Follows directions	0	1	2	Verbalizes spontaneously	0	1	2				
Complies with treatment	0	1	2	Is able to relax	0	1	2				
Is punctual	0	1	2	Exerts self-control	0	1	2				
Attends regularly	0	1	2	Takes notes/completes	0	1	2				
TOTAL		2	0	assignments							
				TOTAL		1	4				

SUMMARY GRAPH

	I	II	III	IV	V	VI	VII
20							
19							
18							
17							
16							
15							
14							
13							
12							
11							
10							
9							
8							
7							
6							
5							
4							
3							
2							
1							
0							

Reprinted with permission from the *American Journal of Occupational Therapy*. Lillie, M.D., Armstrong H.E. Contributions to the development of psychoeducational approaches to mental health service, 36(7):438-443, 1982 p. 441.

Appendix L

THE SUICIDAL PATIENT

Introduction

The problem of suicide cannot be understood apart from the theoretical frameworks that have been summarized in this text. Depending on one's theoretical orientation, suicide will be understood in terms of given compatible assumptions regarding the etiology of dysfunction, the general nature of the person, and activity and remediation. The additional information that follows, however, is provided to help the reader become more familiar with some of the general knowledge that has been gained across the social sciences regarding suicide as a special problem.

We include the following information because we have, in our work with students, found that the new (and sometimes seasoned) therapist often responds to the suicidal patient with much anxiety. The information provided here may help the reader to use and appraise his or her own treatment assumptions and to assist the therapist to understand and respond to the needs of the suicidal patient. We hope this information will be useful, regardless of the theoretical framework favored. We recognize that not every treatment guideline proposed in the ensuing discussion is equally compatible with all treatment frameworks. Where we create disagreement, we encourage the reader to engage in dialogue with colleagues.

The Need for Information

At some point, the occupational therapist is likely to become involved with a patient who is considering suicide. These individuals may be psychiatric patients or persons who are coping with physical loss or limitations, as well as with family concerns. The therapist may be the first to recognize the suicide wish, or the patient may be in treatment because the severity of his or her depression is recognized. We agree with the recommendation of the Center for Studies of Suicide Prevention, National Institute of Mental Health,[30] that all individuals in health fields have core information regarding suicide—information that includes suicide theory, suicide predictors, and basic concepts in suicide prevention.[31] Even if health professionals are not directly providing treatment to suicidal individuals, they need to know the resources available in their own communities; resources that can respond to the needs of the individual during the crisis phase—as well as be available later for support. The student who has not already done so is encouraged to participate in courses or seminars designed to enhance his or her understanding and skills in the area of suicide prevention.

Current Understanding of Suicide

Suicide is the deliberate self-inflicted termination of one's life. In contemporary literature, it is regarded as existing on one end of a broad continuum of what are termed self-destructive or life-threatening behaviors.[40,41,43] It follows that, while taking a gun to one's head is clearly self-destructive, one also can discern the self-destructive potential of forgetting to take one's insulin, if diabetic or drinking alcohol to excess. Many patients who eventually make a clear suicide attempt have a prior history of self-destructive behavior.† Many individuals who ultimately die of disease may, in retrospect, be viewed as having taken quite active steps to hasten their own death. Although the discussion of suicide theory and prevention in this text focuses on the more obvious suicide behaviors and expressed plans to take one's own life, the therapist will undoubtedly encounter equally troubling instances of less clear, yet very self-destructive behavior in the patients for whom he or she cares.

Suicide No Longer Seen as an Indicator of Mental Illness

Although it was once generally believed that individuals did not try to take their own life unless they were mentally ill, that theme is no longer evident in contemporary suicide literature. Rather, the wish to die, even if a transient desire that is not well developed, is conceived or experienced by most persons at some time in their lives. A suicide wish, even if well developed, is not perceived as a sign of mental illness as such. However, when there are physical or emotional problems, the risk of suicide becomes much greater.

Past Perspectives on Suicide

Suicide has been related to many emotional states: depression, anger, guilt, hopelessness and apathy. Suicide and suicide attempts have been conceived as a wish to sleep, a wish for

psychological rebirth, a way to become immortal, and a way to escape the unbearable.†

For a long time, the traditional Freudian psychoanalytical posture regarding suicide dominated the literature and generally dictated the treatment response. Briefly stated, Freud believed that depression is a response to the loss of a significant love object. Object loss may be actual separation from the object, or at a lesser level, inability to be as dependent on the loved person as one wishes; it elicits conscious or unconscious rage. This anger is turned inward against the self in an act of self-destruction.[12,16,35] Currently, less emphasis is placed on the role of hostility, whereas hopelessness and loss of self-esteem are given more focus. Further, as behavioral theory, existential-humanism, social and cognitive psychology continue to affect suicide theory as well as general psychosocial treatment they have significantly modified the view of health, stress, distress, and helping in response to suicide. Overall, there has been more emphasis given to the relationship of the suicidal individual within the whole social milieu, the individual's patterns of coping in all areas of his life, and the conscious and cognitive components of the individual's actions.[15,24,28,38,39,40,41]

Physiological States and Suicide

Although not conclusive, much recent study has been to better understand the relationship of depression and stress on biochemical changes in the body. Those substances of special interest have been the neurotransmitter substances in the central nervous system, especially the catecholamines (norepinephrine and dopamine) and the indoleamine serotonin.[6,14,24] The focus on the biochemical or or-

---

†Self-destructive refers here to behaviors that may lead to death and not to self-mutilating behaviors such as superficial cutting and burning oneself with cigarettes. These behaviors are viewed as having a different psychological purpose.

‡Klopfer[20] discusses the Jungian perspective as one in which attempted suicide is viewed as a move by the ego to start over in a symbolic rebirth. This perspective is not to be confused with a literal interpretation of rebirth through reincarnation. Although not cognizant of Jungian theory, some individuals have, after a brush with death, described the feeling that they had been given a second chance and felt reborn.

ganic manifestations of suicidal depression goes along with the strong re-emergence in psychiatry of interest in the brain, as we have discussed previously in our text.

Orienting to Suicide Prevention

Above and beyond the personality of the suicidal individual, three contextual dimensions of suicide bear directly on the understanding and prevention of suicide:

1. Suicide crisis is an acute, not chronic state, usually measured in hours or days, not months or years. Although many individuals have a life history of self-destructive behavior, or make many suicide threats or attempts during a lifetime, the actual crisis that occurs when one seriously contemplates decisive action is either alleviated or the person makes an attempt, in a short period of time. This perspective on suicide as a crisis problem has significantly affected the current approach to suicide across a variety of theoretical treatment frameworks. This is not to say that all suicidal individuals receive only brief, crisis treatment, as many suicidal individuals experience a suicide crisis in the context of general stress, physical or psychological, that dictates long-term treatment. The acute phase of treatment will focus on the person's present experiencing of crisis. The alleviation of intense symptoms is sought, success is nurtured, and the therapist often becomes more directive and parental.†

2. The death wish is viewed by virtually all students of human nature as ambivalent. The paradigm of suicide is not merely a matter of wanting to die or not wanting to die but rather one in which there appears often to be both a desire to die and a wish to live, or be rescued.

3. Most suicidal events are dyadic, that is, there is often a significant other person about whom the individual is thinking when he or she considers dying. This significant other may be someone whom the person wishes to make take notice or punish, or someone whose burden he or she wishes to lessen. The significant other may be someone already dead whom the individual wishes to join.[35]

Demography of Suicide

Suicidologists have attempted to correlate statistical or demographical data in an attempt to identify high-risk individuals.[7–9,21,22,36,42,43] Authors in this field emphasize that such demographical information may be misleading because 1) it does not accurately reflect failed suicide attempts, and 2) many deaths that were in fact suicide are not identified as such. For example, such deaths may be covered up by family members or members of the community because of the stigma attached to suicide and because of the punitive laws and insurance disclaimers pertaining to suicide.

The following data are frequently cited:

Age: The most statistically significant and consistent differential in suicide rates is between men and women. The rate is from two to seven times greater for men than for women.[21,29]

Sex: The second most significant, relatively consistent factor relates to age. The suicide rate of white males tends to increase consistently with age, the highest rate of suicide being among the eldest males. The suicide rate for white females increases until about the age of 55, then decreases slightly thereafter.[42] It should be noted that although the rate among young people is still very low in comparison to other previously mentioned groups, it has become one of the leading causes of death in this age group.[42]

---

†Therapists who follow a Rogerian, nondirective approach do not necessarily make the shift to a directive approach. They continue to believe in the essential health of the individual and to base their therapeutic actions accordingly.

Race: The suicide rate of blacks is less than half that of whites. Whereas suicide rates for whites increases with age, the rate for blacks increases through ages 25 to 29 and then declines.[36]

Social Involvement: Any factors that lessen social contact tend to increase suicide risk. These factors include death of spouse, living alone, emotional isolation within a marriage, unemployment, and low participation in social groups.[29,43]

Health Factors: Poor physical or emotional health is correlated to an increased rate of suicide. Poor health includes chronic or acute health problem, a history of emotional or mental disorder, and substance abuse. Alcoholism (25% of all suicides have been related to alcohol dependence) and manic depressive episodes have been especially implicated.[8,25,26,33,43]

Judgment: Anything known to decrease the ability of an individual to exert sound judgment increases the risk of suicide. Judgment may be diminished by high emotionality, cognitive dysfunction, organic mental disorder, intoxication, and sleep or food deprivation.[29]

Other factors known to correlate statistically with suicide include a family history of suicide, early parent loss, and a history of previous attempts.[34]

Seeing Beyond Statistics

Although the preceding factors may be of special significance to those attempting to identify high-risk individuals, these findings should not be construed as a means for deciding whether or not an individual will succeed at suicide. When dealing with individuals in one's own practice, statistics may not bear out. Certainly, the emotional character of the individual is of critical importance. However, no pat profiles or statistics can assure us that our patient will be safe from his or her own self-destruction. When an individual's hopelessness is great enough by his or her own measures, suicide looms as a possibility.

Characteristic Emotion and Cognition of Suicide

Depression is frequently referred to as the key emotion of suicide, but depression may be a misleading indicator. Severe depression, as exemplified by both physical and emotional lassitude, may leave an individual too lethargic to carry out a suicide wish. Suicide may be attempted. Depression is lifted and energy returns. Other emotional and cognitive factors that are emphasized in the literature are:[2,17,27,35,36,40,41]

1. *Hopelessness:* A diminished self-esteem most often leads to hopelessness. Not only is the individual in a situation that seems unredeemable, as may occur with chronic illness, he or she frequently feels shame, disgrace, and impoverishment of life itself.[35] Especially significant is the impact of loss— loss of a loved one, a part of the self, or self-esteem. A person who loses the ability to walk and holds no hope that this function will return may see suicide as a way out of a hopeless situation. When a loved one will not come back, suicide may be a means to escape that reality or to try to force the other to realize how much pain he or she has caused.

   Closely related to hopelessness is a disturbance in motivation. Although the dynamics of motivation are subject to interpretation according to theoretical framework, it is evident that many suicidal patients are able to produce actions on their own behalf, but they no longer experience the desire to do so. Suicide preoccupation is thereby an immobilizing influence.

2. *Rigidity:* Frequently, the individual committing suicide is regarded by others as relatively inflexible and unable to shift roles. He or she is unable to perceive alternatives, keeping the self in a mold that others are blamed for creating.

   Rigidity is often demonstrated in the thinking of the suicidal individual. There is a tendency toward polar or **dichotomous**

thinking; that is, the individual tends to think in terms of right or wrong, moral-immoral, always or never.[27] When involved in activity, the person may be able to see only task involvement as resulting in success or failure, not in terms of enjoying the process or the opportunities for socialization that it affords. Such thinking reduces the ability for effective problem-solving, and especially for compromise.

3. *Commitment*: Many suicidal individuals have high goals or aspirations, whether occupational or relational. These expectations cannot be moderated, and when they are not met, a sense of failure develops.

4. *Failure*: The individual feels that he or she has failed to live up to personal, often high expectations, and can perceive no other standards as viable. Failure may be task related (e.g., being unable to hold down the right kind of job or get into the college of one's choice). Failure in a simple task—for example, being unable to complete an occupational therapy project—may be viewed as a blow to the esteem as much as failure in a life task (e.g., gaining employment) when the individual uses idiosyncratic logic. Failure may also be relationship oriented (e.g., failure to be a good mother, inability to sustain the interest and attention of a spouse, or inability to engage with friends comfortably). Guilt is a frequent adjunct to failure. For example, the individual feels guilty because he or she thinks that personal behavior has disappointed others or perceives the self as a burden to others.

5. *Shame*: Individuals experience shame when their failures are made public. When one loses a job or fails school, the failure is no longer private. A loss of self-esteem and a loss of pride develop. This sense of shame may be a distorted response because the individual may assume that others have a negative opinion of him or her when they may not.

6. *Isolation*: Isolation may precede or become an integral part of the suicide picture. The person with few significant others in life is already at greater risk. Additionally, with the loss of self-esteem and hope, the individual emphasizes the relative strength and success of others and his or her own lack of significance. There is also a kind of cognitive isolation in which the individual, even if with others, feels increasingly: "No one can know how I really feel and I am really different from everyone else." Increased withdrawal from others develops, which lessens the potential support others might give and to reduce the opportunity for positive experiencing.

7. *Anger*: Although anger does not necessarily cause suicide, it is often present in the person who attempts suicide. Anger may appear as overt, acting out behavior, or may seem to be hidden. Anger may relate to shame, as when the individual concludes, "Because I am angry, I am not worth being cared about."

8. *Perception of time*: Several authors have noted that the suicidal individual is more present oriented.[3,5,13,27] These individuals find it difficult to project themselves into the future and imagine what would happen "if." In addition, Neuringer[27] found evidence that time, in the present, is perceived as moving very quickly. The self-destructive person feels that his or her present condition is changeless over endless time, while the future is too far away to offer any hope.

9. *Idiosyncratic logic*: The lack of logic or what might be better conceived as idiosyncratic logic has been frequently noted.[1,2,17,27,38] What often seems to occur is that the decision to act is made, and then the individual interprets all subsequent events as pointing to the validity of the decision. Tripodes[38] emphasized that frequently suicide notes dwell on issues or incidents or cite as obvious concerns events that others would regard as irrelevent.[8] The individual writing the note describes himself or herself as different from others and, therefore, not evaluated according to common beliefs. The individual inaccurately perceives a cause-

effect relationship when two events occur together. He or she can not decenter or see how personal perceptions and opinions are different from others and tends to think in terms of absolutes, or tends to perceive all circumstances as having equal importance.[38]

Alverez[1] also speaks about what he calls the private logic of suicide. Suicide may come to represent to the self an act of success where before there had been indecisiveness and powerlessness. It may seem an act of great power and control, despite the fact that it leads to an extinction of power. Suicide may be most difficult to accept by those left behind when it is the choice of an individual whose life, by external measures, seems to be successful. The person may have an internal belief that he or she does not deserve success or happiness; or, success, as culturally defined may seem empty and pointless. When there is no major obvious loss, yet there is a diminution of self and purpose in the eyes of the self, to the outsider the reason for suicide is beyond reason.

Crisis Model Within a Broader Treatment Scope

Life Out of Balance

In general, the wish to commit suicide or the act of suicide is seen as a response to a crisis in which the individual's perceptions about what is wrong with the self and one's own life are not countered by a belief that he or she can somehow change the experience or change his or her feelings.

We might think of living as a balancing act. On the one hand are life's demands as exemplified by personal and role expectation, losses and disappointments. On the other hand are life's rewards or pluses as provided by social contact and interpersonal sharing, personal satisfaction, accomplishments at work and play, increases in status and joys. Balancing these two is the individual's coping capacity, which includes, but is not limited to, his or her capacity for self-observation, insight, and judgment; the ability for perseverance; the person's beliefs about purpose; his or her values; and the repertoire of life skills (Figure L.1).

In a time of exceptional stress, coping capacity may be diminished, or may be perceived as inadequate to deal with all that life demands. When there is a loss of a loved one, of wage-earning capability, or of self-esteem, then not only do demands become greater, but personal resources may dwindle. How often and unfortunate that when we experience the loss of someone we love, it is he or she we identify as the one person who could help us. Added to this is a loss of coping capacity, perhaps due to fatigue or emotional burnout, or perhaps due to a recent questioning of values

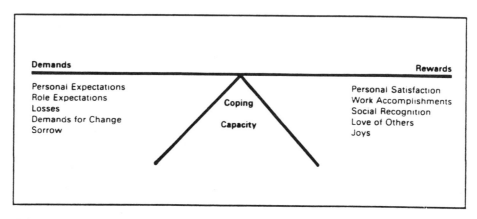

FIGURE L.1   Suicide.

and purpose. The part of the person that normally restores equilibrium—the mediator—is ineffective.

The suicidal person is frequently an individual who has had or is currently identified as having psychiatric problems (see box). As a result, many suicidal crises occur in the context of a broader treatment approach or preventive stance. The individual's coping capacity has already been shown to be less effective, and his or her demands and rewards are in precarious balance.

In two often cited studies Robins et al[33] and Dorpat and Ripley[8] investigated large groups of successful (completed) suicides. Using hospital records and talking to family members, associates and physicians the investigators concluded that 95% to 100% of the individuals were psychiatrically ill. Both studies especially implicated alcoholism and manic depression (bipolar depression). More recent descriptions of practice have also cited schizophrenic process as a primary psychiatric problem correlated with suicide.

It is becoming increasingly clear to health professionals that the now familiar crisis model is not sufficient to deal with suicide. Much more attention is being given to less intensive but longer term follow-up within the community to assist the individual to improve quality of life, to increase his or her awareness regarding avenues of support, and to help the individual avert future crises.

Intervention

Levels Of Intervention

The occupational therapist may become involved in intervention at several levels. When the suicide crisis occurs with an individual who is already in a treatment program (e.g.,

in an inpatient or community mental health setting), the occupational therapist would likely be involved as a member of the treatment team. This involvement would also occur when the individual is brought into a short- or longer-term treatment program at a mental health facility, as a response not only to the crisis but to what is envisioned as more generalized dysfunction.

When the individual is a patient of the occupational therapist, but not within a psychosocial setting (as with home health care or physical dysfunction treatment settings), the therapist's primary role in intervention is to be alert to suicidal messages, to assist in clarifying that a suicide threat exists, and to guide the individual to appropriate treatment.

When the individual receives crisis treatment only, as may occur through a crisis mental health program, the occupational therapist would less likely be involved. Many crisis centers, for example, offer crisis treatment in from one to six individual psychotherapeutic sessions with a staff counselor. More recently, attention has been given to the usefulness of providing community support groups and activities for the individual after the crisis has abated. Although we could find no discussion specific to occupational therapy in this regard, such community follow-up would seem to be a viable avenue for occupational therapy involvement.

Key Aims in Prevention

Attempts to prevent suicide are aimed at picking up suicide messages; providing protection, when necessary; helping the individual more realistically assess his or her demands and alternatives; rebuilding self-esteem through successful experiences; rebuilding a supportive social network; increasing the individual's self-reliance; and increasing the individual's ability to identify and respond effectively to stress situations that trigger suicidal thoughts.

Ambivalence

One important ingredient in prevention is the existence of ambivalence. An individual will almost always be personally ambivalent, even when the wish for death or relief is strong. Most persons have a powerful contradictory instinct for survival. Suicide is not conceived as an easy act to accomplish. Perhaps that is why many individuals contemplating suicide will talk about it or drop hints, knowing that this behavior increases the likelihood of rescue. Although it is generally believed that most persons who commmit suicide wanted to die, the study of attempted suicides does not support this premise.[37,43] Many suicide attempts and actual suicides are carried out with the thought, "I don't care whether I live or die." Often, the emotional stress of the suicide attempt adds to the mental muddling that may well have existed before the attempt.[37] The result is ambivalence that is compounded by confusion. This ambivalence buys time for would-be helpers. How much time is not always clear; however, the helping community must make contact during this period, establish some trust and rapport, and make an impact on the individual so that he or she decides to postpone any definitive self-destructive action and to wait and see what happens.

The Extent of OT Involvement with Suicide

It is not possible to know how many occupational therapists treat suicidal individuals because treatment statistics tend to be gathered using other kinds of diagnostic and problem categories. In our experience, therapists frequently encounter suicidal individuals in psychosocial settings.

Psychoeducational Model of Treatment

Although not describing an occupational therapy program, Kiev[19] offers a model of therapy for suicidal individuals that is consonant with principles of occupational therapy across a variety of treatment settings and frameworks. As Kiev writes,

> Personality changes do not come about in therapy sessions but in real life situations when patients are able to experiment with new ways of being and behaving. This is particularly true for those individuals with chronic difficulties in adjustment and getting along. For this reason, treatment moves most rapidly when patients can focus on concrete problems in work, at home or in interpersonal relationships.[19]

Occupational therapy is not a panacea for suicide, but by providing an opportunity for active involvement, it offers the individual a chance to experience the self more successfully and renegotiate some of his or her cognitive distortions. It must be reiterated that many patients who are suicidally depressed have an apparent problem with motivation. These individuals often avoid occupational therapy as well as other kinds of participation because, as they say, they are too tired or no longer interested in accomplishing anything. If the individual is in attendance within the occupational therapy setting, Kiev's guidelines, which he termed a psychoeducational frame, may be useful. In Kiev's model the individual is helped to accomplish the following:

1. Concretize goals;
2. Ascertain what is standing in the way of goal attainment;
3. Look realistically at the feasibility of goals, including a realistic evaluation of personal skills and abilities and the availability of others;
4. Assess what can and cannot be changed;
5. Determine what assumptions and patterns of behaving are standing in the way of positive change;
6. Establish feasible strategies for achieving goals, based on one's own strengths;
7. Check to be certain that goals suit the self and are not tailored to imitate others;

8. Check to be certain that goals are kept to a reasonable number.[19]

Judging the Self by Personal Standards

Once treatment goals have been established, the individual is encouraged in pursuing these goals to achieve the following:

1. Focus on present and daily events.
2. Look to the self, not others, for approval.
3. Avoid preoccupation with detail and over-attention to mistakes; such preoccupation tends to create tension or tedium.
4. Avoid comparing one's own performance to that of others.
5. Become increasingly self-reliant; self-reliance is seen as essential to self-esteem.
6. Look realistically at failure and rejection. Tolerance for mistakes will be sought, and both success and failure will be judged by personal standards, not the expectations of others. Relatedness to others will be encouraged, but the individual must see that others have needs and demands that do not include him or her.[19]

Cuing into Internal Signs

As therapy proceeds and the crisis passes, the patient needs help to identify and monitor those visceral changes and situational events that tend to signal that he or she is in a situation that feels overwhelming. For example, the patient might be assisted in identifying:

1. Bodily changes that signify stress (e.g., muscles feel tight and the individual feels tired);
2. Problem situations that make him or her feel especially vulnerable (e.g., arguments with a spouse, loss of employment, and frustration during tasks);
3. Personal responses that indicate that he or she is overwhelmed (e.g., the person begins to avoid normal social discourse, avoids calling friends, starts skipping classes, or calls in sick to work).

Maintaining the Therapeutic Relationship

An integral dimension of the treatment process concerns the therapeutic relationship. The therapeutic relationship is not different when working with the suicidal individual; however, extra demands may be placed on the therapist.

Responding to Dependency

Suicidal individuals often wish to have a relationship in which they can be dependent on another person. They frequently look to others for approval and nurturance; they tend to sees others as having high expectations for them; and are frequently angry when others do not allow them the closeness and dependency they seek. With severe depression, this may not be apparent at first as the person may withdraw from others; however, the dynamics will often emerge later on in the therapy process. It may be quite natural to encourage dependency when an individual is in great distress. In fact, when the individual is in severe crisis, appears out of control, or to have a limited ability for sound judgment, many professionals across disciplines take a parental, protective stance. Over any extended period, however, such dependency does not serve the best interests of the patient and tends to wear out treatment staff. Being too dependent keeps an individual from realizing his or her own strengths, from accepting personal responsibility for his or her own well-being, and in a very vulnerable position. The helping staff tend to become drained and frustrated, feeling that they have given all that they can. The therapist needs to realize that in fostering dependency, the ultimate message is not, as we might believe, "I care for you," (though well we may) but rather, "I don't believe that you can take care of yourself."

Staff Feeling Controlled

The individual wanting to be taken care of may intentionally or unintentionally use suicide as a way to mobilize others around him or her. The patient can further keep them there by suggesting, "If you don't take care of me as I have asked, I will kill myself," with the implied, "and it will be your fault." At times, the staff will become angry, feeling controlled or manipulated. In response, they may push away an individual who has a genuine need for contact. For this reason, the treatment staff needs to work with the person to help increase his or her own sense of strength and resourcefulness, to communicate a belief in his or her abilities, and to help the individual to look more realistically at the extent to which others can meet the person's needs. Clearly, a suicidal individual may place excess demands on helping staff, and many suicidal individuals will choose to continue a needy and helpless posture in regards to others. It can be an advantage to work along with other staff in a team approach to provide staff with support and a broadened perspective through their interacion with each other.

When Therapists Avoid the Subject of Suicide

Another impediment to the therapeutic relationship may arise when the therapist is particularly uncomfortable with thinking or talking about death. For example, the therapist may tend to cut off any dialogue in this area. Although in particular instances some therapists refuse to talk about suicide with their patients,† many believe that the suicidal individual needs to be allowed to consider the ramifications of taking his or her life, as one would weigh any important decision. What is essential is that the person look realistically at the decision, and with a lot of distortions and fantasies about what would be accomplished.

---

†Some behaviorally oriented therapists, for example, might refuse to discuss the individual's suicide plans because they would perceive themselves as thereby giving attention to and rewarding suicidal thinking. As an alternative, they would give attention to any verbalization or other behavior in which the individual pursued matters pertaining to his or her own well-being and productivity.

When the therapist's response to the individual's suicide talk is, "Oh, let's not dwell on this; let's think about the positive," the therapist may unwittingly increase the patient's sense of isolation and strengthen the cognitive distortion he or she experiences. The extent to which the therapist believes the patient should be allowed or encouraged to talk about personal feelings will depend in part also on the theoretical treatment base.

Although this text does not delve into the ethics of suicide, there are differing views regarding the morality of suicide, some of which have received much attention in the popular media. Readers wishing to discuss this issue might want to address the following:

1. Can the decision to commit suicide ever be a healthy decision?
2. Should an individual ever be allowed to take his or her own life, if the decision seems well thought through?
3. How far should one go to protect one from oneself—to the point of depriving him or her of their rights?
4. What if the individual is terminally ill? Chronically miserable?
5. If the individual does not have the final word about his or her own life, who should?
6. Who and what determines competence? Incompetence?
7. What if you, with a clear head, decided you had had enough of life?

The interested reader is referred to Brandt[4] and Kastenbaum[18] for provocative discussions of these issues.

Taking a Break From Introspection

Most therapists agree that for an individual to experience the self in a more positive way, the person needs to experience himself or herself through active engagement. Further, most realize that the patient may well profit from a break from thinking about dilemmas that are not going to be quickly resolved. The therapist will need to balance this recognition with the realization that the exhortation to participate in activity may be misinterpreted as a demand to perform, not entirely unlike the demands the individual already puts upon himself or herself, or perceives as coming from others. In addition, many suicidal individuals are not used to talking about feelings, whether about suicide or any other kind of feeling. Rather, the suicidal individual, as part of his increasing disengagement and isolation, may be very uncommunicative. The therapist must be particularly sensitive with this type of patient so as not to inadvertently shut off and shut out the person.

Inadvertently Isolating the Patient

A third difficulty can arise in the therapeutic relationship that is often quite particular to occupational therapy. When the therapist fears the patient's suicide potential, the therapist may be reluctant to allow the patient to participate in occupational therapy, the domain in which the therapist has primary responsibility. Fearing that the individual might use occupational therapy materials to harm himself or herself, or that the patient cannot be adequately supervised in the occupational therapy setting, the therapist suggests that the patient not be allowed to come with the other patients to the clinic. The therapist might offer instead to bring some materials to the ward, or indicate that the patient can participate in occupational therapy after he or she has stopped feeling suicidal. The result can be that the patient is more isolated and has less opportunity to experience the self in a positive way. The therapist also has communicated the belief, "I believe you are out of control," or "I am frightened of being with you."

Maintaining Safety Precautions

Certainly, occupational therapy settings tend to offer a myariad of potentially lethal materials: from machinery to toxic glues, from kitchen knives to potential ropes. It can be very frightening to think that a patient might use something acquired in occupational therapy to take his or her own life, and the instinct might be to prohibit the patient's participation. This decision, however, needs to be considered carefully. Occupational therapy offers an opportunity for the individual to begin to regain a sense of worth and mastery. Monitoring media by making certain that all materials are accounted for before the person leaves the occupational therapy setting may be preferred. It often makes sense to ask a staff member to stay with the individual while he or she is in the occupational therapy setting, not just to watch the patient, but to provide support and encouragement during this stressful time. One may see this as a way of communicating, "I know you are having difficulty with self-control. I respect this, and I will help you with setting limits." In allowing the patient to participate in occupational therapy, the message is given that the therapist sees coping skills and positive potential that the individual may not see in himself or herself. The individual also is given the chance to reestablish social contact and healthy reengagement when the tendency may have been toward disengagement. Although a severe suicide crisis may in some instances be judged as necessitating strong protective measures by treatment staff, when such protection lasts for weeks and months, the situation may need reappraisal.

Other Therapeutic Guidelines

The following guidelines may be useful when working with the suicidal individual in a variety of treatment settings:

1. A patient may select indirect ways to tell you about the suicidal intent. It is difficult

TABLE L.1 MAKING A CRISIS REFERRAL

1.	Know community mental health resources specific to crisis intervention (eg, public facilities, private therapists or physicians).
2.	Describe to the patient the reason for your referral and your choice of referral choice.
3.	Determine if patient is able to follow through with referral; if not, contact the crisis agency and make an appointment; identify yourself, your relationship to the patient and describe his or her needs.
4.	Arrange for the patient to follow through with the referral; the therapist may need to arrange for someone to accompany the patient to the agency.
5.	Consider the patient's needs and the policies of your institution and follow up on the referral.

Adapted from Valente SM, and Hatton CL: *Suicide: Assessment and Intervention, 2e.* Norwalk, CT, Appleton-Crafts, p. 10, 1984.

for many individuals to admit, even to themselves, that they are contemplating suicide. They may fear that if they tell you, you will judge them harshly or reject them or that you will try to stop them. As discussed earlier, however, an ambivalence often comes into play. This ambivalence may be acted out as hints, for example, the individual communicates that he or she is finishing up family business or the patient will not start any new occupational therapy projects. Or, he or she may tell you "good-bye" when you are unaware that treatment was to be terminated. A person-drawing may show the patient fading into nonexistence or engaged in a self-destructive act.† A direct question such as, "Are you thinking about taking your own life?" is considered better than beating around the bush, and may help alleviate the person's anxiety as he or she wrestles with keeping these thoughts a secret.[23] We do not give the person the idea of committing suicide by asking such a question. Certainly, the person may deny being suicidal and have other explanations for his or her behavior, but, we have communicated our willingness to continue to work with him or her in therapy, or to assist the individual to gain access to other resources for treatment.

2. If a patient tells you, even offhandedly, that he or she is considering suicide, take the remark seriously. The information needs to be shared with all involved health professionals. Again, the indirect or casual mentioning of the suicidal wish may be a reflection of ambivalence. Do not assume that the individual has told everyone his or her thoughts; the patient may have selected to share this information only with you.

3. Know your community resources well and know the steps to make a referral. For referrals outside your agency, see Table L.1.

4. Play for time. Recognizing the ambivalence, try to arouse the patient's curiosity and interest, so that he or she continues to postpone any definitive action while waiting to see where therapy might lead. Make provocative references to the next session or the next person the patient will be seeing that are designed not to be coy, but to stimulate his or her curiosity and to concretize the image of self as projected into the future.[2]

5. Facilitate the expression and clarification of concerns. Patients who are very depressed often lack the energy to talk about their feelings and concerns, and they may need much support and encouragement from all concerned to help identify them. It is not just feelings about suicide that may need to be expressed, but concerns about all areas of the individual's functioning. For example, if a patient can talk about fears of failure, confusion about values, or concerns about finding a job or paying bills, there is more opportunity for the individual to clarify his or her own needs and to renegotiate distortions. In oc-

---

†The use of the Machover Figure Drawing Test as a screening device for suicide is described by Richman in his book *Family Therapy for Suicidal People.*[32]

cupational therapy, as patients reenter into active participation, the therapist may find it helpful to assist patients to recognize their own feelings about doing. The individual does not need to examine every one of his or her actions, but he or she does need the opportunity to talk about and learn from experiences.

Expressing feelings may help alleviate stress and may provide an opportunity to reduce feelings of isolation, allow you and others to provide emotional support and physical limits if needed, and begin the process by which the patient can start becoming aware of alternatives for coping.

6. Ascertain the degree to which lethal danger signals are in play (Table L.2). These factors are considered indicative of increased suicide danger, for they decrease the ability of the self to judge a situation accurately, lessen the internal constraints that stop destructive action, or indicate that a choice to act has been made and accepted by the individual.

7. Determine whether the patient has a specific plan to accomplish the suicide; it is thought that the person who has a specific plan is more lethal. If the patient tells you his or her plans, however, at some future time this information may help you or others intervene. For example, if a patient suddenly disappears from the treatment setting, you may have information about where he or she would go. If the person tells you that he or she plans to drive a car into oncoming traffic, the treatment team may act to prevent the patient's access to vehicles.

8. Let the patient know what you intend to do. Although confidentiality is repected, the individual needs to know that you will not keep anything secret that he or she has told you if it is toward the end of aiding the suicide. The patient may get angry with you, but you must emphasize that his or her welfare is the most important issue. If you intend to limit access to tools or materials, you need to let the individual know your reasons.

9. Help the treatment team and the individual assess his or her strengths and resources. Although this evaluation may not occur immediately in the treatment process, occupational therapy provides the patient through a tangible experience, an opportunity to gain insight into personal strengths, limits and resources and start to feel less confused and overwhelmed by his or her own difficulties. The individual may at least feel that he or she has a place to start.

10. Communicate your belief that there is hope but don't negate the patient's feelings nor the gravity of the problem. Communicate that you see the patient as worthwhile and that you believe that viable options exist.

11. Be aware that the suicidally depressed individual may be acutely sensitive to any perceived criticisms from you or any perceived task failures. Try to keep the channels of communication and expression of feeling very open. Structuring for success is appropriate. Learning to deal with failure may need to be saved for the time when at least some equilibrium has been restored.

12. As the patient becomes able, help him or her to explore alternative coping methods. As therapy progresses and the patient is more amenable to trying new behaviors,

TABLE L.2 SUICIDE DANGER SIGNALS

1. Distrust and withdrawal from significant others.
2. Mental confusion.
3. Substance abuse (eg, drugs, alcohol, overuse of medication).
4. Extreme hopelessness.
5. A history of impulsiveness, or current impulsive behavior.
6. Family history of suicide.
7. Pradoxic calm or sudden uplift in mood indicating the decision to act has been made.
8. The existence of a specific plan.

Adapted from Valente SM and Hatton CL: *Suicide: Assessment and Intervention, 2nd edition.* Norwalk, CT, Appleton-Crafts, p. 110, 1984.

role-playing may be useful. Help the patient identify personal and community resources, provide opportunities for task accomplishment, and eventually, provide opportunities for new ways to judge task failure. Help identify how coping skills gained in occupational therapy are the same skills that will assist the person to function in the everyday world. Be aware that the patient's pessimism and low esteem tend to block any easy access to perceiving alternatives. Do not allow yourself to be put off by this attitude.

13. Be aware of the influence and interrelatedness of other patients. A misguided patient or patients may be talked into helping the suicidal patient gain access to restricted materials or into helping the person cover his or her tracks. In addition, when one patient becomes suicidal, it may stir the suicidal thoughts of other patients and provide a type of permission for them to pursue their wishes. When there is a community approach to treatment, the issue of suicide becomes everyone's issue. Priorities may rearrange themselves to allow everyone a chance to explore their own feelings around this issue.

14. Be aware of your own boundaries, and communicate them clearly to the patient. Patients need to know when you are and are not available to them. If an individual or individuals are designated as contact persons to be called on (e.g., by phone) after hours, encourage the patient to use the appropriate channels.

If a patient seems reluctant to end his or her therapy sessions with you, it may be helpful to alert the person 10 to 15 minutes before time is up and ask if there are any issues he or she wishes to raise. It may also be helpful in establishing a sense of completion if you talk with the patient at the end of each session and summarize what has been accomplished.

Termination of Treatment

Although the manner of termination and extent of follow-up depends on the type of treatment program in which the individual has been involved, significant findings may influence programming.

Responding to Suicide as a Life-style

In a study of clients at the Los Angeles Suicide Prevention Center, approximately one half of those who commit suicide were chronically suicidal, tending to be needy, dependent, chronically depressed, and often chronic abusers of drugs and alcohol.[22] These individuals tended to make frequent demands on treatment staff and eventually wore out staff who found them to be incessantly demanding. In response, the center developed a reachout service that they called "Continuing Relationship Maintenance." This program, not considered therapy, per se, was conducted by volunteers, who were supervised by paraprofessionals and professional staff. The individuals, post-crisis, were taught to use community resources and met both individually and in groups to engage in supportive activities. Activities included both social activities and active listening by an attentive volunteer. This experimental program, in a manner consistent with the recommendation of the Center for Studies of Suicide Prevention, National Institute of Mental Health, emphasized the importance of the gradual "amelioration of self-destructive lifestyles" with less emphasis on "active intervention to ensure temporary safety of the patients."[22]

Although occupational therapy and other possible ancillary services were not discussed in this preventive program, it would seem that a role in such a program would be very viable for occupational therapy and consistent with the beliefs and aims of the profession.

Recommended Reading List

Bellak L: Intensive brief and emergency psychotherapy. In Grinspoon L (Ed): *Psychiatry Update, Vol.III*. Washington, DC, American Psychiatric Press, Inc., 1984.

Gaylin W (Ed): *The Meaning of Despair*. New York, Science House, 1968.

References

1. Alvarez A: *The Savage God: A Study of Suicide*. New York, Bantam Books, Random House, 1970.
2. Beck AT: *Cognitive Therapy of Depression*. New York, Guilford Press, 1979, pp. 228–224.
3. Binswanger L: The Case of Ellen West. In May R, Angel E, Ellenberger H (Eds): *Existence*. New York, Basic Books, 1958.
4. Brandt R: The morality and rationality of suicide. In Shneidman E (Ed): *Suicidiology: Contemporary Developments* New York, Grune and Stratton, 1976.
5. Brockopp G, Lester D: Time perception in suicidal and nonsuicidal individuals. *Crisis Intervention* 2:98–100, 1970.
6. de Catanzaro D: *Suicide and Self-Damaging Behavior*. New York, Academic Press, Incorporated, 1986.
7. Diggory J: United States suicide rates, 1933–1968: An analysis of some trends. In Shneidman E (Ed): *Suicidology: Contemporary Developments*. New York, Grune and Stratton, 1976.
8. Dorpat T, Ripley H: A study of suicide in the Seattle area. *Compr Psychiatry* 1:349–359, 1960.
9. Farberow N, Breed W, Bunney W, et al: Research in suicide. In Resnik H, Hathorne B (Eds): *Suicide Prevention in the 70's*. Rockville, MD, National Institute of Mental Health Center for Studies of Suicide Prevention. US Dept of Health, Education and Welfare publication (HSM0) 72–9054], 1973, pp. 45–80.
10. Farberow N, Shneidman E (Eds): *The Cry for Help*. New York, McGraw-Hill Book Company, 1961.
11. Fawcett J, Comstock E, Hendin H, et al: Priorities for improved treatment approaches. In Resnik H, Hathorne B (Eds): *Suicide Prevention in the 70's*. Rockville, MD, National Institute of Mental Health Center Studies of Suicide Prevention. US Dept of Health, Education, and Welfare publication (HSMO) 72–9054, 1973, pp. 45–80.
12. Freud S: *Mourning and Melancholia*. (1917) Vol.4. In collected papers. London, Hogarth Press, Limited, 1949.
13. Greaves G: Temporal orientation in suicidal patients. *Perceptual Motor Skills* 33:1020, 1971.
14. Guttmacher L: *A Concise Guide to Somatic Therapies in Psychiatry*. Washington, DC, American Psychiatric Press, Inc., 1988.
15. Helig S: A personal statement. In Hatton CL, Valente SM (Eds): *Suicide: Assessment and Intervention*. Ed 2. Norwalk, CT, AppletonCentury-Crofts, 1984, pp. 256–261.
16. Hendin H: Suicide: Psychoanalytic point of view. In Farberow N, Shneidman E (Eds): *The Cry for Help* New York, McGraw-Hill Book Company, 1961, pp. 181–192.
17. James N: Psychology of suicide. In Hatton CL, Valente SM (Eds): *Suicide: Assessment and Intervention*. Ed 2. Norwalk, CT, Appleton-Century-Crofts, 1984, pp. 33–53.
18. Kastenbaum R: Suicide as the preferred way of death. In Shneidman E (Ed): *Suicidology: Contemporary Developments*. New York, Grune and Stratton, 1976, pp. 421–441.
19. Kiev A: Crisis intervention and suicide prevention. In Shneidman E (Ed): *Suicidology: Contemporary Developments*. New York, Grune and Stratton, 1976, pp. 445–478.
20. Klopfer B: Suicide: The Jungian point of view. In Farberow N, Shneidman E (Eds): *The Cry for Help* New York, McGraw-Hill Book Company, 1961, pp. 193–203.
21. Linden L, Breed W: The demographic epidemiology of suicide. In Shneidman W (Ed): *Suicidology: Contemporary Developments* New York, Grune and Stratton, 1976, pp. 71–98.
22. Litman R, Wold C: Beyond crisis intervention. In Shneidman E (Ed): *Suicidology: Contemporary Developments* New York, Grune and Stratton, 1976, pp. 525–546.
23. MacKinnon R, Michels R: *The Psychiatric Interview in Clinical Practice*. Philadelphia, W.B. Saunders Company, 1971, p. 208.
24. Maris RW: *Pathways to Suicide: A Survey of Self-Destructive Behaviors*. Baltimore, Johns Hopkins Press, 1981.
25. Maris RW, Dorpat T, Hathorne B, et al: Education and training in suicidology for the seventies. In Resnik H, Hathorne B (Eds): *Suicide Prevention in the Seventies* Bethesda, MD, National Institute of Mental Health, 1973, p. 33.
26. Murphy G: Suicide and attempted suicide. In Winokur G, Clayton P: *The Medical Basis of Psychiatry*. Philadelphia, W.B. Saunders Company, 1986.
27. Neuringer C: Current developments in the study of suicidal thinking. In Shneidman E (Ed): *Suicidology: Contemporary Developments*. New York, Grune and Stratton, 1976, pp. 229–252.
28. Pretzel P: A personal statement. In Hatton CL, Valente SM (Eds): *Suicide: Assessment and Intervention*. Ed 2. Appleton-Century-Crofts, 1984, pp. 249–255.

29. Resnik H: Suicide. In Kaplan H, Freedman A, Sadock B (Eds): *Comprehensive Textbook of Psychiatry.* Baltimore, Williams and Wilkins, 1980.

30. Resnik H, Hathorne B (Eds): *Suicide Prevention in the 70's.* Rockville, MD, National Institute of Mental Health Center for Studies of Suicide Prevention. US Dept of Health, Education, and Welfare publication (HMS) 72–9054], 1973.

31. Resnik H, Hathorne B: The challenge of the seventies. In Resnik H, Hathorne B (Eds): *Suicide Prevention in the 70's.* Rockville, MD, National Institute of Mental Health Center for Studies of Suicide Prevention, [Dept. of Health, Education and Welfare Publication No. (HMS) 72–9054], 1973, p. 3.

32. Richman J: *Family Therapy for Suicidal People.* New York, Springer Publishing Company, Incorporated, 1986, pp. 49–68.

33. Robins E, Gassner S, Kayes J, et al: The communication of suicidal intent: A study of 134 consecutive cases of successful (completed) suicides. *Am J Psychiatry* 115:724–733, 1959.

34. Roy A: A family history of suicide. *Arch Gen Psychiatry* 40:971–978, 1983.

35. Shneidman E: Current overview of suicide. In Shneidman E (Ed): *Suicidology: Contemporary Developments.* New York, Grune and Stratton, 1976, pp. 1–22.

36. Swanson W, Breed W: Black suicide in New Orleans. In Shneidman E (Ed): *Suicidology: Contemporary De-velopments.* New York, Grune and Stratton, 1976, pp. 99–128.

37. Stengel E: *Suicide and Attempted Suicide.* Baltimore, Penguin Books, 1964.

38. Tripodes P: Reasoning patterns in suicide notes. In Shneidman E (Ed): *Suicidology: Contemporary Developments.* New York, Grune and Stratton, 1976, pp.203–233.

39. Valente SM, Hatton CL: Intervention. In Hatton CL, Valente SM (Eds): *Suicide: Assessment and Intervention.* Ed 2. Norwalk, CT, Appleton-Century-Crofts, 1984, pp. 83–148.

40. Victoroff V: *The Suicidal Patient: Recognition, Intervention, Management.* Oradell, NJ, Medical Economics Company, 1983.

41. Weisman A, Feifel H, Henley C, et al: Death and self-destructive behaviors. In Resnik H, Hathorne B (Eds): *Suicide Prevention in the 70's.* Rockville, MD, National Institute of Mental Health Center for Studies of Suicide Prevention. US Dept of Health, Education, and Welfare publication (HMS) 72–9054], 1973, pp. 13–22.

42. Wise MG, Rundell J: *Concise Guide to Consultation Psychiatry.* Washington, DC, Amercian Psychiatric Press, 1988.

43. Worden J: Lethality factors and the suicide attempt. In Shneidman E (Ed): *Suicidology: Contemporay Developments.* New York, Grune and Stratton, 1976, pp. 131–162.

Index